Tom Kitwood on Dementia

A reader and critical commentary

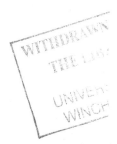

Tom Kitwood on Dementia

A reader and critical commentary

edited by

Clive Baldwin and Andrea Capstick

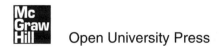

Open University Press

Open University Press
McGraw-Hill Education
McGraw-Hill House
Shoppenhangers Road
Maidenhead
Berkshire
England
SL6 2QL

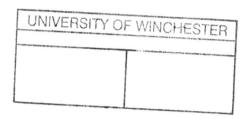

email: enquiries@openup.co.uk
world wide web: www.openup.co.uk

and
Two Penn Plaza
New York, NY 10121–2289, USA

First published 2007

A catalogue record of this book is available from the British Library

ISBN-10: 0 335 22271 4 (pb) 0 335 22272 2 (hb)
ISBN-13: 978 0 335 22271 1 (pb) 978 0 335 22272 8 (hb)

Library of Congress Cataloging-in-Publication Data
CIP data has been applied for

Typeset by RefineCatch Limited, Bungay, Suffolk
Printed by OZ Graf. S.A.
www.polskabook.pl

The **McGraw·Hill** Companies

To my parents, Peter and Irene Baldwin and, as always, Patty and Sarah Rebekkah (CB)

To my grandfather, Jim Proctor, who has lived to tell the tale (AC)

With gratitude and love

Contents

Publisher's acknowledgements

The authors and publisher wish to thank the following for permission to use copyright material:

Kitwood, T. (1970) The Christian understanding of man In *What is Human?* London: Inter-Varsity Press.

Kitwood, T. (1988) The technical, the personal and the framing of dementia. *Social Behaviour*, 3 (2). Oxford: Blackwell.

Kitwood, T. (1989) Brain, mind and dementia: With particular reference to Alzheimer's disease. *Ageing and Society*, 9 (1). Cambridge: Cambridge University Press.

Kitwood, T. (1990) The dialectics of dementia: With particular reference to Alzheimer's disease. *Ageing and Society*, 10 (2). Cambridge: Cambridge University Press.

Kitwood, T. (1992) Towards a theory of dementia care: Personhood and well-being. *Ageing and Society*, 12 (3). Cambridge: Cambridge University Press.

Kitwood, T. (1993) Person and process in dementia. *International Journal of Geriatric Psychiatry*, 8 (7). Reproduced by permission of John Wiley & Sons Limited.

Kitwood, T. (1993) Towards the reconstruction of an organic mental disorder. In Radley A (ed) *Worlds of illness*. London: Routledge. Reproduced by permission of Taylor & Francis Books UK.

Kitwood, T. (1993) Towards a theory of dementia care: The interpersonal process. *Ageing and Society*, 13 (1). Cambridge: Cambridge University Press.

Kitwood, T. (1994) The concept of personhood and its implications for the care of those who have dementia. In Jones, G. and Miesen, B. (eds) *Caregiving in Dementia*. London: Routledge. Reproduced by permission of Taylor & Francis Books UK.

Bredin, K., Kitwood T., and Wattis J. (1995) Decline in quality of life for patients with severe dementia following a ward merger. *International Journal of Geriatric Psychiatry*, 10 (11). Reproduced by permission of John Wiley & Sons Limited.

Kitwood, T. (1995) Findings related to well-being, and Findings related to ill-being. In *Brighter futures: A report on research into provision for persons with dementia in residential homes, nursing homes and sheltered housing.* Anchor Housing Association.

Kitwood, T. (1995) Cultures of care: Tradition and change. In Kitwood, T. and Benson, S. (eds) *The new culture of dementia care.* London: Hawker.

Kitwood, T. (1996) A dialectical framework for dementia, in Woods, R. T. (ed) *Handbook of the Clinical Psychology of Ageing.* Wiley: Chichester. Reproduced by permission of John Wiley & Sons Limited.

Kitwood, T. (1997) Personhood, dementia and dementia care. In Hunter, S. (ed) *Research Highlights in Social Work.* London: Jessica Kingsley.

Kitwood, T. (1998) The contribution of psychology to the understanding of senile dementia, in *Mental Health Problems in Old Age: A reader*, Gearing, B., Johnson, M. and Heller T. (eds). Wiley: Chichester. Reproduced by permission of John Wiley & Sons Limited.

Kitwood, T. (1998) Professional and moral development for care work: some observations on the process. *Journal of Moral Education* 27 (3). Reproduced by permission of Taylor & Francis Ltd.

Kitwood, T. (1998) Toward a theory of dementia care: Ethics and interaction. *The Journal of Clinical Ethics* 9 (1).

Every effort has been made to trace the copyright holders but if any have been inadvertently overlooked the publisher will be pleased to make the necessary arrangement at the first opportunity.

Acknowledgements

This book arose from a suggestion by Rachel Gear of the Open University Press to whom we are indebted not only for the idea but also her support throughout the process. While we take ultimate responsibility for the content of the Reader, we would like to thank Deborah O'Connor, Habib Chaudhury, Alison Phinney and Barbara Purves from the Centre for Research on Personhood in Dementia at the University of British Columbia, Vancouver, for their collaboration in co-authoring Part 3, on personhood. From our own institution, we would like to thank Ruth Bartlett for her work on citizenship and personhood and Errollyn Bruce, who worked with Tom Kitwood, for her support and insightful comments. Our thanks also to Linda Fox for her contribution to the biographical information in the introduction. The work is all the richer for all these contributions. For her assistance in formatting and proofreading thanks are also due to Patty Baldwin. To Andrew Kitwood, our thanks for giving permission on behalf of the Kitwood family to reproduce Tom's work. To the Galerie Becket Odille Boïcos, Paris, for permission to reproduce the work of William Utermohlen. Finally, our grateful appreciation to past and present colleagues at Bradford Dementia Group who have sustained and developed the theory and practice of person-centred care over the years.

About the editors

Clive Baldwin is Senior Lecturer in Dementia Studies with Bradford Dementia Group, University of Bradford. He has been involved in research into ethical issues facing family carers at Ethox (University of Oxford). He has a particular interest in narrative theory and method and how this relates to personhood in dementia. He is a member of the Christian Council on Aging Dementia Group.

Andrea Capstick is Lecturer in Dementia Studies, Bradford Dementia Group, University of Bradford. Together with Tom Kitwood she played a leading role in the development of BDG's educational programme and was the inaugural course leader for the BSc (Hons) in Dementia Studies. She is currently undertaking a Professional Doctorate in Education. She is a member of the Higher Education Dementia Network.

Introduction

Tom Kitwood is one of the leading figures in the development of our thinking on the nature and process of dementia, the experience of dementia and the development of person-centred care. The overall sweep of Kitwood's work is vast and it has rightly been considered to have altered the way both dementia itself and the provision of care services are conceptualized today.

His untimely death in 1998 interrupted the development of this thinking, which has since been carried on by others and incorporated into mainstream service development and evaluation. Kitwood foreshadowed a number of now taken-for-granted approaches to the delivery of healthcare: the application of a bio-psychosocial approach, the development of a values base, the promotion of user involvement and user-focused/directed services and, through the development of Dementia Care Mapping, a focus on evidence-based care and continuous quality improvement.

Kitwood wrote for a variety of audiences and was eclectic in his intellectual sources, publishing in a variety of different disciplinary and professional outlets. With the exception of *Dementia Reconsidered*, there is no one place that covers the breadth and extent of his work – and even then *Dementia Reconsidered* cannot be viewed as all-encompassing or the definitive statement.

In presenting this Reader, we are aware of the joint dangers of eulogy and criticism. As Gibson (1997) said in her review of Kitwood's final book, *Dementia Reconsidered*:

> Just as Kitwood cautions the reader against accepting 'neuropathic ideology', so too should the reader be cautious about uncritically substituting 'Kitwood ideology'. We must remain open to further scientific findings while we engage in critical examination of all new ideas from whatever source, and rigorously test them against experience derived from practice. (Gibson 1997: 29)

In so doing, however, if our analysis here appears often to be concerned with the aporia in Kitwood's theory and their correlates in dementia care practice, this should in no sense detract from our debt to his originality and vision.

For our critical overview we have chosen four areas that, to us, seem to incorporate the majority of Kitwood's ideas in one way or another: his theories of dementia, ill- and well-being, personhood and organizational culture. In so doing, we hope to demonstrate how Kitwood's work is still of contemporary interest and relevance. We also present a briefly annotated bibliography of Kitwood's work on dementia. While this is not a complete bibliography – we have chosen to omit the majority of book reviews – the listing should serve as a foundation for readers wishing to follow up the themes and issues raised in this publication.

Kitwood's work

Kitwood's work on dementia covered a remarkable amount for such a short career. In just 10 years Kitwood, sometimes in conjunction with others, developed working theories of dementia, dementia care and personhood that challenged the prevailing medical discourse and its therapeutic nihilism. He developed a tool, Dementia Care Mapping, to observe well- and ill-being in people with dementia that has become well established and respected internationally, and promoted a person-centred agenda to the point where it is increasingly recognized as central to service provision both in the UK and abroad.

The range of his work, however, also means that there is a good deal of room for interpretation and, as Adams (1996) has rightly pointed out, is difficult to summarize. Not everything was worked out fully and the intersections of different areas of his work were not fully articulated. The question becomes, then, how to interpret his work without imposing that interpretation as the only one.

We recognize that any interpretation of Kitwood's work is open to criticism – our interpretations may not be those of others and we are not so presumptuous as to think that ours, as presented here, is, or should be regarded as, definitive. With Bakhtin we would argue that polyphony – the encouragement of multiple viewpoints – is better than monologue, a single voice claiming to contain the truth. We hope that the way that we have presented Kitwood's work in this Reader will generate debate and a multiplicity of interpretations, within the spirit of his work as a whole. Interpretation is an ongoing process and one of the important points we have tried to make in this Reader – and one that we emphasize here – is that it is the very interpretability of Kitwood's work that makes it so attractive and, in part, explains its influence. Instead of a codification of rules, Kitwood gets us to think about ourselves and our practice by providing us with a framework that allows for, indeed generates, creativity and development.

So interpret we must and it is, we feel, incumbent upon us here to make explicit our position. In so doing, we hope to alert readers to some of the problems and possibilities involved in reading Kitwood and to create spaces in which further questions can be asked about his work. We would strongly encourage the reader to make use of the original sources in each Part alongside our commentary so as to be able to evaluate our interpretation of Kitwood's work and those of others.

As with any body of work developed over time, it is possible to find in Kitwood's work inconsistencies, contradictions, incomplete ideas, omissions and ambiguities. Are such things simply failings to be criticized? Certainly Kitwood has been strongly criticized for his reconsideration of dementia (Flicker 1999) and even those more sympathetic to his overall project thought his work limited because it did not necessarily represent a 'true' picture of dementia:

> Just as a map constructed by poor methods will be of little use to travellers in a foreign land if they do not properly represent that land, so the ideas developed by Kitwood will be of little use to practitioners if they do not properly represent what dementia is really like because they have been poorly developed. (Adams 1996: 952–3)

We shall explore these criticisms later. Here, we want to suggest that many of the inconsistencies etc. to be found in Kitwood's work are explainable, not as failings inherent in the framework he was developing but partly as a result of the time and environment in which Kitwood was working and partly as a function of who Kitwood was and how he worked. While these factors do not explain all the difficulties present in Kitwood's work, they do make many of them understandable.

In what follows we shall examine a number of social, professional and personal factors that impacted on Kitwood's work: ambiguity, audience, rhetoric and the personal. In so doing, we hope to provide the reader with the context and means to understand and interpret Kitwood's work.

Ambiguity

Kitwood wished to change the world by persuasion and sometimes took a fundamentalist approach to this. Fundamentalism, however, is an approach that works best when the message is clear and simple, yet it is possible to identify a number of ambiguities in Kitwood's work when this is viewed as a whole. Of course, the reconsideration of dementia – its theory and its practice – was an ongoing work and it would have been surprising if there had not been developments in Kitwood's thinking. Indeed, had he not died so suddenly and unexpectedly, it is inevitable that his approach to dementia would have developed further. When we refer to ambiguities here, however, we are not referring to the differences between earlier and later work, but themes that were never clearly resolved throughout this work as a whole: for example, his philosophical position in relation to positivism and social constructionism (this is raised in Part 1 with regard to his theory of dementia) and his oscillation between attributing poor dementia care to individuals (a failure of moral adequacy) or organizations – a point that is explored in Part 4.

A second source of ambiguity was the fact that Kitwood wrote for disparate audiences with specific purposes in mind and we cannot always be sure as to those purposes – for example, where he states that carers are 'very poorly prepared, in moral terms, for the task they will face' implying a moral deficiency (Kitwood 1998a: 403). This is not a view he repeated elsewhere and we cannot be sure as to his intention here. It could be he thought that the readers of the *Journal of Moral Education* would be specifically interested in this area of discussion; alternatively, it could be that because it was unlikely that the care practitioners he is writing about would read the journal, he felt freer to describe them in these terms. While some are certain that Kitwood never blamed anyone (Woods 1999), others are less so (Davis 2004). The problem of audience is discussed later.

Ambiguity can also be explained partially by his tendency towards theoretical eclecticism. For example, in his theory of personhood he attempted to bring together the discourses of transcendence, ethics and social psychology. In so doing, he removed the concepts from their original contexts (for example, Buber's I-Thou relationship) without fully appreciating the consequences of this removal. Similarly, he used the term 'depth psychology' as almost synonymous with any form of psycho-analytic or psychotherapeutic approach rather than in the more specialist manner that others might understand it. While there are advantages to theoretical eclecticism – for instance, it may fuel creativity by not being wedded to a single approach and can aid recognition of the diversity of phenomena (Gaston 1995) or allow for greater interdisciplinarity – it can also appear idiosyncratic or inconsistent and, at worst, incoherent.

One of the difficulties that Kitwood faced in developing his ideas was that, at the time he was writing, there was no existing community of people with whom to work through the ideas in a critical but supportive scholarly atmosphere. Most of us, now-adays, have such a community – our colleagues and our peers engaged in similar work in a similar way – but Kitwood often saw himself as, at least initially, virtually alone in pushing forward his alternative theories of dementia and dementia care. Consequently, he lacked (or did not make use of) many of the opportunities to discuss and critique his work prior to publication that we take for granted and this may explain some of the idiosyncrasies and inconsistencies in his work.

While Kitwood, we would argue, avoided incoherency, he did not avoid inconsistency. In presenting some of these inconsistencies later on, we hope to enable the reader to decide how significant they are.

Audience

Kitwood wrote for a variety of audiences. His published work spans professional and academic journals and healthcare, educational and social science publications. His work was aimed at all levels – from family carers to senior medical personnel. In addressing different audiences, he would emphasize different aspects of his theory or practice, omit others and draw in material relevant to the case he was making for that particular audience. On the one hand, this ability to adapt his message to a variety of audiences is a great strength and can help us explain the uptake of his message across a variety of fields. On the other, it presents a number of problems for understanding or interpreting his work as a whole.

First, there is no way of knowing whether, for example, the omission of a certain aspect of his theory in a later article should be taken as an indicator that Kitwood had abandoned that line of thought or simply as a tactical decision not to distract from the main message of that article for that audience. We shall see significant examples of this in Parts 1 and 2 where we explore Kitwood's aetiology of dementia: in some writings he appears to be taking an almost structuralist, social constructionist view of dementia as a result of late-stage capitalism but in *Dementia Reconsidered*, there are only very faint vestiges of such an approach.

Second, by working within different discourses there is an inherent potential for ambiguity and/or apparent contradiction to find its way into the work as a whole. Concepts from differing discourses may sit uneasily together and even terms used across discourses may have different meanings or inferences. Similarly, in addressing different audiences, Kitwood used different languages in order to make his ideas accessible and acceptable to different groups of people. While this can be seen as a great talent, it also creates opportunities for slippage in meaning, thus introducing ambiguity into his work as a whole. The problem here lies in discerning whether such ambiguities and contradictions represent problematic aspects of the work or are the result of translation between discourses and languages.

Rhetoric

Linked to the problem of audience is that of rhetoric – both in the classical sense of attempting to influence the thought and actions of the audience and in the more pejorative sense of undue use of exaggeration or persuasive techniques to bolster an argument.

In the first sense of the word, there can be little doubt as to Kitwood's rhetorical ability. Person-centredness is now clearly and firmly on the agenda as a result of his work (although, not necessarily interpreted as Kitwood intended).

With regard to rhetoric in the second sense, it is clear from a number of writings that Kitwood painted broad brush-stroke pictures to attract attention and to inspire and motivate, for example, his creation of binary opposites such as ill-being/well-being (Kitwood et al. 1995), old/new culture (Kitwood 1995a), Type A/Type B organizations (see Kitwood 1997a: Chapter 7). This tendency runs the same risks as the positivistic attempts of psychiatry to create 'disease categories' (as in the Diagnostic and Statistical Manuals) – a process that Kitwood himself criticized. In both cases, the true picture is likely to be considerably less clear, with overlapping categories, excluded cases and uncertain 'diagnoses'. In other words, we need to be aware with any such argument of the dangers of confusing ontology (what there actually is in the world) with epistemology (a temporary or contingent 'way of seeing' what there is). Kitwood was, of course, crucially aware of such debates in the philosophy of science, but it may be argued that he applied his knowledge of them somewhat selectively in the service of persuasion. In so doing, perhaps Kitwood fell prey to Adams' criticism cited earlier of not representing the landscape of dementia accurately and thus, to a degree, misleading the unwary traveller. Even in presenting empirical data, such as in the *Brighter Futures* report (Kitwood et al. 1995) Kitwood and his colleagues made 'no attempt to disguise their evangelical zeal. Indeed their position is often close to advocacy' (Murphy 1997: 104).

The personal

Personal factors, too, are important in understanding Kitwood's work – as with all of us, personal preferences, enthusiasms, commitments and foibles all played a part in making his work what it was.

Kitwood was a great communicator, able to take his message to a wide range of people and places. He was persuasive and charismatic and no doubt his ministerial training stood him in good stead. His message was also extremely challenging for it provoked reflection not only on theory and practice but on moral character for those involved and it is to his credit that he could popularize these complex and difficult concepts and motivate others to implement, explore and develop them in practice.

Optimism and pessimism also played a part. At times Kitwood took the view that everything was terrible:

> As the twentieth century draws to its close . . . it is becoming clear that the system of liberal democracy, whose organization is allegedly rational and whose economic life is grounded in the pursuit of profit . . . is deeply implicated in many kinds of global injustice; it is not even capable of delivering a secure and prosperous life to all of its own citizens . . . a permanent underclass has been created, cut off from the ordinary privileges of citizenship.

And yet, on the same page, and referring to the same period:

> [. . .] a new and vibrant humanism has been gaining ground, more strongly committed, more psychologically aware, more culturally sensitive, more practical and pragmatic than anything that has gone before. (Kitwood 1997a: 144)

We may speculate as to the impact of this oscillation in Kitwood's work – did he, for example, abandon some of his more radical claims about dementia (for example, that it was an outcome of dysfunctional societal relations) because he felt pessimistic about the possibility of persuading others to this view? We will, of course, never really know, but reading his work with a view to the optimism or pessimism expressed might help us to gain further insights.

Clearly Kitwood's Christian faith – albeit later renounced – had a continuing influence within his work – not only in content (as we shall see in Part 3 on personhood) but also in style. At times his tone could be sermonizing and there are indications of a certain fundamentalism – if you are not for me, then you are against me. Although an avowed humanist in later life, he retained some belief in a spiritual aspect to life – hinted at, though not developed, in *Dementia Reconsidered*. His sense of social justice also survived his abandonment of faith and is clearly evident in his passion and commitment towards people living with dementia.

In some ways there are similarities between aspects of Kitwood's work and that of David Smail – an author of whom Kitwood was obviously aware but did not explicitly draw on in any significant way. Smail is a clinical psychologist who has argued that much distress is caused by societal rather than personal factors (or, to use his own terminology, by distal rather than proximal causes). Smail believes that there is a tendency to psychologize these (societal) problems, seeing their outworkings in the individual (unhappiness, anxiety, depression, distress) as evidence of an individual pathological weakness (see, for example, Smail 1984, 1993). While Kitwood also implied, at times, that dementia was caused by distal factors, he also had a tendency towards psychologizing problems. In his early work this can be found in relation to people with dementia – whose lack of robust personality made them vulnerable to dementia (see Kitwood 1988a) – and in his later work in relation to those who care for people with dementia (Kitwood 1998a). This tendency adds another complicating factor into the interpretation of Kitwood's work – to what extent did he believe in proximal and distal causes and how, then, did he balance these? This reflects the humanist/anti-humanist debate found in *What is Human?* between existential pessimism and humanistic optimism: that is, between seeing people as being determined by social and cultural structures or as autonomous actors in the world. This debate was not resolved in Kitwood's work.

A further aspect that has a bearing on Kitwood's work is a sense of journey or development. Just as his professional and personal life can be viewed as a journey through many landscapes, his academic work in dementia also moved from place to place. This movement allowed him to bring together a wide range of ideas and influences (for instance, from Christianity, the natural sciences, psychotherapy and the social sciences) and to cover a wide terrain, moving from a focus on people with dementia to those who care for them to organizational development and change, to education and training.

It also allowed him to move on from those areas that proved less rewarding or promising. Thus we find ideas that were introduced, played with and then virtually discarded – for example, the psychobiographical approach we find in *Understanding Senile Dementia* is abandoned as a research methodology but its traces survive in the promotion of life history as a way of understanding particular manifestations of dementia. Similarly, the focus on well-being and ill-being (Kitwood et al. 1995) was replaced with an emphasis on psychological needs (Kitwood 1997a).

Kitwood was fascinated by the new. He enjoyed picking up ideas that were stimulating and interesting but would equally drop these as something else came along that attracted his attention. Movement in this sense was, then, not necessarily planned or systematic. Again this allowed him to bring in a wider range of ideas than might have been the case had he been more focused on just one or two aspects, but it may also partly explain some of the underdeveloped or unfinished ideas within his work.

The influence of these personal attributes can, in some way, be traced within Kitwood's work, which is at once both richer and more open to criticism for them. But just as history and personality, for Kitwood, were essential for understanding people with dementia, history and personality also help us understand him as an academic, an iconoclast and a person.

The Kitwood Reader

This Reader is divided into four parts – each considering an important strand in Kitwood's work:

Part 1: Kitwood's critique of the standard paradigm
Part 2: Ill-being, well-being and psychological need
Part 3: Personhood
Part 4: Organizational culture and its transformation

Each of the four parts explores Kitwood's work in the area through a description of Kitwood's position and its development, a critique of that position and an indication of areas that, building on Kitwood's work, could be usefully developed. The readings included in each section have been selected as being representative of Kitwood's thought in each of these areas – although not limited to that area, as many of Kitwood's writings cut across the four areas presented here – and as providing some insight into the development of his thought.

Kitwood reiterated his arguments across articles, with slight changes of expression or emphasis, and individuals may lend more importance to one iteration than to another. The selection of readings here may well not satisfy everyone – but we believe that they cover the main aspects of his thought in the four strands of his work as a whole.

Part 1 traces the development of Kitwood's critique of what he termed the 'technical' or standard paradigm and his 'reconsideration' of dementia within a personal framework. It can be argued that this reconsideration was Kitwood's greatest contribution to improving dementia care as it served to move the debate away from the therapeutic nihilism of the day towards a more human, positive approach to those living with dementia. This is not to say that this reconsideration was without its problems – as we shall see there are tensions within it that Kitwood either did not recognize or chose not to deal with. For example, the tension between the positivist and social constructionist frameworks that sought to explain dementia. We shall argue that while Kitwood's work has been influential in dementia care practice, this has been at the expense of his more radical reconsideration of dementia. For example, the dialectical nature of dementia and theory of rementia have been almost totally ignored.

In Part 2, we explore the development of Kitwood's theoretical work on ill-being and well-being in dementia. In some ways Kitwood's thought in this area accompanied the development of his theory of dementia – initially focusing on the negative aspects of the current situation (ill-being/the limits of the standard paradigm respectively) and moving towards a focus on well-being (within the alternative theory of dementia discussed in Part 1). It is in this section particularly that we see some of the unresolved tensions in Kitwood's work most clearly – for example, that between the individual and the societal levels in the aetiology of dementia. Is dementia a result of individual pathology (whether simply neurological or as a result of individual vulnerability) or a function of a social system that militates against sentience generally (Kitwood 1987a)?

Part 3 focuses on personhood – the bedrock of Kitwood's most well-known work on person-centred care. In this section we outline Kitwood's theory and trace its roots to his earlier work, in particular, *What is Human?* (1970). Kitwood's focus on personhood was developed as part of his larger project to improve the lives of those living with dementia. Thus, rather than theorizing personhood and imposing that theorization on individuals, Kitwood took as axiomatic that personhood as a moral status accreted to every individual. We then discuss some of the criticisms of Kitwood's theory of personhood and look forward to ways in which it might be developed, in particular by viewing it as processual, as embodied and as related to both citizenship and place. As with other the parts in this Reader, we hope to generate questions and idea in the minds of our readers as to how to take forward Kitwood's work, building on its strengths and overcoming its limitations.

Finally, in Part 4, we turn to Kitwood's work on organizational culture and its transformation. In developing his critique of care settings, Kitwood applied his concept of 'malignant social psychology' to organizations and contrasted what he termed the 'old' and 'new' cultures of dementia care, outlining the characteristics of both. Part 4 examines those developments and then details some of the more problematic and challenging aspects of Kitwood's work in this area, namely the social and political context of his thinking, the attribution of blame and the role and nature of education in staff development. We shall see that while taking an organizational view, Kitwood did not explicitly address many of the more structural issues impacting on and within organizations – power, gender, ethnicity, ideology, and so on. Indeed, Kitwood moves between blaming the organization and the individual for poor dementia care. There are significant gaps in Kitwood's work in this area, though others have since taken forward some aspects of it. In 1997 Kitwood had begun to give more attention to organizational frameworks and he had only just started developing this work when he died. If he had lived, it is likely some of the problematic aspects of this work would have been worked through and that we would have seen further developments of his thought in this area.

Endnote

There can be no doubt as to Kitwood's influence on the field of dementia care. Major themes that he developed have been taken up internationally and person-centred care is almost inextricably linked with his name.

But that influence seems very much to be limited to those working in dementia care – rather than those involved in research into the causes and potential cures for dementia. While a bio-psychosocial approach to care is widespread, there is little to support the claim that Kitwood's theory of dementia – as a dialectical process in which distal and proximal causes come together resulting in neurological impairment – has been taken up in any significant manner. Indeed, in 2000 the Annals of the New York Academy of Sciences Volume 924, entitled *Alzheimer's Disease: A compendium of current theories*, carried no mention of Kitwood or his theories whatsoever.

The oversights of the New York Academy aside, person-centred care is now firmly on the agenda with a vast amount of research having been undertaken. Major national policy initiatives have taken up the concept – albeit in a rather restricted fashion, usually interpreting it merely as 'individualized care' – and courses in 'person-centred' dementia care can be found across the world. But herein lies the rub – the very popularity of 'person-centredness' often conceals a rather superficial engagement with the complexity of Kitwood's original theories. There is still much evidence of the language of person-centred care being adopted without the corresponding shift in practice. For example, Kitwood's dementia 'equation', $D = P + B + H + NI + SP$, is taken simply as meaning that we should take into account these factors when working with people living with dementia: the person-centred approach can thus become another way of managing people with dementia rather than a focus for understanding how these factors interact dialectically to create the lived experience of dementia. As Kitwood himself wrote:

It is conceivable that most of the advances that have been made in recent years might be obliterated, and that the state of affairs in 2010 might be as bad as it was in 1970, except that it would be varnished by eloquent mission statements, and masked by fine buildings and glossy brochures. (Kitwood 1997a: 133)

Kitwood, of course, does not have the final word on dementia theory and practice. Things have moved on since *Dementia Reconsidered* and Kitwood's death and it is right that we should move on also. We should perhaps, be a little wary of moving too quickly into new areas of work or new research agenda, without having fully engaged with Kitwood's ideas in their complexity, for his work is a rich source of ideas and possibilities. It is as a contribution to that engagement we present this book. While we suggest where future work might profitably lie, such work must be based on sustained reflection.

It is now 10 years since the publication of *Dementia Reconsidered*, and almost the same length of time since Tom Kitwood's death. It is, therefore, an appropriate time to review his work in the context of the present day, to acknowledge what we have learned from it and to identify the challenges that still lie ahead.

Biography

Thomas (Tom) Marris Kitwood was born in 1937 in Boston, Lincolnshire, the son of a local businessman. He gained a scholarship to Rugby and then studied at King's College, Cambridge. His studies there were interrupted by the then compulsory period of National Service which he described as having spent 'two years carrying a clipboard around Salisbury Plain', commenting also that he would rather have spent the two years in prison. Returning to Cambridge, Kitwood graduated with a BA in natural science in 1960. A committed Christian at this time, he then went on to train for the priesthood at Wycliffe Hall theological college in Oxford and was ordained in 1962. Following this he taught for several years at Sherborne, an independent boys' school in Dorset.

In what was evidently a major life change, Kitwood then moved to Uganda, East Africa, where he took up a post at Busoga Boys' School in the hills above Lake Victoria. Here he continued to teach chemistry and also became school chaplain. Over time, however, he began to have doubts about his Christianity and to explore the possibilities of the more secular faith in human potential that he found in humanism. These doubts were already beginning to be apparent in his first book *What is Human?* (1970). While in Uganda, Kitwood married Jenny Cooper, the daughter of missionary parents and their first child, Andrew, was born there.

Kitwood's time in Uganda coincided with the military coup led by Idi Amin in 1971, during which the democratic Obote government was overthrown. This was a period of widespread atrocities, forced repatriation and exile of native Ugandans. Kitwood helped the Ugandan headteacher of the school in Busoga to escape Amin's brutality by crossing the border into Kenya, but he also realized the impossibility of remaining in Uganda under this regime. Together with his wife and young son, he returned to Britain. It is unclear whether this experience further tested his faith or helped to shape his later political beliefs. On his return, however, Kitwood not only resigned his holy orders, but renounced his Christian belief (although he later developed an interest in Buddhism and Taoist philosophy). He retained from his experience in Uganda a deep interest in what he described as 'negritude' (the black experience) and a lifelong concern with moral and spiritual life. He was a committed socialist and pacifist, active in both the Campaign for Nuclear Disarmament and the local Labour movement.

Kitwood moved his young family (a daughter, Lucy, was born following the return to Britain) to Bradford where he spent three years on a student grant, completing an MSc in the Psychology and Sociology of Education in 1974. His PhD on *Values in Adolescent Life* (1977) was supervised by Professor Rom Harré, whose own work on ethogenic social psychology became a significant influence on his subsequent work. Kitwood took up a Lectureship in Science and Society at the University of Bradford in 1979, and became a Senior Lecturer in Interdisciplinary Human Studies in 1992. He was a chartered psychologist and practised privately as a psychotherapist. His books *Disclosures to a Stranger: Adolescent values in advanced industrial society* and *Concern for Others: A new psychology of conscience and morality* were published in 1980 and 1990 respectively.

Kitwood was a popular and inspirational teacher in Higher Education, who often used experiential methods such as role play in his teaching of 'depth psychology' (psychoanalytic theory). From the mid-1980s onwards he combined this work with a growing interest in dementia and dementia care. His fascination with dementia began in 1985 when he became academic supervisor to a psychiatrist and a clinical psychologist who were doing research in this field. Shortly afterwards, Kitwood was commissioned by Bradford Health Authority to carry out an evaluation of a day care service for people with dementia. From this point on, his interest in dementia deepened and became the centre of his work, and it was this evaluation that led directly to the development of Dementia Care Mapping (DCM), one of his most well-known innovations.

Kitwood worked with a number of academic partners in the early days of his dementia career. Notable among these was Kathleen Bredin, with whom he developed Dementia Care Mapping, an observational method for assessing the quality of care and quality of life for people with dementia in formal care settings. The intention was, so far as possible, to take the perspective of the person with dementia which had, until then, been almost entirely overlooked. With Bredin, Kitwood co-authored the seminal text *Person to Person: A guide to the care of those with failing mental powers*, published in 1991. It was from Bredin's own interest in Rogerian humanistic psychology that many of the key concepts in person-centred dementia care originated.

In 1992 Kitwood formed Bradford Dementia Research Group, as it was then known. The word 'research' was removed from its title in 1994, becoming Bradford Dementia Group (BDG). The group was, at this time, a small research unit within the Department of Interdisciplinary Human Studies at Bradford University where Kitwood was still a full-time lecturer. Much of the group's initial work was connected with the development of DCM, but as time went on its membership grew gradually and the range of projects broadened to include family support work and training courses for dementia care workers. In addition to the core membership based in Bradford, a growing number of associate members outside the University were involved in taking forward its projects throughout the UK and, increasingly, internationally.

The extent to which Kitwood's study of academic psychology (and his particularly eclectic and critical approach to this) underpinned his theoretical work on dementia has received little attention. He was passionately interested in – although by no means a slavish follower of – the work of Freud and the various strands of post-Freudian theory. He made many conceptual links between this body of work and the unconscious psychological defences that he believed to be pervasive in the field of dementia care. Building on this he devised a three-day course, *The Depth Psychology of Dementia Care*, intended as an intensive, experiential route towards a deeper understanding of the experience of dementia. He became increasingly aware of the organizational cultures and attitudes that led to the acceptance of, and collusion with, poor care practice. From this came the idea for the 1995 book, *The New Culture of Dementia Care*, which Kitwood edited along with Sue Benson, editor of the *Journal of Dementia Care*.

The education of dementia care workers was a growing concern for Kitwood during this period, as it became increasingly clear that the skills involved in delivering person-centred care were complex, difficult to implement in practice and did not come naturally to everyone. He was also acutely aware of the need to improve the status of dementia care work by developing programmes of professional development. From 1996 onwards BDG began to offer, in addition to its existing short course, a range of accredited modules in dementia care validated by the university. In 1997 Kitwood (together with colleague Andrea Capstick) made a successful bid to the UK Alzheimer Society for three years' partnership funding to develop BDG's existing accredited distance learning provision. This enabled the group to consolidate its educational work alongside its research and development activities.

In 1998 Bradford Dementia Group, now consisting of eight core members, moved to the School of Health Studies at the University of Bradford. Kitwood was awarded a professorship in the summer of that year, a personal chair awarded on the basis of his work in the field of dementia care and titled the Alois Alzheimer Chair of Psychogerontology. At the time this was one of only two chairs in psychogerontology in England. In September 1998, Kitwood left on a lecture tour to the USA. While he was overseas it was announced that he had won the Age Concern Book of the Year Award for his book *Dementia Reconsidered*. Eric Midwinter, chair of the judging panel, described the book as 'outstanding . . . sound in its theoretical construct, yet fresh and pioneering in its original insights. It is fluently and humanely written and, while clearly and practically focusing on the subject matter, it somehow manages to touch on universals and values that affect all our lives' (Age Concern 1998). Kitwood returned from the USA in time to attend the Age Concern book award ceremony at the end of October and then returned home to Bradford. Tragically, he died suddenly and unexpectedly at home the following weekend at the age of 61, as the result of a previously undetected heart defect. As he had wished, his funeral service was conducted by an officiant of the British Humanist Association, and he was buried in a secular plot.

In little more than a decade, Kitwood had transformed what was initially, for him, an academic sideline into a burgeoning area of research, development and education, in which he had become internationally recognized. By the time of his death the work of BDG was being developed overseas in 14 countries. Since then Bradford Dementia Group has continued to grow and develop under the leadership of Professor Murna Downs. It currently has 20 members and has become an academic division of the School of Health Studies (the Division of Dementia Studies), with a full undergraduate and postgraduate degree programme and a thriving and diverse research portfolio.

A note on the text

The critical commentaries at the beginning of each Part make reference to articles by Tom Kitwood which are reproduced here as readings, and also to the wider body of his published work (see the annotated bibliography, p. 333). To assist the reader, quotations from articles reproduced here indicate page numbers in the original source followed by their location within this text (eg Kitwood 1997a: 128/114). Quotations from other Kitwood publications indicate the page number in the original source only.

William Utermohlen
5 December 1933–21 March 2007

(Cover image: Night by William Utermohlen)

Bill Utermohlen was born into a German immigrant family in south Philadelphia in 1933. He studied art at the Pennsylvania Academy of Fine Arts from 1951 to 1957, then one of the most rigorous art academies in the USA, where he began developing a draftsmanship of exceptional precision and power.

In 1957 the artist came to Europe on the GI bill and travelled through France, Spain and Italy, where, like many painters of his generation, he developed a lifelong love for the work of Giotto and Piero della Francesca. In 1957 Utermohlen enrolled at the Ruskin School of Art in Oxford where he met a young fellow American and struggling painter, Ron Kitaj. In 1962 he settled in London, where he met and married the art historian, Patricia Redmond. In 1967 he received his first important London show at the Marlborough Gallery. London life and London characters have most particularly marked his numerous portraits, which constitute one of the richest aspects of his work. In the 1980s he painted two major murals for two great north London institutions, the Liberal Jewish Synagogue at Saint John's Wood and the Royal Free Hospital in Hampstead.

Apart from the portraits, still lives and drawings from the model, which punctuate his entire career, Bill's art can be arranged in six clear thematic cycles: the 'Mythological' paintings of 1962–1963, the 'Cantos' of 1965–1966 inspired by Dante's Inferno, the 'Mummers' cycle of 1969–1970 depicting characters from south Philadelphia's celebrated New Year's Day parade, the 'War' series of 1972 alluding to the Vietnam War, the 'Nudes' of 1973–1974 and finally the 'Conversation Pieces', the great decorative interiors with figures, of 1989–1991.

In 1995 Bill Utermohlen was diagnosed as suffering from Alzheimer's disease. Signs of his illness are retrospectively apparent in the work from the early 1990s, notably in the 'Conversation Pieces', of which the cover painting, 'Night', is a major example. In the works of 1995–1997 Bill's style changes dramatically. There is a greater concentration on self-portraits in which a variety of states of mind – terror, sadness, anger, resignation – are openly expressed. Although more spontaneous, the surface of these last works is still supported by Bill's innate sense of drawing and structure that underpin the brushwork and give the paintings their true power.

Since their exhibition by the Wellcome Trust in London in 2001 these last portraits have received an increased recognition by the medical community, the press and the public. They have been widely exhibited in the USA in Harvard, Philadelphia, New York and North Carolina. A larger exhibition of his late work was held at the Cité des Sciences in Paris and at the Skirball Cultural Center in Los Angeles in the course of 2007.

The artist's work is represented by the Galerie Beckel Odille Boïcos, Paris.

Part 1

KITWOOD'S CRITIQUE OF THE STANDARD PARADIGM

Kitwood's critique of the standard paradigm

Readings

Kitwood, T. (1989) Brain, mind and dementia: with particular reference to Alzheimer's disease, *Ageing and Society*, 9(1): 1–15.

Kitwood, T. (1990) The dialectics of dementia: with particular reference to Alzheimer's disease, *Ageing and Society*, 10(2): 177–196.

Kitwood, T. (1993) Towards the reconstruction of an organic mental disorder. In Radley, A. (ed.) *Worlds of Illness*. London: Routledge.

Kitwood, T. (1993) Person and process in dementia, *International Journal of Geriatric Psychiatry*, 8(7): 541–545.

Kitwood, T. (1996) A dialectical framework for dementia. In Woods, R.T. (ed.) *Handbook of the Clinical Psychology of Ageing*. London: John Wiley & Sons.

Critical commentary

It was in the mid-1980s that Kitwood became interested in dementia. He had been asked to provide academic supervision to mental health professionals working in dementia and from this he proceeded to develop the theory of dementia (Bender 2003) that can be found in many of his publications (1987a, 1987b, 1988a, 1988b, 1989, 1990a, 1990b, 1993a, 1993b, 1996a, 1997a). While there is much repetition in these publications, each had a slightly different emphasis and it is possible to trace changes over time. It is the purpose of this chapter to describe Kitwood's theory of dementia, tracing its development and placing it in context. Following this, mainly descriptive, process we shall examine some salient aspects of both the theory and its development. In the penultimate section, we shall comment on some of the criticisms levelled against Kitwood in this area and then, finally, look towards the future.

Kitwood's critique of the 'standard paradigm'

Kitwood's theory of dementia stemmed from his initial critique of what he termed the 'standard paradigm', or technical frame, in dementia. Drawing on Kuhn's notion of paradigms in science, Kitwood argued that the paradigm within which most research and practice in dementia operated was medically based, deficit focused and therapeutically nihilistic:

> The accepted wisdom of today's geriatric medicine is that there are several well-defined organic diseases which bring about dementia in old age. Of these, two are said to account for the majority of cases. The first is a condition in which the cerebral grey matter shows degenerative changes very similar, or possibly identical, to those found in Alzheimer's disease in middle life. The second is associated with the destruction of tissue that follows the bursting of small blood vessels in the brain (multiple infarction). (Kitwood 1987b: 117)

Kitwood was to challenge fundamental aspects of the medical model of dementia, arguing, in contrast, that dementia should be seen as a dialectic between the personal, social and neurological. In so doing, Kitwood aimed to move the debate towards the development of a social model of dementia.

The first step in the development of an alternative theory of dementia was a detailed critique of the current position. This critique took on three overlapping and interacting aspects: an exploration of the limits of neuropathological research; a critique of the medicalization and Alzheimerization of dementia; and the problems of diagnostic imprecision.

Limits of neuropathological research

In *Explaining senile dementia: The limits of neuropathological research*, Kitwood endeavoured to provide a detailed critique of the neuropathological evidence with regard to dementia. Selecting four papers, three of which he held to be definitive in their field, Kitwood challenged both their findings and their assumptions. Kitwood summed up his argument against the standard paradigm in dementia research thus:

1 Many people show psychological symptoms of dementia in old age.
2 In clinical terms, the dementias fall into a small number of overlapping syndromes, only loosely correlated to recognizable neuropathology as identified by post-mortem.
3 The neuropathology found post-mortem can be roughly classified into two main types: Alzheimerian and multi-infarct, although many brains show a mixture of both.
4 The neuropathological processes identified in the demented are present, to some degree, in many well-preserved old people.
5 Some people become demented with very little accompanying neuropathology and, in general, the correlation between degree of dementia and the severity of neuropathology found post-mortem falls far short of a basis for sufficient explanation.
6 Those in whose brains a neuropathological process is far advanced cannot sustain normal cognitive, emotional and behavioural functions. Probably there is a threshold beyond which a demented state is inevitable, although this may vary from person to person (Kitwood 1987b: 133).

In short, the standard paradigm fails to provide an account of why some people experience dementia with very low, or no, neurological damage and why some people with a high degree of neurological damage do not experience dementia.

Furthermore, the standard paradigm is limited in three significant ways: first, by its inability to incorporate psychological factors into the aetiology and progression of dementia; second, by its conflation of two distinct discourses regarding the mind and the brain; third, by its means of maintaining its own validity.

The first of these, the failure to incorporate psychological factors into the explanation of dementia, is, for Kitwood, both an a priori and empirical failing. It is an a priori failing because it is irrational to rule out such factors without considering them when there are gaps in the explanatory force of current theory. It is an empirical failing, in that if neuropathology alone cannot account for 'the change from normal to demented functioning in an individual' even 'granted a certain degree of degeneration of grey matter' (Kitwood 1988a: 127/113–114), then there must be some explanation outwith neuropathology, i.e. psychological factors. Just as psychological factors had been found to be relevant in other diseases such as cancer, 'psychology seems to be implicated proximally in the causation of dementia, even if it contributes to the distal causation as well' (ibid.).

The second limitation to the standard paradigm is that which comes about through the conflation of two discourses: 'one related to a person's behavioural and cognitive impairments, and the other related to processes occurring in the nervous system' (Kitwood 1996a: 270). In this conflation, explanatory power is lost because one discourse takes precedence and the nuances and the complexities of reality are obscured from view. By focusing on the neurological processes, the standard paradigm excludes the contribution of psychology to the understanding of dementia, for example, explanations of such phenomena as pseudodementia and rementia (see later).

The third limitation to the standard paradigm is the way in which it seeks to deal with evidence that does not fit neatly into the paradigm (see Kitwood 1993a). Kitwood argues that such evidence is accommodated into the existing paradigm through ad hoc adaptations to the theory. There are four such problems for the standard paradigm:

- *pseudodementia* – that is, the presentation of a range of symptoms that look extremely like those of Alzheimer's disease but are reversible – for example, dementia-like symptoms found with depression, uraemia, chronic constipation and pneumonia
- *apparent precipitation* – that is, the onset of a dementing illness fairly quickly after one or more life crises
- *catastrophic decline* – related to the previous point, but referring to a dramatic downturn after a life change, for example, following hospitalization for assessment, being taken into respite care or moved into a residential or nursing home
- *moderate* or *transitory 'rementia'* – that is the (at least partial) recovery from dementia (Kitwood 1993a: 147–151/55–57).

It is worth quoting Kitwood at length:

It is difficult, although not impossible, to explain phenomena such as these in terms of the 'standard paradigm', with its linear causality.

X → neuropathic change → dementia

The pseudodementias have to be presented as a fundamentally different set of conditions from true SDAT [senile dementia of the Alzheimer's type], originating solely in neurochemistry, although some of the symptoms of the latter are closely 'mimicked' in the former. The apparent precipitation of SDAT is explained in terms of a theory of 'unmasking': that is, the person already 'had' the dementia, although it was not apparent until after the crucial life events. Here the arbitrary sliding of the term dementia between neurological and psychological frames of reference is par-ticularly apparent. Catastrophic decline has to be accounted for in roughly the same way (the dementia was in fact already far worse than had been realized); for unlike the case of multiple infarction, it is implausible to suggest that massive Alzheimer-type degeneration of the grey matter can occur over a space of 3–6 months. Rementia has to be reframed in terms of a precarious distinction between remedi-able and non-remediable symptoms, or on the assumption that the original diag-nosis was incorrect. 'Benign senescent atrophy' remains uninterpreted, but it is possible to postulate a shrinkage of grey matter, without the actual death of nerve cells.

It may well be the case, then, that the 'standard paradigm' can now only be upheld through the rather dubious procedure of 'saving the appearances'; or, to use Popper's term, through a succession of ad hoc modifications. (Kitwood 1989: 6/25)

While the standard paradigm exhibits these anomalies, its dominance also has three undesirable outcomes. First, in being the established framework within which to address dementia, it effectively excludes alternative approaches and thus inhibits the development of both knowledge about dementia and new ways of providing dementia care; second, it excludes the person with dementia, seeing only the dementia rather than the person (see Kitwood 1993b); and, third, it leads to a 'pervasive (and perhaps unjustified) pessimism, as epitomized in such images as "the prison that waits" or "the living death" (Kitwood 1996b: 91).

While we are fundamentally in agreement with this critique of the standard paradigm, it is important to note two caveats to Kitwood's presentation of the argument.

First, in stating that a single discourse can hide the complexities of reality from view, Kitwood seems to be accepting dementia as a biomedical reality (if only partially under-stood in these terms) thus endorsing a positivist view of dementia, a view that is at odds with the social constructivist stance he takes on the aetiology of dementia (see Part 2) where dementia is viewed as a result of dysfunctional social relations.

Second, in criticizing the standard paradigm for being upheld only by a series of ad hoc modifications (Kitwood 1993a), Kitwood misrepresents the philosophy of science. Citing Popper, Kitwood implies that the 'ad hoc modifications' are indicative of a failure of the standard paradigm and are designed to cover up inherent difficulties with the standard paradigm that in essence would falsify the theory that dementia is simply a biomedical phenomenon.

In other publications, however, (see Kitwood 1987b) Kitwood cites the work of Lakatos (Lakatos 1970) as opposing Popper's falsificationism and as pointing to the resistance to change in established research programmes. This, however, is to misrepresent somewhat Lakatos' argument. In contrast to Popper, Lakatos argued that ad hoc modifications are part and parcel of scientific development and a research programme (in the widest sense of that term, that is, an underlying explanatory theory that generates facts and hypotheses) should not be rejected simply because such adaptations need to be made, either on the basis of theoretical difficulties or indeed factual counterevidence. According to Lakatos, research programmes consist of a 'hard core' or irrefutable centre. So far Kitwood is in accord with Lakatos. Lakatos, however, goes on to argue that this hard core is surrounded by a 'protective belt' of potentially refutable explanations of anomalies. This protective belt serves as a means to manage anomalies, some of which will be appropriated into the research programme, others of which will be eliminated through ad hoc modifications. If we apply this sort of analysis to the case of dementia, the hard core – the standard paradigm – can be seen as being protected by these ad hoc modifications until such time as they are refuted or become irrefutable, rather than being falsified by the anomalies that Kitwood raises.

In other words, a Lakatosian analysis would tend to support the continuation of the standard paradigm in the face of anomalies, rather than the abandonment of that paradigm because there are anomalies. We shall see later, however, that Lakatos can also be enlisted in support of the development of an alternative paradigm because multiplicity of research programmes is preferable to univocality.

The medicalization and Alzheimerization of dementia

The second strand to Kitwood's critique was to explore the construction of dementia as a disease – the medicalization or 'Alzheimerization' of senility. Although this was a theme of which Kitwood spoke, it is not well represented in his publications (see, for example, Kitwood 1996a, 1997a). In *Dementia Reconsidered*, he says: 'At a popular level, the definitional issues have been clouded by what might be termed the "alzheimerization" of dementia. Twenty-five years ago the name of Alois Alzheimer was known only to a small handful of specialists, and the main dementias of old age were often labelled as senility. Today Alzheimer has become a household word' (Kitwood 1997a: 22).

This process was not, according to Kitwood, a result of further data regarding the phenomenon but an outcome of a series of pragmatic decisions: both financial and political. Through the corralling of research monies and successful lobbying the Alzheimer's movement (an alliance of scientists, government representatives, members of the public and the media) two processes were established. First, Alzheimer's became almost synonymous with dementia, virtually replacing the previous, less obviously medical, term senile dementia. Cognitive decline was therefore no longer to be seen as a normal part of aging but as a pathological process.

Second, it helped to extend the boundaries of Alzheimer's to include a wider population by removing age as a primary criterion of disease (see Fox 1989). Originally, a distinction was made between pre-senile and senile dementia, depending on the age of the patient. It was Kraepelin, the head of the research laboratory in which Alois Alzheimer worked, who proposed that the pathological changes noted in the brain by Alzheimer be classified as a disease separate from senile dementia (Alzheimer's observations, it must be remembered, were of a middle-aged woman). Pre-senile dementia thus became Alzheimer's disease. It was not until much later (mid-1970s; see Fox 1989) that senile dementia and Alzheimer's disease were tied together, based on the pathological changes in the brain and not on age of onset. Senility was thus dissociated from the idea simply of growing old and identified with a disease process. There was thus a 'unifying construct' around which to focus the varying interests of members of the alliance. In short, dementia and aging became medicalized and Alzheimerized (see Adelman 1995; Bond 1992; Fox 1989; Lyman 1989).

This biomedical view includes, according to Lyman (1989), three features: dementia is pathological and individual; is somatic or organic in aetiology, caused by progressive deterioration of the brain; and is to be diagnosed, treated and managed according to medical authority.

Problems of diagnostic imprecision

The third strand of Kitwood's critique is the difficulty of accurately diagnosing dementia. For Kitwood, there were a number of contributory factors to this difficulty:

- The kind of evidence that is considered as relevant to making a diagnosis.
- The weight given to problems of memory.
- The bluntness of such tests as the Mini-Mental State Examination.
- Confounding factors such as possible depression, that also may affect cognitive functioning.
- The limits of CT scanning (see Kitwood 1997a: 26–27).

We can also add to these possible confounding factors the definitional problems outlined earlier (see 'Limits of neuropathological research') and the conflation of various phenomenon under the rubric of Alzheimer's disease (see earlier in the current section).

Furthermore, a definitive diagnosis of Alzheimer's disease requires post-mortem examination through which the pathological damage – the plaques and neurofibrillary tangles – can be identified. Although this is allegedly 'hard evidence' (see Kitwood 1987b), there are a number of problems with this approach. First, the research indicates that there is a degree of overlap between the characteristics of the brains of those with dementia and those without, suggesting that the issue of diagnosis on the basis of post-mortem evidence is not as clear-cut as it is generally assumed to be. The psychological condition of dementia can accompany varying degrees of pathological damage. What degree of damage beyond that to be expected in old age is required in order to support a diagnosis of Alzheimer's disease? Second, post-mortem evidence indicates that some brains show a mixture of indicators (Alzheimer's disease and multi-infarct dementia) thus confounding the picture of diagnostic clarity: for the purposes of diagnosis, which indicators are given preference? Third, even if there is a correlation between pathological changes in the brain and the signs and symptoms of dementia, it cannot be assumed that one is causative of the other. According to Kitwood (1987b), the hypothesis of exclusive neuropathological causation would be falsified by a single case 'where there is unequivocal evidence of dementia without associated neuropathology' (p. 128) and he claimed that such a case had already been presented in the research he was reviewing.

Dementia remains a somewhat difficult diagnosis to make – in 2004 one-third of GPs surveyed reported limited confidence in their diagnostic skills with regards to dementia (Turner et al. 2004). New diagnostic techniques – for example, cognitive rating scales, brain imaging and radiological tests (see Alzheimer's Australia 2004) – have enabled practitioners to be more accurate in their differential diagnoses. Despite these developments, however, conceptual and diagnostic problems still remain (see Hohl et al. 2000 and Knopman et al. 2001 for examples).

Dominance of the standard paradigm

If, as Kitwood argues, the standard paradigm, the technical frame, is so fundamentally flawed – conceptually and empirically – the question that arises is why the paradigm has attained, and continues to maintain, ascendancy in dementia research and practice.

Several factors can help explain this:

1   There is a general dominance of the scientific paradigm in Western society – the scientific methods and technical reasoning developed from the Enlightenment onwards have been firmly established and have a momentum that clearly achieve results. Thus alternative approaches may appear to be irrelevant or absurd.

2   There are vested interests in maintaining this approach – from the technical training and experience of medico-scientific professionals to the activities of drug companies.

3   The technical frame provides a kind of distancing between health professionals and their patients, which in an environment that is under-resourced and under-supported, 'helps make their working life more bearable, and rationalizes the woes that they encounter day by day' (Kitwood 1988a: 128/114).

4   For relatives and carers the technical frame may enable them to cope with the feelings of grief, fear, anger, guilt and inadequacy they feel as it is easier to describe the afflicted person as 'having' a disease than 'having to face the immensely threatening possibility that there might have been, and might still be, psychologically malignant processes going on within the family, including even their own relationship to the dementing person' (ibid.).

5   On a more macro-level, Kitwood postulated that the technical frame aids 'a widespread and collusive denial of what is involved in ageing and dying in the modern world' (ibid.). In other words, the framing of dementia as a technical problem allows us, at some level, to believe in the possibility of a cure and thus deny it as an inevitable and existential problem (see Kitwood 1993a).

6   The technical frame also helps us not to think of the problem as a structural one, that is, many of the problems faced by older people are a function of their structural position – 'a disastrous disempowerment through lack of income, work role, and mobility; great personal insecurity; a progressive loss of social connections; and for some an entry into a barren world where there is little genuine love and intersubjectivity, where they are related to mainly as a stereotype' (1988b: 174). While it is conceivable that we might arrange things differently, this would require fundamental transformation.

An alternative theory of dementia

Following, or rather alongside, this critique of the standard paradigm, Kitwood developed an alternative theory of dementia. In order to be a credible alternative, this theory should:

- overcome the conflation of discourses, with the resultant dominance of one or the other
- be able to explain what the standard paradigm could not – for example, individual differences in the onset and progression of dementia and phenomena such as pseudodementia and rementia
- be empirically testable
- be more encompassing of potential factors – that is, include psychological factors – involved in the onset and progression of dementia
- be based on, or at the very least, substantially incorporate, the intersubjective experience of dementia
- be practically useful, pointing clearly to what we should and should not be doing in care practice.

Dementia reconsidered

Kitwood first of all sought to bring together, into a theoretically coherent framework, the two discourses of neurology and psychology. He did this by postulating that every event or state a person experiences psychologically is also an event or a state in the neurophysiological system. For example, a psychological desire has a concomitant phenomenon within the neurological functioning of the brain. This is not to say that such desires, for instance, are reducible to the activities of neurones, or that these desires cause these activities. Rather, that psychology and neurology are attempting to describe what is happening in two different ways, but are referring to the same event or state. An analogy would be two theories of light – one describing light in terms of particle theory, the other in terms of wave theory. Both have their strengths and weaknesses but are, essentially, describing the same phenomenon, that is, light.

These events – whether viewed as psychological or neurological – occur within an 'apparatus' or structure which sets limits to what the brain can do. This structure has two crucial aspects: the developmental aspect, that is, the development of the brain as a result of learning and experience throughout the lifecourse (for Kitwood such development is not limited to the earlier years of life); and the pathological aspect indicated by such things as the loss of neurones and interneuronal connections through specific disease processes.[1]

Dementia is thus a function of the interrelationship between psychological and neurological events within the parameters set by the configuration of an individual's brain in terms of its developmental and pathological aspects. This interrelationship is the basis of the 'dialectic framework for dementia'.

Having established this framework, Kitwood then seeks to explain the dementing process. In *The dialectics of dementia* (Kitwood 1990a) he proposes three basic 'equations':

1   Senile dementia is compounded from the effects of neurological impairment (NI) and of malignant social psychology (SP).

2   Neurological impairment in an elderly person attracts to itself a malignant social psychology.

3   Malignant social psychology, bearing down on an aged person, whose physiological buffers are already fragile, actually creates neurological impairment.

In these equations there is a dynamic between social psychology (SP) and neurological impairment (NI), these being the only two aspects of the equation at this time. In this 1990 article, Kitwood does not detail his arguments on the third of these equations. Indeed, he says that the third is not crucial to the theory – we will return to this later in this chapter.

The theory of dementia that was included in *Dementia Reconsidered* takes up the first two of these equations and details the elements of malignant social psychology that contribute to the trajectory of dementia (see Part 2 on 'ill-being, well-being and psychological need').

A further aspect to this alternative theory of dementia, presented in 1993 (Kitwood 1993a, 1993c), is that the dementing process depends not only on psychological and neurological factors but also on other personal and social factors: that is, personality (P), biography (B) and health (H). Dementia is thus a configuration of five factors:

$$D = P + B + H + NI + SP \quad \text{(Kitwood 1993c: 541/67)}$$

For Kitwood (1996a) following Mischel (1977) and Burkitt (1993), personality is regarded as 'resources for action' rather than a series of 'traits'.[2] According to this view, each person develops his or her own unique repertoire of resources according to the opportunities that life provides and which are related to broader factors such as locality, culture and class. These resources can be both positive, such as fortitude, or more negative, such as avoidances and blocks. (It is important to understand the role of these resources when we come to discuss Kitwood's aetiology of dementia.)

Related to personality, but not coterminous with it, is individual biography. We cannot, according to Kitwood, understand the phenomenon of dementia particular to an individual without having some sense of his or her life story and, in particular, the experience of loss within that biography.

The third factor, physical health, is important because some degree of confusion can be directly induced by problems at a metabolic level – for example, toxins in the system – and other health problems, such as loss of mobility, sight or hearing, affect the opportunities for interaction and maintaining competence. Such deteriorations in physical health are often attributed to a progress of dementia when such attribution is inappropriate. Hence the configuration:

$$\text{Dementia} = P + B + H + NI + SP$$

The exact configuration of these factors will be unique to the individual and it is in this way we need to understand Kitwood's emphasis on the uniqueness of persons and the individuality of care required to maintain personhood. The dementing process is thus presented as an 'involutionary spiral', unique to the individual as illustrated in Figure 1.1.

The dialectics of dementia

Kitwood's alternative theory of dementia has, in some ways, proved massively popular. His 'equation' $D = P + B + H + NI + SP$ is cited as the basis for person-centred care, that is, care that takes into account the individual's history and personality. But Kitwood's theory of dementia involved more than simply an argument for a more holistic approach to dementia care – the dementing process was seen as a dialectic where each of the factors in the equation interacted with the others to *create* dementia. In this theory, dementia was not the background 'given' against which person-centred care (that is, accounting for P, B, H and SP) was to be implemented, but was a function of both care and neurological impairment. This is reflected in, on the one hand, the mass of literature on the benefits of person-centred care and, on the other, the almost total lack of any research on the relationship between care and neuropathology. For example, are there any significant neurological differences between those who receive sustained, high-quality person-centred care (in Kitwood's sense of maintaining person-hood through positive social relationships) and those who are merely warehoused until death?

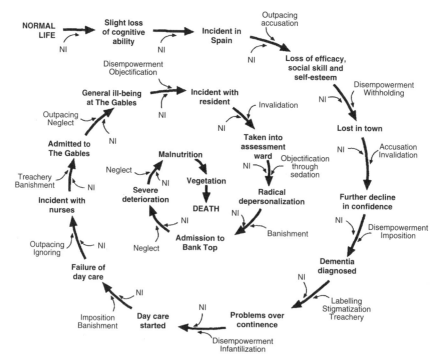

Figure 1.1 The involutionary spiral of the dementia process 1997. (Figure 3.3 from Kitwood 1997a: 52)

Ambiguity and inconsistency

In the introduction to this Reader we raised the issue of ambiguity and inconsistency within Kitwood's work. Here we would note the ambiguity in his position regarding the aetiology of dementia (raised again in Part 2 under ill-being and the onset of dementia) and his position within positivist and social constructivist philosophies.

At times, Kitwood seems to hold the view that dementia is the outworking in the individual of societal dysfunction – witness his statement in 1987:

> . . . all the possibly dementogenic factors that we might seek to identify, whether personal dispositions, life events, or social-psychological processes, are themselves situated in a broader pathology of social relations. They can be viewed as necessary consequences of a society with fundamentally unresolved injustices, although I shall not argue this point here.

> In the case of late capitalism the whole social process works against the development of sentience. Virtually all the major institutions, whether of education, industry, commerce, law or government, operate with an extremely restricted conception of what it is to be human. (Kitwood 1987a: 91)

And this is represented in his 1990 version of the 'involutionary spiral' (see Figure 1.2), where social factors are linked to further neurological impairment.

However, by 1993 Kitwood had removed those links (Kitwood 1993b: 105). Having said that, we cannot be sure the removal of these links was because Kitwood had changed his mind on the aetiology of dementia or for some other, more tactical reason – that by not focusing on this macro-social constructivist approach to dementia he hoped to persuade others of the credibility of other, perhaps more immediately important, aspects of this theory.

This ambiguity then leads us on to the question as to Kitwood's stance with regard to the competing philosophies of positivism and social constructivism. On the one hand, his approach seems to be firmly in the social constructivist camp – that social factors are dementogenic. On the other, however, there seems to be an acceptance, in his later works, of neurological impairment as an objective factor in and of itself. This ambiguity is suggested – but not discussed – by Harding and Palfrey in their book *The Social Construction of Dementia: Confused professionals?*, in which they claim that Kitwood was a social constructionist, yet later, without acknowledging their own inconsistency, criticize him for accepting the medical model (see Harding and Palfrey 1997: 60, 64).

Criticisms of Kitwood's theory

Kitwood's reconsideration of dementia was not received with universal acclaim. Indeed, reviewing *Dementia Reconsidered* in the *British Medical Journal*, Flicker (1999) criticized Kitwood for:

- not providing supporting evidence for his claims
- not requiring rigorous testing

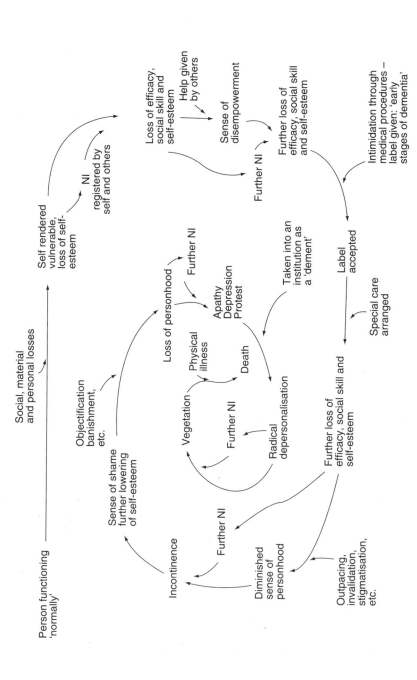

Figure 1.2 The involutionary spiral of the dementia process 1990. (Figure 2 from Kitwood 1990a: 192)

- being selective and anecdotal in his presentation of evidence
- failing to take note of more recent work in neuropsychology.

Flicker is not alone in criticizing Kitwood in this way. Adams (1996) criticized him for his lack of evidence and both Adams (1997) and Murphy (1995) raised issues about the lack of robust methodology in Kitwood's work.

The criticism of lacking empirical evidence is only partially valid – and only then in a relatively weak form. It is true in that in many places Kitwood makes a claim that he does not immediately support by reference to empirical research. This 'failing', however, should not automatically or even necessarily be interpreted as an inherent flaw in Kitwood's opus for the following reasons.

First, at the start of an emerging theory or discipline, it is often difficult to find empirical work to substantiate one's claims. Empirical work often, if not predominantly, follows from theoretical work rather than vice versa and so we should not be surprised that at the outset Kitwood did not have empirical data to draw on. For example, until it was theorized that the Self did not disintegrate with the onset and progression of dementia the data that now support that theory were not available because they were not being looked for or were being interpreted within a different theory.

Second, the criticism cannot be held to apply to Kitwood's work per se. Kitwood published a number of articles in which he reported on empirical work where it was available. In his critique of the medical model, he closely examined research reports in order to support his emerging theory of dementia. In his theorizing about 'rementia' he drew on research undertaken by others (see, for example, Kitwood and Bredin 1992a: 278–279/135–136). As he developed his theories he engaged in and reported on a number of empirical studies (Kitwood 1990a, 1990b, 1995b; Kitwood et al. 1995) and the development of the Dementia Care Mapping tool provided a wealth of data on well-being and ill-being among people with dementia in institutional settings.

Third, Kitwood was aware of the need to provide supporting evidence if his theories were to be accepted. Indeed, he explicitly laid down an empirical challenge:

> The quality of care can be assessed empirically . . . As care improves the long-term patterns of dementia may prove to be very different from those described in the older literature, and epitomized in the standard stage theories. We may reasonably expect to find far less vegetation – possibly none at all. There should be a much higher level of sustained well-being, and in a proportion of cases the kind of long-term therapeutic changes that I have described. Dementia will then be a different set of clinical conditions from those we have inherited, and which are described in the standard textbooks of today.

> All of this is open to further investigation, by the accepted methods of social science. Popper suggested that a good scientist should be willing to make risky and falsifiable statements, ahead of actual testing. So here is mine. If it is found that better care, as operationally defined, is accompanied by no change in the overall long-term pattern, the account of dementia that I have given will have been falsified. If, however, the kind of changes that I have reported from one small study, and those that I have predicted, are indeed found, we can no longer regard the

disease processes that accompany dementia as autonomous, the 'standard paradigm' will have been falsified. The door would then be open for radical reconstruction of the whole field, giving dementia care an immensely more important place. (Kitwood 1997a: 101)

It is our contention that there is now more than enough empirical evidence if not to falsify the standard paradigm, certainly to lend credence to Kitwood's theories. And, with Woods, we would agree that even were Kitwood 'ever an arm-chair theorist, the armchair was located firmly in the day-room of a residential home in the midst of people with dementia' (Woods 1999: 5).

The criticism regarding methodology is, perhaps, more valid as Kitwood did not always explicate his methods as clearly as he might. For example, in *Brighter Futures* (Kitwood et al. 1995), there is a lack of discussion regarding the statistical methodology (Murphy 1997); in *Understanding senile dementia* (Kitwood 1990b), the description of the methodology – vital to generating credibility for the psychobiographical approach – appears, as Kitwood acknowledged, 'highly subjective and undisciplined' (p. 19/122) without regard to the methodological literature that might have supported his case; and in *Positive long-term changes in dementia* (Kitwood 1995b), even Kitwood acknowledged that, 'Doing research in this kind of way is far from ideal, and it is possible that there is considerable distortion' (p. 135). There seems, in Kitwood's work, an ambivalence towards methodological issues. On the one hand, he made the challenge to falsify his theory through empirical research; on the other, he was not enamoured with what he called 'dreary empiricism'. Through his background in the natural sciences he knew of the benefits of importance of methodological rigour, yet in his work on dementia he was often more inclined to the intuitive and particular.

Having said this, however, we do not think that the situation regarding methodology fatally undermines Kitwood's work. What Kitwood did, regardless of his own methodological failings, was to develop a research paradigm – as per Lakatos – that generated questions, research programmes and activities and data that contributed greatly to our understanding of dementia and the practice of dementia care. Having done this, perhaps it is left to those who follow to develop the methodological rigour that will confirm or falsify Kitwood's theories.

Rementia

Linked to the reframing of dementia is the concept of 'rementia' – the possibility that individuals might, if circumstances were favourable, regain some of their lost abilities. This rementia, as conceived of by Kitwood, is more than a generalized feeling of wellbeing – as it has sometime been interpreted – but a claim that good dementia care, upholding the personhood of the individual with dementia, may result in the slowing, halting or even reversal of cognitive function (measurable through tools such as the Mini-Mental State Examination). Going further, rementia might also involve some degree of neurological repair – a distinct challenge to the medical model of progressive and inevitable decline.

The idea of rementia stems directly from viewing dementia as a dialectical process. If, as is suggested, dementia is a function of the interaction of personal, social and neurological factors, then changes in any of these will have some impact on the dementing process. Positive changes, such as what came to be termed 'positive person work' should, according to Kitwood's challenge, result in positive changes in cognitive functioning: that is, rementia. This can be represented as in the adaptation of Kitwood's involutionary spiral of the dementing process in Figure 1.3. The social, material and personal losses are still operating to render the self vulnerable but social relations are countering the neurological impact of such losses rather than facilitating them.

In *Dementia Reconsidered*, Kitwood claimed that the idea of rementia had moved from being 'tantamount to heresy' when he first proposed it, to being accepted by many people (1997a: 4). Although Kitwood claimed some evidence for the idea of rementia (for example, Brane et al. 1989; Karlsson et al. 1988; Roach 1985), his view that it had become accepted by many seems somewhat optimistic if research publications on the subject are any indication of interest. Although there have been one or two studies that have provided some research evidence for the phenomenon (for example, Moniz-Cook et al. 2003; Sixsmith et al. 1993), the concept of rementia has not been taken up in any significant way in the literature of dementia.

The future of dementia theory

It is perhaps a little premature to discuss the future of dementia theory when the alternative theory put forward by Kitwood has not really been tested and implemented only in a diluted form. Even so, we would like, at least tentatively, to suggest that there is scope for further developing Kitwood's ideas in three ways.

First, Kitwood's work on the interplay of social and psychological factors in the aetiology of dementia was not fully worked out and there would seem to be potential here to develop these ideas and extend our understanding of the social model of dementia. This is a theme we return to in Part 2.

Second, philosophical developments may lead us to understand dementia differently. For example, Deleuze and Guattari (2004) write of the process of deterritorialization whereby certain framings of ideas, people, ways of being (and so on) are undermined by reconfigurations of those elements that frame them in those particular ways. Dementia is still predominantly framed in terms of configurations of neuropathology, decline, loss (of cognitive faculties, self, engagement, and so on), disease and suffering – that is, in relation to what is framed as 'normal' and 'healthy'. But there is, according to Deleuze and Guattari, nothing given about any configuration and thus it is possible to reconfigure the framing of dementia using different elements. Of course, some work on this deterritorialization has already taken place with the development of different models of dementia (the social model, the disability model and, more recently, the citizenship model) and the increasing vocality of people with dementia themselves. But still much work needs to be done. We are not advocating necessarily that dementia is demedicalized (in the sense of a return to seeing it simply as a function of the aging process) but that in order to further deterritorialize dementia it is necessary to delink it from ideas of loss – a much deeper cultural association.

Indeed, some authors have argued that we should view dementia as a window into 'otherness' with all the benefits that brings:

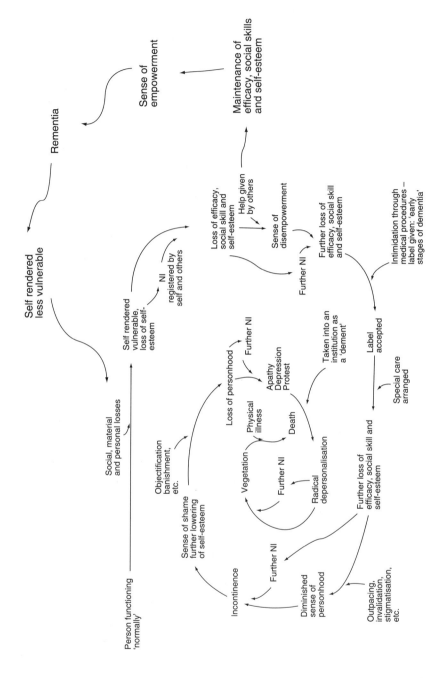

Figure 1.3 The rementing process. (adapted from Figure 2 Kitwood 1990a: 192)

Can we find meaning in dementia by turning the gain-loss paradigm on its head and by recognizing that there lie hidden riches if we look at dementia through a different prism, beyond loss and gain? That is, if we open ourselves to understanding dementia in a new light we may find that we 'gain' insight into its 'otherness.' This otherness is grounded in the realm of imagination and in a human thirst to be creative. It is an attitude that allows life to be lived in amazingly diverse and rich ways that defy the normal or consensual path of life. This otherness allows for the road less traveled, allows us to live our life in the way important to us, not necessarily in the way prescribed for us. (Shabahangi 2005: 4–5)

Such a cultural shift would, in our view, allow other ways of being in the world to be fully valued and the uniqueness of persons to be celebrated.

Leading on from this, we might, third, begin to explore the contribution made by people living with dementia to the lives of others. In research undertaken by one of the authors (CB), a number of carers reported ways in which their relative (living with dementia) contributed to their lives and their families in terms of enhancing the quality of relationships:

She's part of the home, she's part of the family and she enriches us in ways that are phenomenal sometimes, this is the lady who has never been particularly fond of babies but she met her two great nephews, one is 1 and one 4, she's met one of them before, they've come from Australia, and she was enthralled with the baby. She's never loved babies in her life but at this moment in time babies are what fits, she likes little babies and you can't, to have that amount of pleasure given you, it makes everything worthwhile. (daughter caring for her mother)

Similarly, some carers say that their relative with dementia has contributed to their (the carers') spiritual life and that new meanings and levels of relationships have been made possible because of the dementia. While not wanting to deny the pain many families experience, we want to suggest that, at the least, dementia can be seen not simply as tragedy but a combination of tragedy and opportunity for growth.

All of this, of course, is only possibility. To retheorize dementia in terms of rementia, 'otherness' and contribution is contrary to the prevailing cultural focus on loss and tragedy. Much work needs to be done in order to develop a 'progressive research programme' – in the Lakatosian sense of a programme that generates new facts – along the lines indicated here. Again, citing Lakatos in support of our argument, we should not allow the current paradigm (whether the standard paradigm or a negative social model) to hold itself as arbiter of what is acceptable or appropriate as a research programme. Multiplicity of research programmes is more likely to contribute to the growth of knowledge than univocality.

Concluding remarks

In presenting his alternative theory of dementia Kitwood always had in mind the development of care practice. We shall see in Part 3 how his a priori commitment to viewing individuals as persons – regardless of their capacities – helped inform his theory of personhood. Similarly, the theory of dementia also had the goal of improving the way people with dementia are treated.

By viewing dementia as a dialectical problem, Kitwood drew attention to the problematic aspects that the cognitively intact bring to the caring relationship. In viewing dementia as a problem of others (that is, we are basically sound, undamaged, competent and kind while those with dementia are damaged, derailed and deficient – see Kitwood and Bredin 1992a), the possibility that the actions of the cognitively intact may contribute to the progression of dementia is excluded from consideration.

By viewing dementia as a two-way process Kitwood sought to provide a framework that provided practical benefit: by understanding our role in the dialectic of dementia, it is possible to act and provide care in a way that supports personhood and thus maintains the well-being of the person living with dementia. It is to the issue of well-being and psychological need that we turn in the following section.

Notes

1   Kitwood represented these factors in the fashion of an equation:

$$\frac{\psi \equiv b}{B^d, B^p}$$

where ψ represents psychology and b represents the functional state of the brain, B^d represents the developmental aspect of the brain and B^p the pathological. Why Kitwood chose to represent his argument in this pseudoscientific fashion is unclear as such 'equations' seem to have generated distraction from his argument rather than clarity.

2   It is interesting to note here that Kitwood was not always consistent about this. See the critique offered in Part 4 on 'organizational culture and its transformation'.

1.1

Brain, mind and dementia: with particular reference to Alzheimer's disease (1989)

ABSTRACT

A new theoretical framework for understanding and working with the dementing illnesses of old age is presented, and explicated with particular reference to senile dementia of the Alzheimer type. For several reasons the commonly accepted model, which assumes a simple linear causal relationship between neuropathology and dementia, is inadequate. A more comprehensive model, grounded in a monistic view of the mind-brain relationship, must take into account not only the psychological states that correspond to particular brain states, but also both developmental and pathological aspects of brain structure. Using this we can describe the dementing process, 'normal' psychological functioning in old age, pseudodementia and 'benign senescent forgetfulness'. Further, the scope for some degree of 'rementia' is explored.

Introduction

It is now becoming clear that virtually all the losses and difficulties of later life are socially constructed: that is, they are a consequence not of the ageing process in itself, but also of the norms and collective arrangements that are taken for granted as applying to old age. There is one form of distress that is faced with particular dread, especially now that life expectancy has been prolonged. It is that of 'going senile': in other words, developing one of those dementing illnesses whose course seems to be little more than an inevitable path to degrading incapacity and, if life continues for that long, eventually to a near-vegetable existence. This dread has a clear basis in reality; for although the figures on prevalence are notoriously inconsistent (due, among other things, to the use of diverse diagnostic criteria), it seems likely that among all those aged over 65 in the industralised societies some 7% will develop a dementia, and among those over 80 the figure may be as high as 20%[1]. Empirically, it is now generally agreed that there are more and less helpful ways of 'managing' a dementia; or, to be more accurate, 'managing' the person who is dementing. But the overall conceptualisation of these conditions is far from adequate to their complexity, or to the needs of the sufferers themselves.

In much of the literature on dementia, especially that which adopts a medical-science, or 'technical' frame, data are commonly presented in such a way as to imply that there is no need to take the psychological level seriously, other than as a source of clinical indicators. It seems to be assumed that once the pathology present in the brain has been clearly described, one can find there a sufficient explanation of the dementing condition. The commonly assumed causal frame, then, which constitutes the 'standard paradigm' for aetiology, is linear:

$$X \rightarrow \text{neuropathic change} \rightarrow \text{dementia.}$$

In the case of the dementias associated with multi-infarction, the nature of X seems to be fairly well understood; successive minor failures of blood supply cause death to the nerve cells and the accompanying tissues. In the case of senile dementia of the Alzheimer type (SDAT) X remains mysterious, and there is controversy over whether it represents one or several causal agents. In all dementias the fundamental problem is usually held to be a failure of cognition, associated especially with the short-term memory. Disturbances of mood and behaviour are seen as secondary, either as accompaniments or consequences of the cognitive deficits. The 'standard paradigm' originates in medical science research and is applied in a great deal of clinical psychiatry. Among many nurses and other caregivers, however, I suspect that often it is accepted only superficially, and with a good deal of 'doublethink'.

As I have tried to show elsewhere[2] the 'standard paradigm' faces a twofold difficulty, and this is particularly severe in the case of SDAT, with which we are principally concerned in this paper. Empirically, the correlations between the degree of dementia (as measured by behavioural and psychometric indices) and the extent and type of neuropathic change found *post mortem* are far less strong than seems commonly to be assumed, leaving some 80% of the variance unexplained in moderate or severe dementia; or, putting matters another way, there is a considerable overlap between the observed condition of the brains of mentally well-presented and of demented elderly people. Also in the scanning of the brain using computed tomography (CT), it is now widely accepted that measures of atrophy do not correspond closely to cognitive dysfunction, nor do they lead to sound prognoses in relation to dementia. CT has great value for the purpose of screening out other possible causes of impairment, such as infarction or brain tumours, but is of only very limited use in the positive diagnosis of SDAT. One research group has even gone as far as to suggest that besides the familiar 'benign senescent forgetfulness' we should now recognize a new term: 'benign senescent atrophy'. This points to those cases where CT provides clear evidence of deterioration in brain tissue, but there is no evidence of dementia at a clinical level.[3,4]

There is a second point, less widely acknowledged. The view of the relation between brain and mind that seems to be widely held by psychiatrists in the field is one of strong, or type-type identity. This postulates that whenever brain state Q exists, so also does psychological state P, and that whenever psychological state P exists, so also does brain state Q. This view is exceedingly difficult, if not impossible, to justify with logical rigour, and it seems wiser to assume a less stringent relationship such as that of supervenience; accepting the radical differences between the psychological and natural scientific types of language.[5]

The conceptual confusion to which I am referring is revealed in another way in the literature on SDAT. The term dementia, as commonly used in geriatric psychiatry, oscillates uncomfortably between neurological and psychological referents. Dementias are often classified on the basis of lesions found *post mortem* in relatively small samples; and hybrid terms creep into usage, such as 'hippocampal dementia'.[6] For the two reasons given above, this simply will not do. On the one hand it is necessary to describe and if possible explain the lesions, using concepts belonging to the appropriate natural-scientific disciplines. On the other hand, it is necessary to retain dementia as a psychological term, covering a range of conditions that can only partially be distinguished at a clinical level – all of which involve progressive impairment of such faculties as memory, attention, planning, judgement and emotional response, together with the disappearance of selfhood; dementia means, literally, a 'loss of mind'. The collapsing of the neurological and psychological frames into one could only be justified if two conditions obtained: type-type identity between brain and mind, and very high empirical correlations between dementia and neuropathology. There are some indications of a recognition of this in recent research; and one of the tendencies of the last few years has been to move away to some degree from neuropathology to clinical phenomenology, both in identifying SDAT and in understanding its progress.[7]

The relation between brain, mind and dementia, however, remains obscure. This paper is an attempt at a basic clarification. It is grounded in the practicalities of work with SDAT sufferers, but is also (I hope) consistent with the findings of medical-scientific research.

Further problems for the 'standard paradigm'

There are, as we have seen, two very serious obstacles in the way of accepting the 'standard paradigm' as applied to any dementia: the one logical, and the other empirical. But in addition, there are several types of phenomenon that are extremely difficult to accommodate. Four are particularly relevant to our discussion.

(i) *Pseudodementia.* As is well known in the clinical field, it is possible for a person to present a range of symptoms that look extremely like those of Alzheimer's disease, and yet for these to be reversible.[8] The commonest cases are those associated with depression, where the lifting of mood is also accompanied by a more-or-less full return of normal psychology and behaviour. Furthermore, dementia-like symptoms are often found with conditions such as uraemia, chronic constipation and pneumonia; with the retention of anaesthetics in the nervous tissue after an operation; and with the accumulation of drugs in the body of a person whose rate of metabolism is rather slow. The crucial point is that here – as indeed with some cases of severe anxiety or depression in earlier life – there is clear evidence of cognitive impairment without, apparently, irreversible damage to brain tissue.

(ii) *Apparent precipitation.* From our own studies[9] it seems that in a substantial proportion of cases (perhaps around 30%) a dementing illness of the Alzheimer type sets in fairly quickly after one or more major life crises. Our evidence for this is derived almost entirely from retrospective accounts given by spouses, daughters and sons, and of course it is open to criticism on the grounds that it involves their own 'search after meaning', and hence a good deal of distortion. Even if such evidence is not to be taken literally, however, it certainly should be taken seriously. We have found the onset of Alzheimer's disease to be associated in the minds of relatives with a variety of crises, such as bereavement, physical illness, severe family conflict, uprooting, assault and loss of major roles. Our evidence is tentative, because it derives from work that is still in its very early stages; but there are some clear pointers in the same direction in the literature; for example Amster and Krauss.[10]

(iii) *Catastrophic decline*. This phenomenon relates closely to the second, but is distinguished from it in that it refers to a dramatic downturn after a dementing illness was already clearly in evidence. The most common examples are those following admission into an institution run on a rigid regime, poorly resourced, and with a staff whose own morale is low. Sad to say, there are still plenty of such places, reflecting the workhouse of another era. After entering such an institution, a person who was still in the 'borderlands of dementia' might become globally impaired, with complete loss of recognition of relatives and friends, within so short a period as 3–6 months. Possibly this phenomenon has not been sufficiently researched in a systematic way, although it is well known to those who have been involved for some time in dementia care. A tentative explanation has been offered by Barnes, Sack and Shore,[11] in their theory of a 'cycle of dementia': successive disconfirmations and disempowerments occur social-psychologically, to a person who is already, but not disastrously impaired in cognition.

(iv) *Moderate or transitory 'rementia'*. It is time that a term such as this found its way into the discourse surrounding Alzheimer's disease, for it signifies a phenomenon that is crucial for clear understanding of the nature of this condition. In medical science it is now recognized that treatment with certain drugs, such as THA (tetrahydroaminoacridine), may bring about some degree of (possibly temporary) recovery from dementia in some patients, possibly about one third in a typical sample.[12] Parallel phenomena of recovery without drugs are well-known to caregivers, and there are occasional reports in detailed case studies, such as that of Roach.[13] Under certain circumstances sufferers from Alzheimer's disease who had, apparently, gone far down the path of behavioural and cognitive impairment, can regain some of their lost faculties. The conditions for this seem to include a very high ratio of caregivers to sufferers, close personal attention, and a general climate in which care can be expressed physically, together with free expression of the emotions. The best-known indicator of rementia is the re-gaining of urinary and faecal continence, but it is possible also to observe moderate recoveries of memory, social skill, and ability to complete simple tasks, together with a general reduction of signs of anxiety. Even more puzzling than the modest improvements to which I have been referring, are those occasions on which sufferers in the early stages of SDAT are able to exhibit short-lived and fragile restoration of near normal function. It is as if the dense overcast layer surrounding the psyche parted for a few moments, revealing sunshine and blue sky beyond. The family care-giver reports 'Suddenly it was as if I was with the old, familiar [John, Joan . . .], and I remembered how it used to be with us – I had almost forgotten.' In some cases this phenomenon seems to be evoked by particular persons.

'My daughter came to visit, and for half an hour he was almost like he used to be. After she had gone, he was as confused as ever.' Also in some cases it is evoked by the opportunity to carry out long-practised, and highly skilled tasks.

It is difficult, although not impossible, to explain phenomena such as these in terms of the 'standard paradigm', with its linear causality.

X → neuropathic change → dementia.

The pseudodementias have to be presented as a fundamentally different set of conditions from true SDAT, originating solely in neurochemistry, although some of the symptoms of the latter are closely 'mimicked' in the former. The apparent precipitation of SDAT is explained in terms of a theory of 'unmasking': that is, the person already 'had' the dementia, although it was not apparent until after the crucial life events. Here the arbitrary sliding of the term dementia between neurological and psychological frames of reference is particularly apparent. Catastrophic decline has to be accounted for in roughly the same way (the dementia was in fact already far worse than had been realised); for unlike the case of multiple infarction, it is implausible to suggest that massive Alzheimer-type degeneration of the grey matter can occur over a space of 3–6 months. Rementia has to be reframed in terms of a precarious distinction between remediable and non-remediable symptoms, or on the assumption that the original diagnosis was incorrect. 'Benign senescent atrophy' remains uninterpreted, but it is possible to postulate a shrinkage of grey matter, without the actual death of nerve cells.

It may well be the case, then, that the 'standard paradigm' can now only be upheld through the rather dubious procedure of 'saving the appearances'; or, to use Popper's term, through a succession of *ad hoc* modifications. There is a different, and possibly more fruitful way of making sense of the wide range of phenomena associated with SDAT, which brings the psychological and neurological aspects more closely together. The central hypothesis is not remarkable, although its implications are profound. It is that in all cases of SDAT we are dealing with a combination of structural damage and functional change in brain tissue, and that the pathology found in the brains of SDAT sufferers after death is not primarily causal, but epiphenomenal or consequential; however, the presence of neuropathic change itself sets limits to brain function, and increasingly so as the condition progresses. If so, SDAT is very far from being the straightforward 'organic mental illness' (in the old-fashioned sense) that it is usually claimed to be.

The relationship between mind and brain

It is obvious now that there can be no 'purely organic' mental disorders, clearly demarcated from those which are functional, and this is acknowledged in the approach adopted in DSM III.[14] But what is still far from clear is how the psychological and material (neurophysiological–neuropathological) levels are to be brought together into a single framework. Very few people today find ontological dualism of the Descartes kind – the postulation of two fundamentally different substances, matter and mind – convincing. A basic commitment to monism, however, does not entail that one can dispense with the psychological level, as some psychiatry seems implicitly to claim. An approach is required that does justice to the validity both of mental descriptions, which we clearly need for our life as social beings, and those other descriptions cast within the frameworks of the various natural sciences.

We may begin in the following way. For every psychological (ψ) event (e.g. having a desire) or state (e.g. feeling elated) in an individual, there is a corresponding biochemical-electrical brain state (b). Or, as some philosophers would say, the one is identical to the other, but the descriptions employ different frameworks: the one intensional and the other extensional (within which law-like generalizations may be stated).

In short, then, $\psi \equiv b,$

b might loosely be termed a 'functional brain state'. It exists within, or is instantiated by, a brain in such-and-such a structural condition.

The microstructure of the brain arises, as is now clear from neurophysiological and related sciences, in part from the various interneuronal connections that exist and in part from those enduring chemical changes which are associated with long-term memory. There is, no doubt, a genetically given basis to all this, on which a structural development is brought about through a whole range of learning experiences. In the case of experimental animals, principally rats, the evidence for structural change accompanying learning is very strong.[15] With humans the subject-matter of cognitive psychology is finding the logical counterpart of certain structural patterns in brain tissue; and it also makes good sense to say that selfhood in all its complexities (and, perhaps, fragmentations) corresponds to a structural configuration in the brain. In this sense brain structure, then, is continually changing. We may well suppose that when a person undergoes intensive psychotherapy and acquires a different sense of self, or takes a degree in middle life, moving from concrete to formal-operational thought in some field, new interneuronal connections are made, and hence a new pattern of brain structure has emerged. For obvious reasons, it is extremely difficult to ascertain the nature of these changes in detail in human beings; but if monism is correct it follows that all relatively enduring psychological developments must have their counterpart in brain structure. In other words, in the brain enduring function gradually becomes structure. Function might be regarded as 'fast process of short duration', and structure 'slow process of long duration'.[16] Unfortunately, however, that does not exhaust the story of brain structure, because we have also to reckon with the fact that the tissue is subject to lesions of various kinds, including those which are associated with the two most common forms of senile dementia: Alzheimer-type degeneration, and multiple infarction. Overall, then, brain structure involves two main aspects. These might be termed 'developmental' (B^d) and 'pathological' (Bp). We may express varying degrees of neuropathology as Bp_1, Bp_2, etc. If our concerns were primarily 'technical', this would need to be expressed much more precisely, and with reference to type and location.

Thus the full situation, whether in mental health or mental illness, and whether the brain is in good or bad repair, may be represented as follows:

$$\frac{\psi \equiv b}{B^d, Bp}.$$

The horizontal line here signifies 'carried by', or 'permitted by', a brain in such-and-such a structural condition.

It would seem to follow that a formulation of this kind should be reckoned with in all psychiatry, whether of those who are, in traditional terms, functionally or organic-ally ill. However, it is reasonable to suppose that some mental disorders (such as a mild reactive depression or a short psychotic episode) involve changes primarily at the level of brain function rather than structure, and so might be represented as

$$\frac{\psi' \equiv b'}{B^d}$$

(since Bp here is an irrelevant term).

For most people, most of the time, the structural brain state (B^d, Bp) does not determine in a positive way what is the case functionally. So long as the tissue is fairly intact, the brain state simply sets certain limits, allowing a very wide (but not infinite) range of possibilities. Presumably, however, if the brain is damaged through an external event, or if a neuropathological process of some severity sets in, the range of functional possibilities becomes more restricted. The limiting condition, of course, is actual brain death, where the functional brain state as indicated either in the ψ or b frames is zero.

The most puzzling thing (as ontological dualists might agree) in explaining the relationship between mind and brain, is the nature and direction of causation. Speaking loosely, it is obvious that events at the mental level can bring about changes at the neurophysiological level; and vice versa. A clear example comes from the threshold of the mental hospital. Two persons are experiencing severe anxiety, complete with a range of physiological symptoms, such as palpitation, sweating, restlessness, etc. One spends an hour with a therapist, and emerges in a much calmer state. Undoubtedly biochemical changes have occurred; and yet the external cause was an interaction that was purely symbolic. The second person is given an injection of a tranquillising drug, and left to rest a while; and the results are rather similar to those in the first case. In the terms of already used in this paper, the proper way to represent these events is:

$$\psi \equiv b_{time\ 1}$$
$$\downarrow \leftarrow \text{causal agent.}$$
$$\psi \equiv b_{time\ 2}$$

Clearly it is a shorthand to say

$$\psi_{time\ 1} \rightarrow b_{time\ 2},$$

for the first example, or

$$b_{time\ 1} \rightarrow \psi_{time\ 2},$$

for the second, postulating purely mental causes in the former, and purely chemical causes in the latter. If we choose to use the mental language, we can talk in a loose way about mental causes, although the language is not such as to lead to the postulation of causal laws. If we choose to use a natural-scientific language (from biochemistry, neurophysiology, etc.), again we can speak of causes, and we might indeed find some causal laws. However, it would be mistaken to suggest that, at any one point in time, a mental event or state causes a neurophysiological event or state; we are simply dealing with alternative descriptions of the same reality.

Application to the psychiatry of old age

Let us return now to the four components which, I have suggested, are necessary for conceptualising the mind-brain relationship for the purpose of psychiatry. We can characterise what may be the case in 'normal' old-age psychology, in benign senescent forgetfulness, in pseudodementia, and in senile dementia of the Alzheimer type.

First, then, let ψ_a signify normal psychological functioning in old age. 'Normal' here is used in a fairly weak sense, implying that a person is able to go about the business of life, can perform the necessary cognitive tasks, can relate well enough with others, has an intact sense of self, etc.; there may also be certain interests, preoccupations and concerns that relate specifically to the predicament of old age. Accompanying ψ_a there is also a set of functional brain states typical of later life: b_a. Possibly the neurotransmitter balance is different, from that of earlier stages, or the overall level of activity is less, but the brain function is not impaired in any serious way. Structurally, there has been only a relatively small amount of degeneration of grey matter (P_1) such as is well within the range for well-preserved old people, and which brain function can, so to speak, tolerate. The situation, then, may be represented as shown below:

$$\frac{\psi_a \equiv b_a}{B^d, Bp_1}.$$

We come now to the case of 'benign senescent forgetfulness', where the self is clearly intact and mood shows no abnormality, but there are unusually large deficits of memory, especially short-term. This can be distinguished from the above in that now, it seems, there are structural impairments in the brain tissue (P_2); corresponding to 'benign senescent atrophy':

$$\frac{\psi_a \equiv b_a}{B^2, Bp_2}.$$

The case of pseudodementia in old age stands in a marked contrast to this, because here, undoubtedly, there are brain-functional changes that entail cognitive deficiencies, and that special kind of 'loss of self' that represents the psychosis peculiar to old age: in short, $\psi'_a \equiv b'_a$.

However, since pseudodementia is (by definition) reversible, it is not accompanied by appreciable structural damage to the grey matter. The condition, then, may be represented as shown below:

$$\frac{\psi'_a \equiv b'_a}{B^d, Bp_1}.$$

Now we come to the crucial case, senile dementia of the Alzheimer type. Here there seems to be not only immediate functional impairment ($\psi'_a \equiv b'_a$), but also some degree of neuropathic change. In the early stages of the illness the structural state of the brain still allows a range of functions – as is evidenced by the wide variability in cognition and behaviour over a short period in a single SDAT patient. The condition may be represented as shown below:

$$\frac{\psi'_a \equiv b'_a}{B^d, Bp_2}.$$

Finally, in very severe dementia, where a person is seriously impaired in almost all function, having also lost virtually all of his or her everyday sense of selfhood, and in that sense has moved into a kind of deep psychosis (ψ''_a), we have:

$$\frac{\psi''_a \equiv b''_a}{B^d, Bp_3}.$$

When the illness has progressed to this degree, *and only then*, is it possible to suppose that something approximating to the widely accepted standard causal paradigm is in operation.

A scheme such as the above is only a first approximation, and no doubt needs a good deal of refinement. But its immediate usefulness is that it allows us to rationalise the field in a new way, one that has many implications for research and care-giving. Seeing Alzheimer's disease not as a direct consequence of Bp, but in the more complex terms of ψ, b, B^d and, Bp, potentially explains one of the most notorious features of the condition – the wide range of presenting symptoms. Simply, there can be great variation in $\psi \equiv b$, and in B^d, while the brain has a common form of pathology: the degenerative changes associated with the neurofibrillary tangle, and so on. Further, we can make sense of an observation that is almost the converse: similar symptom patterns are sometimes observed in dementias that are found, *post mortem*, to be associated with different underlying pathologies of the grey matter, or with no pathology beyond the norm. Here there are, presumably, similarities in $\psi \equiv b$, and in B^d, strong enough to override variations in Bp.

Earlier in this paper I mentioned four types of phenomenon that are difficult to explain in terms of the 'standard paradigm', and thus far only one – pseudodementia – has been dealt with in terms of my more elaborate scheme. Apparent precipitation can be accepted as a true (although of course partial) explanation in aetiological terms. For what we are dealing with here is, presumably, a fairly sudden deterioration in $\psi \equiv b$, the consequence of a registration, whether consciously or 'organismically', of difficult and stressful life events. The hypothesis would then be that there was, initially, a reaction of a mild pseudodementia type; but at that stage it was taken as sufficiently close to a normal reaction for it not to arouse great attention or concern. In other words, the early stages of SDAT might be explicable purely in neurochemical terms, with varying degrees of neuropathic change occurring slowly, possibly both before and after the critical events. There is some direct empirical support for this view, from studies that show neurotransmitter deficits in SDAT sufferers. However, the correlations with clinical indices (as also with neuropathology) are rather low. At this stage no clear conclusions can be drawn.[17] Catastrophic decline might also be explained along similar lines. For it seems extremely unlikely, from what is known about the general progress of SDAT, that major degenerative changes of the Alzheimer type could occur in the grey matter within a mere few months. It is much more reasonable to suppose that such a rapid advance in a dementing condition occurs because of a deterioration at the psychological (and concomitantly, brain-functional) level; the dementing person feels betrayed or abandoned, perhaps; and an iterative 'cycle of dementia', involving progressive changes in neurochemistry, rapidly ensues. Transitory or partial 'rementia', too, does not have to be explained away. With those whose brain structure has not deteriorated too far, some function can be restored; there may be certain situations which are registered psychologically as highly comforting or pleasurable, which stimulate almost immediately a change both in the balance and degree of neurotransmitter activity. We do not know whether cells on the threshold of degenerative change can be returned to health, but there is no sound reason in biology for assuming that functional change is always the consequence of prior cellular pathology.

Conclusion

The scheme that I have presented in this paper is extremely bland, and it needs to be developed a good deal before its explanatory potential can be evaluated. Even at this stage, however, it does suggest a new way of ordering the data, both neurological and clinical, relating to SDAT, and it points to where there may be major lacunae in research. Also, and of more immediate relevance, it implies a way of 'being with' those who suffer from SDAT, a way which affirms their personhood even when their competences are very seriously impaired. In this closing section, then, I should like to draw attention to three implications from what I have been proposing.

First, studies of brain micro-structure have generally failed to take into account what may be of crucial importance in determining whether or not a person develops a dementing illness in later life. This is B^d, the developmental aspect. At present there is no non-invasive method available for examining B^d in human beings, although there is a vast literature pointing to its significance in experimental animals; here it is clear that experience is translated directly into interneuronal connections. However, what we can do in our own case is to deal with B^d indirectly, through that other descriptive frame, the psychological. The question then becomes whether certain kinds of psychological 'strength' might be sufficient to enable an individual to remain intact as a social and communicative being, despite the presence of pathological processes in the brain. Because the correlations between dementia and pathology are rather low, this seems at least plausible. My own hypothesis is that one of the crucial factors is the extent to which the 'experiential self' has or has not been well-developed: that is, an integrated centre, grounded in feeling and emotion.[18] For this can remain when the 'adapted self' (derived from role-performance and meeting others' expectations) declines – as is very often the case for people in later life.

Second, there is a serious problem in relation to SDAT (but by no means unique to it) in that a case generally comes to the attention of health or social service professionals only when the person has gone a considerable way down the road of deterioration – often when his or her behaviour has become a nuisance or a threat of some kind. At this point the possibility of doing radical developmental work has long passed. According to the 'standard paradigm', the sufferer is midway in some ineluctable process, on which it is only possible to gaze with compassion and dismay, 'managing' it with kindness and skill. However, as with a range of illnesses, it seems highly likely that there is a period when the organism is in a metastable state, with the possibility either of passing back into health or forward into major pathology. Murphy and Brown[19] studied this phenomenon, and noted that in their cases the onset of illness was often preceded by an affective disturbance such as depression. There is surely a lesson here for our understanding of SDAT. Perhaps a new priority in work with older people is to be sensitive to the possible presence of that metastable state, which would be related as much to disturbance of mood as to cognitive deficit. At this stage work on ψ (hence b) is possible, and also perhaps on B^d, whatever are the tendencies in the area of B_p.

Third, the main emphasis in current psychological work related to SDAT is cognitive, reflecting to some extent a fashion that prevails in psychology as a whole. For example, much attention has been paid to charting the nature and development of deficits in information-processing; and in remedial work techniques such as Reality Orientation have been widely used, in the attempt to help a confused person retain his or her bearings in the everyday world. There is ground, however, for questioning this emphasis. We know from phenomena such as pseudodementia, and the small success in the area of rementia (whether through drugs or other means), that when the biochemical environment is modified, cognitive function may also be radically changed. When this is translated out of the b into the ψ framework, it is tantamount to saying that to some extent cognition is dependent on the emotional ambience. Perhaps, then, more attention should be given to the nuances of the SDAT sufferer's emotional state. Caregiving involves something far more skilled than attempting to adjust the dementing person to our (cognitive) reality; it involves the immensely subtle task of attuning ourselves to his or her (emotional) reality. Some of the drug trials give hopeful indications of what can be done through exogenous alteration of the brain's biochemistry, though probably securing only temporary relief. However, if we accept the identity $\psi \equiv b$, an endogenous restoration is also perfectly conceivable. In the long run, it would be far more therapeutic to stimulate the body's own neurochemicals, through means that are fundamentally psychological. At present we have only tiny and exceedingly transitory indications of how this might be effected. The task (as indeed with the great breakthroughs in technical innovation) is to explore all possible ways of turning such indications into clear and consistent signals. If there were success here, the problem of SDAT would still be very far from being solved. But we might have found ways of keeping the sufferer in the world of persons, and mitigating a kind of psychological pain whose persistence and intensity we can scarcely envisage. The full solution can only come when we have dealt also with brain structure, in both its pathological and developmental aspects. Perhaps the fact that developmental change in later life has been generally neglected is itself a reflection of negative and empirically unjustified images of 'normal' old age. As these images change in society at large, so will the norms of caregiving; also, of course, of psychiatric practice.

Notes

1   Ineichen, B. Measuring the rising tide. How many dementia cases will there be by 2001? *British Journal of Psychiatry*, 150 (1987), 195–200.
2   Kitwood, T. The technical, the personal and the framing of dementia. *Social Behaviour*, 3 (1988), 161–180.
3   Jacoby, R. J. and Levy, R. Computed tomography in the elderly. 2. Senile dementia: diagnosis and functional impairment. *British Journal of Psychiatry*, 136 (1980), 270–275.
4   Jacoby, R. J. and Levy, R. Computed tomography in the elderly. 3. Affective disorder. *British Journal of Psychiatry*, 136 (1980), 270–275.
5   Davidson, D. 'Mental events', in Foster, L. and Swanson, J. W. (eds), *Experience and Theory*, University of Massachusetts Press, Boston, 1970.
6   Ball, M. J., Blume, W., Fisman, M., Fox, A., Fox, H., Hachinski, V., Kral, V. A., Kirsher, A. J. and Merskey, H. A new definition of Alzheimer's disease: a hippocampal dementia, *Lancet*, 5 January 1985, 14–16.
7   Reisberg, B., Ferris, S. H., Shulman, E., Steinberg, G., Buttinger, C., Sinaiko, E., Borenstein, J., de Leon, M. and Cohen, J. Longitudinal course of normal aging and progressive dementia of the Alzheimer's type: a prospective study of 106 subjects over a 3.6 year mean interval. *Progress in Neuro-Psychopharmacology and Biological Psychiatry*, 10 (1986), 571–578.
8   Arie, T. Pseudodementia, *British Medical Journal*, 286 (1983), 1301–1302.
9   Kitwood, T. Understanding senile dementia: a psychobiographical approach. *Free Associations*, forthcoming. Text available on request.
10 Amster, L. E. and Krauss, H. H. The relationship between life crises and mental deterioration in old age. *International Journal Aging and Human Development*, 5 (1974), 51–55.
11 Barnes, T., Sack, J. and Shore, J. The cycle of dementia: *Gerontologist*, 13 (1973), 513–527.
12 Summers, W. K., Majovski, V. Marsh, G. M., Tachiki, K., King, A. Oral tetrahydroaminoacridine in long-term treatment of senile dementia, Alzheimer type. *New England Journal of Medicine* 315 (1986) 1241–1245.
13 Roach, M. *Another Name for Madness*, Boston: Houghton Miffin, 1985.
14 Lipowski, Z. J. Organic mental disorders – an American perspective, *British Journal of Psychiatry*, 144 (1984), 542–546.
15 Diamond, M. C. The ageing brain: some enlightening and optimistic results *American Scientist*, 66 (1978), 66–71.

16 Jahoda, M. *Freud and the Dilemmas of Psychology*, London, Hogarth Press, 1977.
17 Rossor, M. N., Iverson, L. L., Reynolds, G. P., Mountjoy, C.Q. and Roth, M. Neurochemical characteristics of early and late onset types of Alzheimer's disease. *British Medical Journal*, 288 (1984), 961–964.
18 Kitwood, T. in *Social Behaviour*, 1988, *op. cit.*
19 Murphy, E. and Brown, G. W. Life events, psychiatric disturbance and physical illness. *British Journal of Psychiatry*, 136 (1980), 326–338.

1.2

The dialectics of dementia: with particular reference to Alzheimer's disease (1990)

ABSTRACT

A new theory of the dementing process in old age is presented in outline. Its main focus is on the dialectical interplay between neurological and social-psychological factors, with special emphasis on aspects of the latter which deprive a neurologically impaired individual of his or her personhood. The account of dementia so derived is more comprehensive and less deterministic than those which are based on the simpler versions of a 'medical model'. Also, it opens up the way for a more personal and optimistic view of caregiving.

Introduction

In an earlier paper in this journal I presented some of the reasons why we need a new conceptualisation of the major dementias of old age, and Alzheimer's disease in particular.[1] The 'standard paradigm' which underlies so much present thinking about dementia, particularly within medial science, is both faulty and deficient. Its basic assumption of a straightforward linear causal relationship between neuropathology and dementia will not suffice for aetiological purposes; also it carries far too negative and deterministic implications for the nature of caregiving.

In that paper I indicated some of the components necessary for developing a richer account of dementia, focusing on the states of the individual. In particular, I suggested that there must be a direct engagement with the sufferer's psychology (ψ), which corresponds, under another description, with the functional state of the brain (b); hence $\psi \equiv b$. Also, not only do we need to deal with the extent of the neuropathology that affects the brain (Bp), but also with the structure established through development and learning (B^d). Thus the basic framework for understanding dementia and related conditions is

$$\frac{\psi \equiv b}{B^d, Bp},$$

rather than simply Bp. And, of course, the more that evidence points to a failure or imbalance in neurotransmitter activity as being the crucial factor in dementia (at least of the Alzheimer type), the more pressing becomes the need for a reconceptualisation along the lines I have outlined.

I wish now to take the arguments from my previous paper a good way further, and present the framework for a new theory of dementia. The focus here is on the dementing process rather than on the demented state, and on the social-psychological milieu in which that process takes place. There are vast implications for the nature of caregiving, and indeed for our whole attitude to dementia.

A note on method

The theory that I shall be outlining here has a strong empirical foundation, and it is informed by a method, albeit of a kind that some might judge to be unorthodox. The primary data come from two main sources. One is the following up in detail of the psychobiographies of individuals who have developed a dementia, through extended semi-structured interviews with one or more family members. These accounts, although slanted in certain ways (for example, by a bereaved person's desire to make sense of what has happened), show clearly how the dementing illness is intricately woven into the pattern of life-history and social relationships. The second source of data is a close involvement with, and observation of, dementing persons themselves, in such contexts as their own homes, day hospitals, community care schemes and residential accommodation. Recently I have begun a study of the microstructure of dementia care interaction, and this heightens awareness of aspects of social psychology that are commonly overlooked.

My research method, then, consists here essentially in the collection of vignettes from real life, and interpreting their significance in social-psychological terms. Selection and judgment are, of course, involved, in the attempt to draw out features that have general significance. The test of validity is whether the vignettes carry conviction to those who know the field well from a practical standpoint, even though they may not themselves have ordered their knowledge in a systematic way.

The prevailing style of research, both in the social and natural sciences – or at least the ideal towards which investigations commonly aspire – is one in which 'variables' are isolated, and their causal relationships explored. Generally the aim is to hold some variables constant, while the interdependence of a few others (ideally, two) is explored through experiment or naturalistic observation. This certainly has been the pattern in the majority of research on dementia, both in medical science and in psychology. There are, however, some serious difficulties, which have not been sufficiently acknowledged. Persons who are unwell, especially in later life, are hardly ever the carriers of simple disease entities; the 'variables' are multitudinous, and they are interrelated in many complex ways. The tendency of much research, then, is to focus on those variables that are readily accessible and fairly easy to measure, and to ignore the rest. Small signals are indeed detected, but a vast amount simply remains as noise. This sets serious limits to conventional research on dementia, which still rejoices in correlation coefficients of the order of 0.3. An alternative to this strategy is to be more like an engineer than a laboratory scientist. The engineer aims to find predictable patterns, using materials in their complexity, and in contexts close to those of everyday use. The results are less precise than those of pure science, but they are more comprehensive; and they have a direct bearing on the practicalities of design. So here my aim is to stay close to dementia in the real context of everyday life, and thus to provide an account that could never be derived from the method of isolating clear variables. The result is a dialectical theory, through which the dementing process may be more fully understood; some of the implications for action are plain.

Why do elderly people become demented?

If the standard 'paradigm' is taken as sufficient it should, in principle, provide a full explanation of the course of a dementing illness. Where variance is not accounted for, this is to be written off as due to the imprecision of present research methods. This seems to be what logic requires. In fact, however, it is rare to find that the 'standard paradigm' is taken so seriously by those who are involved from day to day in caregiving. Many nurses, social workers, speech therapists, occupational therapists and others who work closely with dementia sufferers seem to operate with a kind of 'doublethink'. The 'standard paradigm' is what they officially believe, on the basis of what they have read or been taught. But also they hold, unofficially and intuitively, a more optimistic and less deterministic theory about dementia; usually they cannot articulate it clearly, but it is this that informs their practice. In a sense even the evidence from medical science is on their side, because some 70% of the variance between neuropathology and dementia is not accounted for.

Now unofficial theories of the kind I have referred to are not based on mere common sense or ignorant prejudice – to be corrected by the findings of rigorous research. Generally they have a rich grounding in the data of real life: the minutiae of caregiving, the close involvement with dementia sufferers as they vary in mood and competence from day to day. These data, the facts of lived experience, are of a very different kind from those obtained from, say, psychometric testing, brain-scanning or histopathology. They are less highly systematised, but no less valid. To return for a moment to the comparison between the engineer and the pure scientist: the engineer's main interest is the actual performance of buildings, bridges, roads, pipes, etc. under the highly complex conditions of use. Abstracted knowledge about, say, the crystal structure of cement with various aluminium contents, is extremely valuable, but it is only one type of resource for understanding better how artefacts behave in the real world.

The theory that I am advancing, then, is grounded in everyday life rather than in the laboratory of the psychologist or the medical scientist. What it lacks in precision it gains in comprehensiveness. It can be summed up in three 'basic equations'.

$$SD = NI + MSP \tag{1}$$

Senile Dementia is compounded from the effects of Neurological Impairment and of Malignant Social Psychology.

$$(NI)_a \leftarrow MSP \tag{2}$$

Neurological Impairment in an elderly person attracts to itself a Malignant Social Psychology.

$$\text{MSP } (\varphi)_a \rightarrow \text{NI} \tag{3}$$

Malignant Social Psychology, bearing down upon an aged person, whose physiological buffers are already fragile, actually creates Neurological Impairment.

Our main focus in this paper will be on the first two of these 'equations', for the truth of which there is abundant evidence. I am advancing the third only tentatively, because it is extremely difficult to test with the research methods that are presently available. Suffice it to say that it is entirely consistent with much that has been discovered in the growing field of psychophysiology. Here some of the stress-related antecedents of illnesses such as cardiovascular disorder, ulceration of the gastrointestinal tract, respiratory disorders and cancer, have certainly been uncovered. It could, then, only be on the basis of gross prejudice that the possible truth of equation (3) would be ruled out *a priori*. The hypothesis is that a degenerative process in nerve tissue might be instigated or accelerated by certain kinds of stress; with the failure of auto-immune reactions as an intervening process; the occurrence of dementia in conjunction with AIDS may provide a parallel. In summary, then, the truth or otherwise of the third equation is not crucial to the theory; but if it were true, the theory would have even greater force.

One core assumption is built into this account of dementia, and it is worth highlighting at this point. It is that human beings are far more deeply affected by the social psychology that surrounds them than is commonly recognised. In particular, the maintenance of self-esteem is essential for good learning, efficacy and constructive relationships with others. Conversely, when self-esteem is lacking or damaged, a person is disastrously incapacitated in many ways, and easily falls into a cycle of discouragement and failure. All this holds true without there being any question of permanent destruction of nervous tissue; but, of course, the quality of an individual's self-esteem has its counterpart at the neurochemical level. Each aspect of the malignant social psychology is, in some way, damaging to self-esteem, and tends to diminish personhood; that is why it merits the epithet 'malignant'. When a person has been subjected to a predominantly malignant social psychology for several years, the effects may indeed be devastating. Remarkably, the greater part of medical science research on dementia seems to overlook this altogether.

The malignant social psychology – in more detail

The presence of processes and interactions that tend to depersonalise a sufferer from dementia is plain enough to see, and many sensitive caregivers are aware of it to some degree. Ten aspects of this malignancy are illustrated below, but probably this is far from exhaustive. In the examples, Mr D or Mrs D stands for the dementia sufferer and C (or C_1, C_2 etc.) for non-family caregivers.

(1) *Treachery* Some form of dishonest representation, trickery or outright deception is used by others, in order to get the dementia sufferer to comply with their wishes.

Example. Mrs D, a childless widow, has no close relatives in the district. Her neighbours report that she is behaving oddly, and wandering in the street at night. Her nearest relatives, who live some way away, are asked to intervene. They visit her, and tell her that they are going out for a drive, as they have often done. The drive ends up at the geriatric assessment ward of the local mental hospital, and she is admitted.

(2) *Disempowerment* Things are done for a dementia sufferer; even though he or she is able to do them, albeit clumsily or slowly. There is a consequent loss of confidence, a de-skilling process, a diminution in the sense of agency.

Example. Mr D is having his dinner; it is clearly a struggle, but he is beginning to succeed, both in cutting up the food and in getting it to his mouth. C, who is getting impatient, says, 'Come on Mr D, let me do that for you'. C cuts up the food and feeds Mr D spoonful by spoonful. Mr D is thus robbed of his own action.

(3) *Infantilisation* This is a more extreme and persistent form of (2), but accompanied by messages, subtle or otherwise, that the dementia sufferer has a mentality and capability very much like that of a young child.

Example. Mr D has always been rather helpless at home, with his wife being 'strong' and motherly. Now he is extremely confused. She speaks to him in exactly the kind of voice she would use with a three-year-old. When he tips over the milk jug, she smacks him lightly and says, 'Jack, that was a naughty thing to do. If you behave like that, I won't let you have tea in the sitting room any more.'

(4) *Intimidation* The dementia sufferer is made afraid by such processes as headscans or psychological assessments, these being carried out in a somewhat impersonal way, by professionals who are powerful and competent. Sometimes intimidation includes threats, or actual physical assault.

Example. Mrs D is persuaded, through her husband, to take part in a programme of research into dementia. She is brought into the research unit at the hospital, and given various physical tests. She is clearly frightened and dismayed. After half an hour of further waiting, she becomes extremely aggressive, and insists on being taken home at once.

(5) *Labelling* A confused elderly person is given a diagnosis, such as 'primary degenerative dementia', or Alzheimer's disease. Expectations of progressive decline and derangement are set up and a self-fulfilling prophecy comes into play. The sufferer is treated differently, in many subtle ways, from this time forward.

Example. Mr D's condition is diagnosed by a consultant as Alzheimer's disease. His wife, who has no strong affection for him in any case, obtains the relevant information, and begins to write him off, consenting to poor-quality care and provision for him. He rapidly deteriorates.

(6) *Stigmatisation* This is an aspect of labelling, but it also carries connotations of exclusion. The dementia sufferer becomes strange, alien, a diseased object, an outcast.

Example. Mrs D is known to be behaving strangely, and the ambulance has been seen coming to collect her to take her to the day hospital. The neighbours cease to show friendly concern and begin to look the other way. Relatives come to visit less frequently. The gossip goes around that Mrs D is 'going senile'. Children are warned to keep out of her way.

(7) *Outpacing* It seems that a dementia sufferer often functions mentally at a much slower rate than those who have no impairment. However, caregivers often continue to go at their normal pace, and so fail to establish good contact.

Example. Mr D has given friendly signals to C_1, who sits down beside him, and develops a conversation with him. Mr D begins to relax and to express to C_1 what he is feeling. C_2, who is bored, comes to sit with them, and begins a new conversation, at a familiar pace, mainly with C_1. Very soon Mr D goes quiet. He complains: 'I am beginning to fade away here, and I don't like it'.

(8) *Invalidation* In order to feel alive, grounded, in touch, we need our experience – especially our emotions and feelings – to be understood, accepted by another. We also need the kind of response that takes our experience into account. All this may be described as the validation – the making real or valid – of our subjectivity. Invalidation occurs when the subjectivity of the dementia sufferer is ignored or overlooked.

Example. Mrs D sits up in bed one morning, and says to her husband (also in bed): 'Who are you?' He is taken aback, and somewhat affronted. He retorts back to her, aggressively, 'And who are you, then?' (He has taken no account of her sense of strangeness and her need for reassurance.)

(9) *Banishment* The dementia sufferer has become intolerable to others in some way. He or she is removed from the human milieu, either physically or psychologically, rather like being 'sent to Coventry'. The result is a deprivation of sustaining human contact.

Example. Mrs D, a former school teacher, is one of two very confused people in a residential home. Also, from her style of speech, etc. she is clearly of a different background from the other residents. They tend to avoid her, and word has gone round the home that she is 'an upper class loony'.

(10) *Objectification* The dementia sufferer is not treated as a person; that is, as one who is an autonomous centre of life. Instead he or she is treated in some respects like a lump of dead matter, to be measured, pushed around, manipulated, drained, filled, dumped, etc.

Example. It is a kind of 'ward round', a review of the people in one area of a long-stay institution. Mr D is brought into the room where the consultant and a few others are sitting. Various questions are asked about him. Is he still wandering? How is he sleeping now? How has he responded to the new medication? Have we managed now to deal with the problem of his aggression? Mr D is present in the room for ten minutes, and eventually he is escorted back. Not one question or comment was addressed directly to him.

Episodes such as those I have used above as illustrations are remarkably common in the lives of older people who are confused, who inhabit 'the borderlands of dementia'. In itemising the malignant social psychology I have deliberately laid aside the effects of institutionalisation *per se*, with its well-known tendency to deprive individuals of their former identity, and to reconstruct them within the institutional frame. Of course, the processes that I have described do occur within long-stay institutions, but they are certainly not specific to them. My general point is that the malignant social psychology is so much a part of the taken-for-granted world of later life that it generally passes unnoticed. Possibly it is particularly prevalent and accepted in medical settings, and this may be one reason why medical science thus far has given it so little attention.

We come now to the question that is implicit in the second of my 'basic equations'. Why should neurological impairment in elderly people attract to itself a malignant social psychology? In some respects this is a subset of the larger question of why any form of disability or vulnerability – especially in the mental sphere – should have such a dynamic. However, some features may be unique to frailty in old age. There seem to be four related reasons to account for equation (2).

The first is that many caregivers and service-providers are extremely lacking in inter-subjective insight. There is a simplistic view that good caregiving is just commonsense, or perhaps 'doing unto others as you would be done by'. In fact, of course, these ideas are very far from the truth. Good caregiving requires a person to 'be there' for the other in a way that far transcends commonsense, and understanding and helping very differently from the case of a person who had a full range of mental competences. High levels of empathy and imagination are required, as also a kind of flexibility of thinking that sits loose to literal, concrete interpretation. At present these qualities are remarkably lacking in the everyday world, and they do not feature strongly in the training of many of the professionals with whom a confused person might come into contact. The norm of everyday life is to be lacking in insight, and this will not suffice as a basis for work with those who are confused.

A second reason for the malignant social psychology is the busy-ness and pressure which many caregivers are facing. To be effectively caring for a dementia sufferer takes a great deal of time and high-quality attention. It requires a person to slow down inwardly, and to cultivate a kind of inner quietness, so that the messages given by the sufferer may be attended to without distraction. Unfortunately, under the conditions that we have at present, many family caregivers are carrying very heavy practical burdens, and often suffering from exhaustion and depression, so that they cannot give of their best. Also the short-staffing in the medical and social services for older people is such that quality care is often virtually unattainable. My tenth vignette, which seems to show the medical profession in a very unfavourable light, should of course be seen in this context.

Third, there is a tendency not to believe in the sufferer from dementia as a person, and so not to treat him or her with the respect that properly accords to persons. At the very least, to be a person is to have the status of a sentient being, to be recognised as having value, and to hold a distinct place in a group or collective of some kind. The failure to recognise dementia sufferers in this way probably derives in part from widely held stereotypes, epitomised in such phrases as 'the person who used to be there has already gone', or 'there is a death which leaves the body behind'. If such beliefs determine the kind of mental set that a caregiver has, he or she becomes attuned to those pieces of evidence that suggest non-personhood. Evidence that points in the opposite direction is ignored or overlooked.

Fourth, and rather more speculatively, we must move on to the ground of depth psychology, for it may be that there are some unconscious motives which also engender a malignant social psychology. As humans, we are highly intelligent beings, and perhaps unique among the animals in knowing clearly what the future may hold for us. We know that we, too, will age and die, unless a sudden death first overtakes us. Living with this knowledge, we carry defences against the anxiety it might arouse. To be with, say, a severely handicapped child may provoke fear and anguish, but at least the caregiver can say, inwardly, 'I will never be like that'. But to be with a confused elderly person is to be reminded, painfully, of one's own possible future. This is particularly poignant for older people who have no neurological impairment; to have to be with someone who is extremely frail, or 'senile', is to be close to one of their most pressing fears. It is not surprising, then, that subtle processes occur which enable people to keep dementia sufferers at a psychological distance, and to avoid engaging with them in their full capacity as persons. The psychodynamics of caregiving is a complex matter, and it is very likely that collusive defences (people 'unconsciously agreeing' to ward off reality in certain ways) are well established in the field of dementia care.[2]

I have used the very strong term 'malignant social psychology' in each of the 'basic equations', and now it is necessary to guard against a possible misunderstanding. There is no suggestion here of a general pattern of conscious, deliberate, malicious intent on the part of family members, caregivers and other professionals. On the contrary, what is so clearly in evidence is a great deal of goodwill, kindness and commitment, although under difficult circumstances and often with far too limited resources. The social psychology is malignant because of its effects upon the person who is neurologically impaired; that is all. If an accusing finger is to be pointed, it is to the general failure of our kind of society to provide well for the vulnerabilities of later life, and the inadequate preparation of those who are going to be working with confused elderly people. Behind both of these there is the generally low standard of respect for persons which society takes as 'normal'. If our norms are in some respects an improvement on those of the nineteenth century, this simply shows how far we have to go.

A dialectical model of the dementing process

The first two of the 'basic equations' from p. 180 can be used to generate the outlines of a full account of a dementing illness in the context of everyday life. It begins with a period of 'normality', and follows the sufferer through various stages of deterioration, until the point of death. A portrayal of the dementing process in this kind of way is not totally new.[3] However, so far as I am aware, no model has been developed which pays close attention to social psychology, or which conceptualises clearly how neurological and psychological factors come together. A typical dementing process might take the form shown in Figure 1.

The starting-point, then, is a time in which a person is functioning satisfactorily in middle or later life: that is, without excessive stress, and with no evidence of neurological impairment. In the terms of my earlier paper his or her state can be represented as

$$\frac{\psi_a \equiv b_a}{B^2, Bp_1}.$$

There is a sufficient competence in the practicalities of living; the person occupies several roles with reasonable success; a fair range of interpersonal relationships are

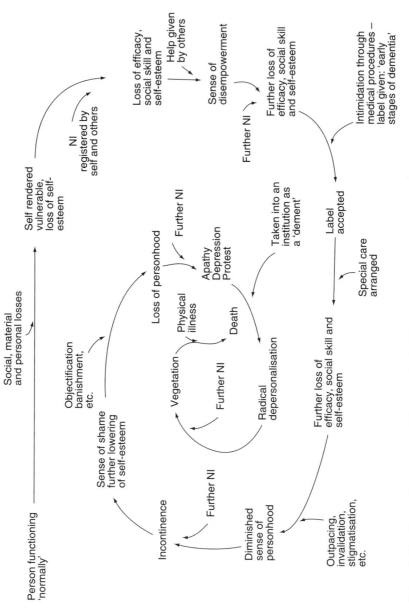

Figure 1 The dementing process. (NI = neurological impairment.)

intact. This 'normality', of course, may not necessarily be one of great psychological health as judged from some standpoint in psychotherapy, but it is sufficient for maintaining the person in a tolerable state of well-being for the present.

We must also, however, take into account the life-changes that typically occur to people in our kind of society when they move into their sixth decade and beyond. Almost every individual during this period of life undergoes a complex mixture of losses, which impose great strain on the psyche (and hence, concomitantly, on the physiology that carries it). Some of these losses are 'social': most obviously, those associated with an occupational role and with parenting. Some of the losses are material, ensuing upon the reduced income that most people have in their retirement, especially after the first ten years or so. Some of the losses are 'personal', including bodily energy, physical appearance, sexual prowess, eyesight, hearing and health. Also, the majority of people experience major bereavements during this period, particularly through the death of siblings or spouse; and as the population ages, the death of a son or daughter is becoming more common. These losses are interrelated in many ways, as has been well documented.[4] Thus many older people are caught up in a cluster of deprivations, and most of the losses will never be made good. The self, then, is rendered vulnerable, and the overall state of many individuals is, in the terms of my earlier paper, one that is approaching

$$\frac{\psi'_a \equiv b'_a}{B^d, Bp_1}.$$

If an ageing person is able to 'work through' and accept the losses, carrying out the 'grief work' that is entailed, his or her psyche is likely to recover a state of 'normality', perhaps with some significant new learning, to which there will be a corresponding modification of brain structure. It seems, however, that many individuals simply have to face without insight a succession of losses such as might devastate many younger persons; they do not have the resources, either in themselves or in their social milieu, to enable them to do the necessary grieving and bring about an inner restoration. Thus they remain in a precarious psychological state. The high prevalence of depression among older people, which is treated at present mainly by biochemical means, is ample evidence of this point.[5] All this, surely, is part of the background to any comprehensive theory of dementia. Yet it is hardly acknowledged within the 'standard paradigm', with its very heavy emphasis on structural pathology in the brain.

Now let us suppose that around this time, which for many persons is one of great psychological vulnerability, there is also a significant deterioration of brain tissue. Typically this manifests itself in unusual deficits of memory, or getting lost in familiar places, or being unable to complete tasks involving a modicum of skill. Whether or not the person acknowledges consciously what is happening, the impairment is registered at some level. In line with what psychotherapy seems to suggest, the most healthy way forward would be to acknowledge and accept what is happening, to 'relax into' the situation, while at the same time doing as much as possible to maintain competence and well-being. This would be done with an openness to others, so that help would be received with goodwill, but only where absolutely necessary. In fact, however, it is more common for a person to engage in a tactic of defensive denial, so that the fact of disability is not clearly acknowledged. This means that such alienation as is already present is now increased. Often this is enhanced by blindness, ignorance or defensive denial on the part of family members, who also have a personal investment in not facing up to the situation. The consequence is a diminished contact between the neurologically impaired person and those others who might best be able to help maintain his or her well-being.

This, then, is the predicament of a person who is on the threshold of the dementing process. Probably he or she already carries the burden of multiple losses, and now comes the problem of an actual disability. Whether the latter comes about gradually, as is believed to be the case in Alzheimer's disease, or through a succession of miniature catastrophes to the blood supply, is of relatively minor importance. The crucial issue is the gravity of what the person is having to face, and the personal and inter-personal resources available for dealing with it.

Now the dementing process, as classically described, gets under way, in the kind of pattern portrayed in Figure 1. Various aspects of the malignant social psychology come into play, augmenting the direct effects of neurological impairment. In the terms of my earlier paper, the malignant social psychology brings immediate effects on ($\psi \equiv b$), while concomitantly the pathological process is destroying brain structure. It is indeed a vicious circle, because each loss of competence, however caused, tends to recruit more of the malignant social psychology. As the sufferer is continually invalidated, objectified, etc. he or she loses more and more of that vital contact with others on which personhood depends. Often confusion is compounded by depression. If, at some point, the person is also taken into full-time institutional care, there is a further stripping away of identity. This is enhanced in those cases where the sufferer is virtually abandoned, presumably because relatives and former friends find visits arouse unbearable pain or guilt. Thus, through the cumulative effect of those processes, there is not only a disability, but also a radical depersonalisation. In a more resourceful, caring and insightful world, the effects of neurological impairment might be offset by a particularly generous and benign social psychology, so that the sufferer would be stabilised and sustained. However, this very rarely happens under our present-day conditions of psychogeriatric medicine and care.

The details of the dementing process are, of course, not generalisable in a simple way. The relative parts played by the neurological impairment and the malignant social psychology vary from one person to another; also, the precise nature of each of these two components is unique to each case. The point is that the framework offered here makes it possible to map out, with any individual, the course of the dementing illness. This can be done in a way that is much closer to real life than those rather abstract schemes which aim to classify the various 'stages of dementia', as if the dementing process were a simple consequence of an advancing pathology in the brain tissue.[6]

One of the most serious anomalies confronting the 'standard paradigm' is that of those individuals who do, apparently, suffer from dementia, and pass through all its well-known stages, but whose brains are found, on *post mortem* examination, to have no deterioration beyond what is normal for their age. These cases have been known about since the first major neuropathological investigations,[7] and they are reported in the literature right through to the present day.[8] However, they are not generally acknowledged in simple textbooks, or in media accounts of dementia, where it is typically presented as the perfect example of an organic mental disorder.

How are these instances, which are a kind of scandal for the 'standard paradigm', to be explained? One tactic would be to suggest that the paradigm is basically correct, but that existing research methods in medical science are not sensitive enough to detect the neuropathology in all cases. The difficulty here is that this admission would cast doubt on the validity of much of the work that is now widely accepted. The other tactic – and it is the one adopted more commonly – is to say that these were cases of pseudodementia (usually associated with depression), and that they were incorrectly diagnosed as true dementias. The difficulty here is that, if so, present diagnostic methods are extremely imprecise. From the standpoint I have been taking in this paper, the latter explanation may well approximate to the truth. However, to describe a person as 'having' a pseudodementia is crude, overcondensed and reified, a flagrant example of the tendency of psychiatry to make entities out of processes. It is possible, rather, to give a detailed description of the kind of process which engenders the dementia-like conditions. It is evident that each aspect of social psychology, as registered, will have its counterpart in brain chemistry. There is no need, moreover, to make such sharp demarcations between depression and dementia, since there is a wide range of possible neurotransmitter imbalances and deficiencies. We can easily understand how a psychologically fragile older person might become demented in a true clinical sense, without significant neuropathology. There is still truth in the old idea that someone can be driven demented.

Thus far, in explicating this view of the dementing process, I have drawn only on the first two of the three 'basic equations' on p. 180. In other words, I have stayed with the commonly held view that the neurological impairment is *sui generis*, following a causal dynamic that is fundamentally distinct from the social psychology. Thus I have offered a kind of minimal presentation, following a tactic of playing safe. Let us consider now, however, the possibility that the third equation is also true, at least for some persons and for some conditions: that is, that degeneration of nervous tissue can actually be brought about as a result of an elderly person being continually and disastrously damaged at a psychological level. In the terms of my earlier paper, this is to suggest a movement from disorder that is simply functional to actual structural damage:

$$\frac{\psi' \equiv b'}{B^d, Bp}$$

If this turns out to be the case, the dementing process would have more causal linkages than indicated in Figure 1, and have a form such as is shown in Figure 2. It should be noted that there is no suggestion here that the causes of neuropathology in Alzheimer-type degeneration might be found exclusively within the psychological domain; simply that this is one of several possibilities, perhaps becoming more salient as the dementing process advances.

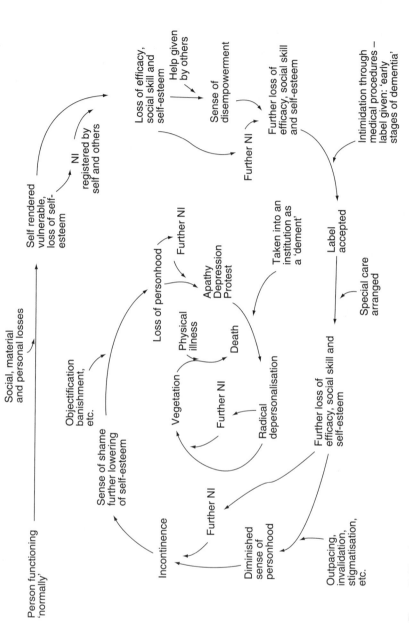

Figure 2 The dementing process, assuming some psychogenic causation of NI.

Whether or not the third equation is true, the theory of dementia which I have been putting forward is dialectical, in the following sense. It looks at process, and envisages this as involving a continuing interaction between different tendencies (T_1, T_2, etc.), to produce a succession of states (S_1, S_2, etc.); each state is transformed by further interaction with one of the tendencies. Thus the dialectical process would have a form such as that shown in Figure 3.

In the case of a pure multi-infarct dementia, it is sometimes possible to chart some of the relatively stable states or syntheses in the dialectical process. In the case of dementia of the Alzheimer type, this is generally not so; the dialectical model still applies, but some of the stages are infinitesimal. Geriatric medicine generally, both physical and psychiatric, might fare better if it abandoned simplistic notions of disease entities and linear causation, and adopted a dialectical view of state and process.

An objection answered

The account of the dementing process presented here has, it may be argued, far greater explanatory power than a simple medical model. In principle, it takes into consideration all that the latter does, but a great deal more besides. Also, this account has relatively few anomalies. Thus there is a strong *prima facie* case that we should shift to looking at senile dementia in the kind of way I have suggested, while not sacrificing any of the insights which medical science can offer.

Now, however, there is an objection to be faced. It is that a dialectical theory such as this is far too vague to be helpful or illuminating; more precisely, it is so ill-defined that it is immune from the kind of rigorous testing that might falsify it. In other words, it fails to meet Popper's criterion of genuine science. This is a very serious point. It must be conceded at once that the theory needs to be subjected to a more sustained encounter with the evidence, and perhaps modified and developed as a result. However, it is the form of the theory that is the more crucial issue.

Let us return to a comparison made earlier in this paper. The laboratory scientist seeks to obtain 'noise-free' knowledge in settings that are 'pure'. The engineer, however, is involved principally with the performance of complex structures in real-world settings. Suppose, then, that an engineer were called in to explain why a particular bridge had failed. (The prime aim, of course, would be to obtain sufficient knowledge to prevent other bridges from undergoing a similar type of failure.) Ideally, it would be necessary to investigate all possible sources of weakness in the structure itself. But the engineer would also need to examine the part played by a whole range of

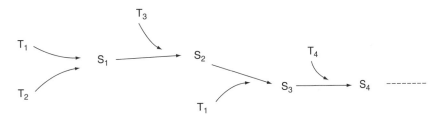

Figure 3 A dialectical process.

situation-specific and conjunctural factors: the type and flow of traffic, the weather conditions, the nature of the terrain supporting the weight of the bridge, and so on. Also simulations might be used, either physical or theoretical, to supply a kind of interactive knowledge which pure science could not provide. Eventually the engineer might be able to approximate to a full explanation of why the bridge had failed. The explanation would certainly include reference to some general principles, but it would also take unique features of bridge-and-setting into account. The form of the explanation would almost certainly be dialectical, and might be incapable of representation except through a computer. It would not be falsifiable in the strict Popperian sense, because the subject-matter is far too complex and impure to fall within one or more precise law-like generalisations. However inconvenient this may be for those who would like the world to be simpler, this is usually how an engineer has to work. Understandably, then, engineering design usually insists on very large margins of safety.

If these points apply to the failure of inanimate structures, they do so with much more force in explaining the failure of a living organism, whose complexity is many orders of magnitude greater, and to which our relationship is personal. In accounting for dementia, then, we can see how impotent is the work of medical science alone, and how faulty is the form of explanation which it generally provides. The work of the engineer, rather than the laboratory scientist, provides a better model, although this must be transcended by inter-subjective understanding. We need at least the outlines of a comprehensive explanation, even if it lacks precision at certain points.

Now although we are not dealing with the kind of explanation to which the methodology of pure science strictly applies, there is a kind of Popperian test which may in due course serve to evaluate the merits of a dialectical account such as I have offered. If dementia is simply the result of an ineluctable process of degeneration in nervous tissue, as the 'standard paradigm' implies, then changing the social psychology would have no radical effect on the course of the affliction. If, however, a dialectical account is nearer to the truth, we may expect some surprising outcomes when the social psychology is changed: then a truer dialectic would come into play, because it involved contradictory rather than mutually reinforcing tendencies. It would be naïve to suggest that this could be subjected to controlled experimentation. However, as the social psychology improves, we might expect dementias that are arrested or even reversed to some degree; and elderly people who, although suffering from severe handicap, are not undergoing the drastic personal deterioration which forms a central part of the classical description of dementia. I suspect that some of the best caregivers have seen this happening at times, and this is one reason why they hold only loosely to the medical model. The crux of the matter is this: if such benign outcomes do occur consistently, the 'standard paradigm' is confirmed as false or seriously deficient. If they do not, the dialectical model presented here is probably false; although it does not follow that the 'standard paradigm' is true.

Towards a new emphasis in dementia research

Medical science, in its whole approach to dementia and in its search for remedies, is in many respects at an impasse. No doubt it will continue to shed light on the nature of the changes at a cellular and subcellular level that accompany dementias of different kinds; perhaps it will also uncover genetic predispositions and bio-chemical anomalies. At the level of cure, all that can be realistically expected from medical science in the foreseeable future is the possibility of a little retardation, palliation, or temporary reversal. Nevertheless, almost any minor advance of know-ledge makes news; people are looking eagerly for miracle solutions, of a purely technical kind.

I have been suggesting, however, that one way out of the impasse is to adopt a much larger framework for the understanding of dementia, because this is the way the evidence from real life is pointing. It is necessary to come close to the actual experi-ence of those who are old and confused, who have had to face various kinds of loss, and who are often subject to the effects of a pernicious ageism. From the standpoint of the 'standard paradigm' there is a disease process in the brain of someone who, *as a person*, remains unknown and irrelevant. Vaguely, on the margins, there is the question of biography and life-setting; also there are various forms of care, some good, some bad. None of this, however, forms an essential part of the story, and it is not deemed to be worth rigorous analysis. Evidence here remains as anecdote or example, rather than being incorporated fundamentally into the theoretical frame. The dialectical theory that I have presented in this paper, in contrast, brings social psychology right into the picture; it is every bit as significant – and in some cases possibly more – than the neuropathology. This is not a merely sentimental move; in my earlier paper I attempted to show how a careful approach to the mind-brain problem makes this absolutely necessary.

At the very least, the determinism and pessimism that seem to be built into the 'standard paradigm' are unjustified at the present state of knowledge; so much of the social psychology still remains unexplored. The neurological impairment that usually accompanies dementia is, so far as we know, irreversible. Meanwhile, there is much in the prevailing social psychology that is undoubtedly pathological; and as many people are beginning to realise, it is time for it to be opened up fully for creative change.

Notes

1   Kitwood, T., Brain, mind and dementia: with particular reference to Alzheimer's disease. *Ageing and Society*, **9** (1989), 1–15.
2   Menzies, Lyth, I., *Containing Anxiety in Institutions*. Free Associations Books, London, 1989.
3   Barnes, E. K., Sack, A. and Shore, H., Guidelines to treatment approaches. *Gerontologist*, **13** (1973), 513–27.
4   Burnside, I. M., Loss: a constant theme in group work with the aged. In Zarit, S. H. (ed.), *Ageing and Death: Contemporary Perspectives*. Harper and Row, New York, 1971.
5   Wattis, J. and Church, M., *Practical Psychiatry of Old Age*, ch. 4. Croom Helm, Beckenham, 1986.
6   Rosen, W. G., Mohs, R. C, and Davis, K. L., A new rating scale for Alzheimer's disease. *American Journal of Psychiatry*, **141** (1984), 1356–64.

7   Tomlinson, B. E., Blessed, G. and Roth, M., Observations on the brains of demented old people. *Journal of Neurological Science*, **11** (1970), 205–42.

8   Homer, A. C., Honavar, M., Lantos, P. L., Hastie, I. R., Kellett, J. M. and Millard, P. H., Diagnosing dementia: do we get it right? *British Medical Journal*, **297** (1988), 894–6.

1.3

Towards the reconstruction of an organic mental disorder (1993)

The argument of this chapter is as follows. Senile dementia has been constructed by a cluster of discourses, of which the dominant one is grounded in medical science. This discourse, however, is far less coherent than it is commonly taken to be. Our understanding of dementia and dementia care can be reconstructed in relation to a discourse which gives central place to personhood and interpersonal relations. The creation of such a discourse challenges both material interests and psychological defences.

In the whole field of modern psychiatry, as it has developed since the founding work of Kraepelin and others around the turn of the century, senile dementia stands as one of the most puzzling of all afflictions. Superficially the primary degenerative dementias appear to be paradigmatic of the category 'organic mental disorder', and this is how they are generally presented in standard textbooks and popular accounts. In fact, however, when the details are scrutinized, almost nothing – not even the alleged organicity – is assured. The discourse generated by medical science is so dominant, and supported by such power and prestige, that its anomalies, self-contradictions and non sequiturs are obscured from view. A tremendous amount of social construction and repair work has been necessary to keep this discourse from falling into ruins.

These problematic features of senile dementia are not simply an intriguing puzzle for sociologists of knowledge. The 'regime of truth' surrounding dementia has a direct bearing on the lives of many millions of people throughout the world, as the great demographic shift towards an older population takes its course. A typical urban area in the industrialized world, with a population of 250,000, is likely to contain some 2,000 sufferers from moderate, and 1,000 from severe dementia; the great majority of these will be in the over-eighties age range (Ineichen, 1987). There is much controversy about how people who have a dementing illness should be treated medically and cared for socially. If we can grasp the nature of the discourses surrounding dementia, the understanding and actions which they both do and do not permit, the psychological defences and material interests which are involved, this may be highly liberating. The dominant discourse may, perhaps, be prized open, and new possibilities envisaged for easing this vast burden of human suffering.

The dominant discourse

By the middle part of this century the main dementing illnesses of old age were becoming well known. As compared to today they were not so salient in psychiatry, because the proportion of people in the older age range, and particularly the 'old-old', was still relatively small. It was widely believed (although without adequate supporting evidence) that the underlying cause of dementia was often the 'hardening of the arteries', and hence an insufficient supply of blood to the brain. Around this time the rest of the dementing conditions that were not associated with some clear pathology such as brain tumour were loosely grouped together as senility; it was recognized that there were various concomitant lesions in the grey matter of the cerebral cortex. Alzheimer's Disease was the name given to a relatively rare clinical entity, where a somewhat younger person (typically in his or her fifties) underwent a rather rapid dementing illness; post-mortem investigations had shown that in the brains of such persons some of the cortical tissue had degenerated drastically.

From the late 1960s, when the ageing of the population was being clearly identi-fied as a problem, and when methods of examining brain tissue were well-developed, a number of major studies were carried out on the brains of people who had lived on into old age. These studies showed that the lesions present in the grey matter of many of those who had a dementing illness were very similar, if not identical to, those that had been identified as typical of Alzheimer's Disease. A consensus grew up that among all cases of senile dementia some 50 per cent were associated with Alzheimer-type degeneration, 10–15 per cent with failure of blood supply (due mainly to small infarcts), and 10–15 per cent with lesions of both types (Albert 1982). The remainder were accountable to tumours, infections, hormonal disorders, metabolic imbalances, hydrocephalus and other conditions.

Henceforth the largest category of senile dementias was renamed as Alzheimer's Disease. It now appeared as if the primary cause of what had previously been called senility had been identified: it was a disease process in the brain, and not ageing per se. With multi-infarct dementia the process was well understood, but for Alzheimer's Disease the underlying cause or causes were obscure. It was soon after these dis-coveries that Alzheimer societies began to be formed in a number of countries. The announcement of a disease entity seemed to provide an explanation, a focus for shared concern and mutual support.

As research on the brain intensified, with the aid of several new investigative techniques, dementia became more clearly demarcated from ageing per se. In some respects this must be regarded as a progressive move. It was now the clear responsi-bility of doctors to do all they could to make accurate differential diagnoses when a person presented symptoms of cognitive impairment. Also it became harder to dismiss a patient or a concerned relative with such platitudes as 'It's just old age'. (Evasions of this kind are, in fact, far from having disappeared, and may be expected to return in force wherever medical services are under heavy economic pressure.)

Although the 'medicalization of dementia' brought about a certain clarification it had other consequences, arguably less benign. The prime task for doctors, in dealing with those who were confused, was to ensure that all treatable causes had been identified and dealt with. This, however, accounted for only a very small proportion of all patients. The majority of the rest were consigned to the category 'primary degenerative dementia', with its two main subdivisions. In the case of Alzheimer's Disease it was (and still is) largely a matter of diagnosis by default. In the case of multi-infarction, on the other hand, some positive diagnostic evidence was available through methods of scanning. But with both types of dementia, the implication was that the condition was hopeless from the standpoint of medical science. Drugs were available, of course, for dealing with accompanying physical ailments, and there were antidepressants and tranquillizers. There was, however, no fundamental medical treatment for the brain pathology. Senility had been a vague term, blurring the distinction between those who were relatively well-preserved and those who were not. 'Primary degenerative dementia', in contrast, was presented as a clear diagnostic category, laden with doom. Its effect, it may be argued, was to exclude and stigmatize, to banish the dementia sufferer from the world of persons. Various ideas about the 'stages of dementia' were advanced, each one claiming that the end-point of a dementing illness was a state near to that of a vegetable.

From this time forward medical science, in whatever of its main branches – epidemiology, aetiology, genetics, neuropathology, pharmacology – accepted the 'organicity' of the main senile dementias as unproblematic. The core assumption, which still underpins the whole discourse, is one of simple linear causation. It may be expressed as:

$$X \rightarrow \text{neuropathic change} \rightarrow \text{dementia}$$

In the case of multi-infarct dementia the nature of both X and the neuropathic change are fairly well understood. General health considerations, at least, can be brought to bear in the attempt to prevent X (failure of blood supply at the capillary level) from occurring. In the case of Alzheimer's Disease there have been many advances in elucidating the neuropathology, with a growing consensus that there may, in fact, be several more-or-less distinct conditions. The identity of X remains mysterious, although many hypotheses have been put forward, and there is controversy over whether one or several causal agents are involved. Biomedical research in the field is extremely active, involving huge commitments of money by drug companies. Within this general frame, however, scientific investigation seems to be largely at an impasse.

Medical science, then, created a powerful discourse about dementia. It was 'technical' in its orientation: that is, it viewed the human being, for the purposes of research, as an extremely complex mechanism, and the problem was to discover precisely why and how the mechanism had broken down. The crucial question of how brain and mind are related was largely ignored or bypassed.

The subsidiary discourses

Under the tutelage of the dominant discourse, and backed by such potent images as 'the death that leaves the body behind', several other discourses took form. One of these had a strongly sentimental character. It was often cast biographically, with accounts about how a person had been before, and how he or she had deteriorated as the disease took over. Frequently these accounts were accompanied by anecdotes about the dementing person's habits, both endearing and annoying, and expressions of the carer's grief. As Gubrium (1986) has shown, sometimes whole life histories were re-cast in the terms provided by the dominant discourse. The sentimental discourse was expressed also in a view of caregiving. The dementing person was taken as being, in many respects, like a child; the task was to keep that person, as far as possible, in good physical health, fed, toiletted, clean and comfortable, protected from harm. In this discourse the carer had a basic stance on the sidelines, an impotent witness to the ravages brought about by the disease, as it pursued its relentless course. Humour, courage, and an almost superhuman endurance were involved, and often religious faith was seen as playing an important part. But the task of the caregiver was assumed to be essentially hopeless.

At the professional level – in the work of nurses, careworkers, occupational therapists, clinical psychologists and others – another subsidiary discourse took form. It was that of 'behavioural management', claiming the branch of psychology that was, allegedly, the most strictly scientific as its main resource. The strongest emphasis was on things done by dementia sufferers that were troublesome for caregivers: incontinence, wandering, sleeplessness, aggression, sexual disinhibition and so on. The general aim was to re-shape behaviour into a more acceptable mould, through methods derived from operant conditioning. The resonances of behaviourism are to be found again and again in the standard care manuals, and in the talk of professionals, especially those at high level. Even Reality Orientation, which was originally conceived as a way of engaging the subjectivity of dementing persons (Folsom 1967) has often been assimilated to a behavioural discourse. In all of this there is a curious irony. The research literature shows very little evidence of constructive change that can be clearly attributable to behavioural methods per se; where success is reported, it often seems necessary to adduce explanations that include the dementia sufferer's subjectivity (Bredin 1991). The behavioural discourse serves as a kind of rhetorical adornment to care practice.

Contradictions and appearances

The intensive medicalization of dementia led, then, to the formation of a discourse which had a dominant and determinative place. It appeared convincing, and was backed by institutional prestige and powerful material interests. In its shadow, and not contradicting it in any serious way, there arose a number of subsidiary discourses, such as the sentimental and behavioural ones we have examined. Together, these discourses from the stock-in-trade of the standard care manuals, the stories written by family members, and the material published by the Alzheimer Societies. The lay world was presented with a bland and impenetrable facade, as if 'the truth' about dementia had been established.

Much of this, however, is illusion. In fact the dominant discourse is far from being coherent, even in its own terms. Serious anomalies and inconsistencies continue to appear; these are contained or assimilated in a way that bears a strong resemblance to the tactic of 'saving the appearances' that was adopted when the Ptolemaic system of astronomy was falling into disarray during the sixteenth century. We have already seen how the problem of brain and mind tends to be bypassed, although this must, surely, be the cornerstone of any theory in psychiatry. But there are four other areas of contradiction with which the dominant discourse cannot adequately deal (Kitwood 1990a).

The first of these has been present throughout the whole period of intensive study of brain tissue. It is that the correlation between the degree of dementia (as assessed clinically or through standard tests) and the measured extent of the damage to the grey matter is much lower than generally believed. This is true whatever neuropathological indicators are taken. In the most famous of all the studies in this area, that of Blessed, Tomlinson and Roth (1968) the correlation coefficients were in the range 0.6–0.8, which appears convincing, especially considering the relative crudity of the measures. But the authors themselves pointed out that when cases where both degree of dementia and extent of neuropathology were low, the correlations approached statistical insignificance. This was not an isolated finding. Right through to the present day postmortem investigations have produced evidence of a similar kind, whatever indices of brain damage have been used. The most serious anomalies of all arise in those cases where a person completes, apparently, the entire course of a dementing illness, going through its stages as classically described, and then the brain is found to have no neuropathic changes beyond what might be expected for one who is not cognitively impaired. These cases are known to all the major research groups in the field (e.g. Homer *et al.* 1988).

How are these anomalies to be accounted for? One move is to point out that the methods of measurement are fairly crude, and indeed may not be sensitive to the earliest stages of neurological damage; thus the correlations would not be expected to be high. This may well be true; but if so, the assertion that dementia is caused by neuropathic change is made on the basis of faith and not of factual evidence. An alternative move is to claim that there are many problems in making a clear diagnosis; the most powerful anomalies (high dementia, low neuropathology) were in fact instances of a reversible 'pseudodementia', whose symptoms are remarkably similar to those of a true primary degenerative condition. This move 'saves the appearances' in one sense; but the cost is to undermine the validity of one of the key variables: that of 'degree of dementia', however that may be determined. Thus we reach the *pons asinorum* of dementia research. Is the ultimate criterion of dementia to be what is assessed clinically, or is it to be one or more of the various forms of neuropathology? The tendency of late has been to choose the former (McKhann *et al.* 1984). This is honest and courageous, but it leaves the anomaly unresolved.

The second major contradiction relates to aetiology. According to the dominant discourse the causes of primary degenerative dementia are entirely physical, as befits an organic mental disorder. Psychological factors such as personality or stress reactions play no part in causation. Yet the psychobiographical study of dementia is not consistent with this view. When relatives are asked to reconstruct the story of a dementing person's illness, in many cases they point to a particular event, or cluster of events, and assert it was from that time forward that the person changed, or began to go downhill. The phenomenon of 'apparent precipitation' is well known in the field of dementia care, even if not in psychiatry.

In our own research (see Kitwood 1990b), psychobiographical data were collected on forty-four persons, and in twenty-seven of these the relative pointed to one or more critical life events as precipitants. The crucial life events fall into the following categories: 1. Retirement, redundancy or major role loss; 2. Bereavement; 3. Rejection or disgrace; 4. Stressful conflict; 5. Geographical change; 6. Accident; 7. Assault or burglary; 8. Major physical illness or operation. To give one example, related to categories 1, 2 and 3; a man who had once been a professional musician had a small organ in his house, which he used to play regularly: the neighbours complained that they were being disturbed, and in a fit of pique he decided to sell it. According to his wife, on the day the organ was taken away, her husband got lost in town, and he began to dement from that time forward. In the research literature there are a few studies which point in a similar direction, such as that of Amster and Kraus (1974), who used a standard life events method.

It may be objected that it is naive to accept at face value the retrospective accounts given by family members. Perhaps a relative, in dealing with a tragic loss and all the accompanying complexities of emotion, is striving to find a pattern and a meaning, and attaches causal weight inappropriately to particular events. Or it might be claimed that some events are genuinely causal, but have directly physical explanations. For example, major surgery such as hip replacement might involve the migration of small blood clots to the brain. To write off relatives' psychological explanations as fundamentally wrong does, however, seem to be arbitrary, especially as some recent research has attested to a remarkable accuracy in carers' observations on those they are looking after (O'Connor et al. 1989). Moreover, it is wholly consistent with medical science to hold open the possibility that loss, change and disruption might, for some personality types, be dementogenic. Depressive reactions may be involved, and the weakening of the immune system as in other major organic disorders such as cancer. Only gross prejudice would uphold the view that there could be no psychogenic aspects in the aetiology of dementia. The burden of the proof is shifting onto those who believe there are none, to bring forward their evidence and reasons.

The third anomaly in the dominant discourse relates to a very well-known fact which simply stands on its own, unassimilated. It is that some persons who are dementing relatively slowly undergo a rapid decline in mental abilities when their life-situation is changed, or when some serious disruption occurs. Typical precipitants here are being hospitalized for assessment, being taken into respite care, or entry into a residential or nursing home. It is not uncommon for a person whose existing support system is unable to continue, and who is then taken into an institution, to deteriorate drastically, even to the point where close relatives are no longer recognized, within so short a period as three months.

These phenomena, and especially the cases where no physical trauma is involved, require explanation. Now it is possible, of course, that rapid deterioration of the kind we are concerned with here has been caused directly by an advance in brain pathology, which simply 'happened to' occur concomitantly, and then acted as a primary cause of mental decline. Such an idea is not consistent, however, with the best evidence available from neuropathology. The crucial case is Alzheimer's Disease of the early-onset type, where it is known that the pathological process is relatively rapid; but here it typically takes years rather than weeks to run its course. Also, to suppose that the deterioration is merely coincidental in every case requires a credulity that borders on superstition. It makes much more sense to suppose that 'psychological factors', in the sense of how the dementia sufferer apprehends his or her life-situation (albeit with impaired cognitions) play a key part in the course of a dementing illness.

There is yet a fourth problem for the dominant discourse. It is one which challenges it deeply, especially the idea of 'stages of dementia' which are related to the structural damage in the brain. Those who specialize in the care of dementing persons, and who are well-enough resourced to aim for excellence, repeatedly testify that some persons cease to deteriorate when their life-situation has become stable, and even undergo a degree of 'rementing', or recovery of powers that were lost (e.g. Bell and McGregor 1991). Research evidence of a systematic kind is just beginning to appear in the literature. Rovner *et al.* (1990), for example, report a comparative study of two groups of residents in institutional care. One group was given far more attention than the other, and an enriched programme of activities. After a year, the first group showed relatively little cognitive decline, whereas the second group showed the sort of decline that might typically be expected. Also, at an individual level, there are now some reports of rementing (e.g. Roach 1985, Hope 1986). Much systematic research is needed on this important topic. Great advances would be made if it could be determined with which types of person, and with which dementing illnesses, and under what conditions, stabilization or rementing tends to occur. Even now, however, the phenomena must be acknowledged; an adequate theory of dementia must, surely, provide a place for them to be accounted for.

Anomalies such as the four discussed here can, of course, be neutralized by those who are determined to 'save the appearances' at all costs. Difficult evidence can be ignored, or explained away through what Popper called 'ad hoc modification'. It is clear, however, even now, that the main primary degenerative dementias, at the very time when they are most decisively claimed to be diseases, do not meet three of the classical criteria for calling a clinical entity a disease. There is no unique set of symptoms which clearly mark each disease off from other conditions. In no category is there a definite disease course, or set of alternative courses. And crucially, there is not a pathology which is found in every positive case, but not found in cases where the disease is not present. All the boundaries around senile dementia are, in fact, extremely vague. And, paradoxically, the entity which is most emphatically proclaimed to be a disease – Alzheimer's – is actually the least defined. The dominant discourse undoubtedly solves many practical problems, especially in providing a focus for biomedical research. What it does not do, however, is to provide the basis for a coherent explanation of the dementing process. The idea that it does so is an illusion.

'Saving the appearances' – another way

The dominant discourse, founded as it is on medical science, clearly faces great challenges to its coherence. This will continue, so long as it takes no account of how brain and mind are related, and so long as it resolutely excludes psychological considerations at its core. Any reconstruction of theory must be such that the anomalies are dealt with better, while full place is still given to the corroborated findings of medical research.

Such reconstruction is possible. Let it be assumed that there is a basic identity between brain and mind, but a complementarity of descriptions. Thus for every mental event or state there is a corresponding functional brain event or state, 'carried' by a brain that is in a particular structural condition (Kitwood 1989). Granted this, we may look at the dementing process in terms of three categories. The first is the structural condition of the brain, arising both from the establishment of interneuronal connections and from any processes that have damaged or destroyed nerve tissue. This category is measurable in principle, although in practice it is far beyond present instrumental capability. In all persons, so the evidence suggests, the structural state of the brain is undergoing decline in the long term; there is a progressive fall-out of neurones, and pathologies of both the Alzheimer type and the infarct type are present to a small degree. The second category is hypothetical. It is the highest level of mental functioning that is possible when a person's brain is in a particular structural state. Presumably this category follows the first closely; that is, the upper limits to mental functioning are set by the structural state of the brain. The third category is the actual mental functioning of the person. Aspects of this are testable, even at the present state of the art; for example through measures of cognitive capability, and performance in activities of daily living. The actual functioning of all persons lies below the maximum that is possible. How far it lies below is hard to say, but some of the evidence from recovery after stroke or other forms of brain damage suggests that the distance may be considerable; in other words, the normal brain has very large reserves.

Using these three categories, the course of a dementing illness may be represented as shown below.

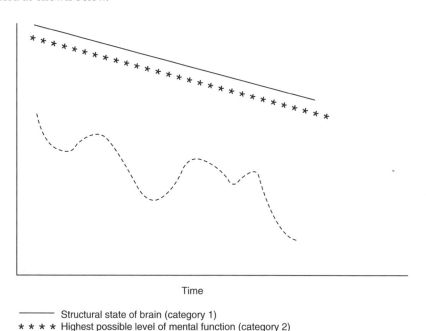

Time

————— Structural state of brain (category 1)
* * * * Highest possible level of mental function (category 2)
- - - - - Actual mental functioning (category 3)

Figure 8.1 Brain structure, brain function and the dementing process.

If these ideas are correct in principle (and there is no evidence to suggest that they are not), there are two important consequences. The first is that anyone who assumes that the line representing the third category is tracing the 'true course' of dementia, as directly determined by brain pathology, is making a grave error. In fact this error is made repeatedly, and the findings of medical science are called in as testimony to its truth. The second consequence is that a space is opened up for exploring ways in which a dementing person's actual functioning may be enhanced or diminished through non-neurological factors. These factors may be termed psychological and social-psychological, and of course have their counterparts in functional states in the brain. The theoretical space referred to here is represented on the diagram by the gap between lines 2 and 3.

The person who is missing

Throughout the many debates on the causes and treatment of senile dementia, and indeed in much of the literature on dementia care, certain questions are very rarely asked. Who is the dementia sufferer? What is the experience of dementing really like? How can those who have a dementing illness be enabled to remain persons in the full sense? That they are experiencing subjects, with cognitions, intentions, desires, emotions, there can be no doubt. In the dominant discourse, however, and in some of the subordinate discourses also, dementia sufferers are present largely as an absence. Those who are recognizable as persons are the carers. The dementia sufferers themselves are not; rather, they are defined out of the world of persons, even to the extent of it being claimed, almost literally, that those in the later stages are already dead.

The crudity that results from framing dementia solely in terms set by the dominant discourse is manifest in many of the writings published by the Alzheimer societies, and in many of the standard care manuals. The following is a real example, although no reference is given out of respect for the author's sincerity and commitment to caring. She describes her mother as having been aggressive for a period of 6 months during 'the disease', and attributes this to an affectation of the parts of the brain that supposedly 'control aggression'. She states that she knew her mother was not trying to hurt her; it simply was because her brain was disturbed. But the author goes on to say that the aggression was shown when she and her mother were alone, and never in the company of others. The inconsistencies here are glaring. Bound as she is by the dominant discourse, the author has no possibility of framing her mother as a social and historical being, living in an interpersonal milieu; who deals with her emotional distress in the context of impaired cognitions and impoverished personal resources; and who needs care which takes these things into account.

The exclusion of the person, of which this is typical, is not the whole story. In and amongst the practicalities of care work a different kind of discourse is often generated, in which the personhood of the dementia sufferer is indeed acknowledged. Such a discourse is not underpinned by theory, although it moves in a direction that is compatible with an interpersonal psychology of action. Careworkers often seem to operate with a kind of 'doublethink'. On the one hand, there is what they 'know' as standard theory, based on the dominant discourse; and on the other there is what they 'know' through experience. The inconsistency is not unduly troublesome, because it is the latter which informs their actions from day to day, while the official theory is largely bracketed.

The move towards a personal discourse comes about also in another way. Although behaviourism and Reality Orientation have had so great a place, various other kinds of dementia care intervention, more respectful of the dementia sufferer's subjectivity, have also been making their appearance at the margins. Validation Therapy, for example, rests on psychodynamic premises; it suggests that some of those who are in the 'old-old' age range have unresolved developmental and personal issues. As with Erikson's theory of life stages, then, one of two alternatives is possible: the person either deals with the issues (and here the 'therapy' may help), or goes into a dementing process that ends in vegetation (Feil 1982). There are many difficulties here, especially the lack of social considerations, but at least dementia is set into a personal and biographical context. Another form of intervention, so-called Resolution Therapy, has a Rogerian base. It suggests that there is meaning to be found in a dementing person's utterance, however bizarre or confused it may seem to be. The task, then, is to acknowledge the underlying feelings as real, and try to meet the need that is being expressed (Stokes and Goudie 1990). Examples such as these – and there are several others (Jones and Miesen 1991) – point to the beginnings of a reaction to the dominant discourse, an attempt to reinstate the dementia sufferer as a person.

Why, then, is the dementing person so excluded from discourse, and why is there an actual resistance to his or her reinstatement?

One factor, almost certainly, is the prevailing pattern of organizational power and prestige, a pattern that has become deeply entrenched over several centuries. The dominant discourse gives certain professional groups, and psychiatrists in particular, a control of the field. The subordinate discourses provide a place for those with less prestigious roles; both discourse and role are cemented into place. The interests vested in this tacit agreement are numerous: occupational definitions, careers, promotions, investments, publications, the allocation of funding for research. The opening up of a new kind of discourse, one which actually challenges that which is dominant at present, would allocate to psychiatry a far less central role, and elevate the work of humbler professions, particularly the front-line careworkers themselves. The whole structure would be shaken to its core.

The resistance seems to occur also at a psychological level, involving forms of defence which operate below the level of consciousness. The concept of psychological defence, referring to ways in which an individual wards off anxiety, is well known and validated. Perhaps, however, there is another and more powerful tactic: that of collusive defence (de Board 1978; Menzies Lyth 1988). The suggestion here is that in organizations people unwittingly agree together to define their field of work in such a way as to exclude from consideration aspects of that work which would be too painful or anxiety-provoking to take into account. In other words, they create a discourse which systematically defends its participants from psychological threat; and practices develop which are in harmony with the discourse. In the case of dementia the threats principally concern dependency, frailty, loneliness, abandonment, madness, dying and death. In this general area lie some of the darkest fears that confront the human race. It is not surprising that an apparently coherent cluster of discourses has developed around dementia, in such a way as not to engage with these things at all. One token of this whole avoidance is the typical lecture on dementia given to lay persons by an 'expert'. The 'disease', its epidemiology and stages are described; then at some point slides are shown, showing the microstructure of damaged grey matter, and the cross-section of a severely atrophied brain.

The dementing person reinstated

It is clear, then, that both sound theory and good practice require a serious and sustained attempt to understand dementia from within, and hence to create a new discourse, an interpersonal psychology. The fact that no one has yet returned from a demented state to tell us what it is like is certainly a drawback; one which does not apply, for example, to severe depression. Yet this particular 'world of illness' is not wholly inaccessible. Some of its aspects have been described by those in the early stages of a dementing process, urgently demanding that their experience be taken with full seriousness (e.g. Davis 1990). The further recesses, too, can be explored to some extent, when the methods of the poet, the anthropologist and the depth psychologist are combined (see Kitwood and Bredin 1992 for an account based on detailed observational research). Three aspects of a dementia sufferer's experience may be central to the creation of this interpersonal psychology.

1. A loss that can never be 'made good'

Life may be regarded as a process of loss and change, with corresponding 'grief work' to be done. This applies of course to bereavement, but also to losses of many other kinds. In later years loss has a special poignancy, because often there is no prospect of an external restoration. Great personal resources are necessary if this is to be faced without despair (Nemiroth and Colarusso 1985). Those who are dementing may be encountering all these 'ordinary' losses. But in addition they are having to deal with a double loss that is far more devastating: this is their drastic decline in mental capability, and with that a failure in the actual capacity to assimilate the loss. 'Grief work' means making a great readjustment, a reorganization of both life in the world and of inner mental processes, so as to take the new situation into account (Worden 1983). Dementia sufferers can no longer carry out that work. This is why validation therapy, with its emphasis on internal assimilative change, is so often impracticable. The main hope for those who are dementing, in dealing with their losses, is that there will be a coherent external world; with support, comfort, reassurance, stability that can be apprehended directly. For those who have no impairments, memories of good experience and of sustaining relationships can remain, while internal change takes its course. Those who are dementing are more at the mercy of impulse and disorganized fragments of memory. They need a living, palpable interpersonal reality.

2. Actions which fall short of the mark

In the terms set by the dominant discourse, those who have a dementing illness tend to present a range of problems of behaviour. The problems are of course, construed as such from the carers and the professional's point of view. But if we take the dementia sufferer's standpoint, we may usually see these behaviours as actions which are either not recognized, or incomplete because the 'action plan' cannot be retained. Wandering, masturbatory acts, screaming and shouting may, for example, be desperate ways in which a person who is drastically deprived of human contact provides self-evidence that he or she is still alive. Hiding and losing objects may be part of a person's attempt to 'make things safe' when there is an overpowering sense that things are continually being taken away. Some incontinent behaviour may be construed as an enactment of the letting go of hope and self-respect. Aggression may at times be a last bid for recognition by someone who craves desperately for it, but who cannot use acceptable means to gain it. The practical task, then, is to enable a dementia sufferer to retain, as far as possible, his or her sense of agency, and to 'fill out' those pieces of an action which are missing due to cognitive impairment. When a person has very serious deficits in memory and other powers, it may well be that he or she can produce little more than a gesture. The carer's task here is a highly creative one: to acknowledge the gesture, to honour its possibilities, and to enable it to be converted into an action that has meaning in the interpersonal world.

3. On the threshold of unbeing

For many dementia sufferers, especially those who are in the more traditional types of formal care, many hours pass by, day after day, with only the very minimum of human contact. Whatever contact there is may be largely instrumental, concerned with such practical tasks as feeding, clothing and toiletting. In all of this there is very little to replenish the sense of personhood. Someone whose memory is intact can draw on internal processes to retain the sense of personhood in times when contact is scarce or lacking; the continuing thread of selfhood survives in periods of deficit. A dementia sufferer does not have this resource, and so sometimes goes to desperate lengths to stay in the world of persons. If he or she remains passive for too long, the very basis of selfhood is stripped away.

The dementing process has sometimes been likened to a dismantling of the person, a return to a state that resembles, in some respects, that of infancy (Norman 1982). This is valid, but possibly its significance has not been appreciated, because often the dismantling has been construed solely in terms set by the dominant discourse.

We need, rather, to draw on the work of those who have taken a much less mechanical and individualistic approach to understanding our human nature. Winnicott (1965), for example, from a myriad of observations in his clinical work, traced the emergence of personhood in the infant. He suggested that subjectivity arises as fragments of intense experience begin to coalesce, until in due course the continuing thread of selfhood is formed. Also the infant acquires a sense of agency when a gesture meets a facilitating response: one that converts it into an action. In due course these joint actions are taken in, and become the infant's own resource of action schemata. Around these experiences, the infant has to deal with emotional issues that may be near to overwhelming: in particular the many ways in which social living makes the point that he or she is not the centre of the world. The infant, then needs to be held, both literally and psychologically.

In dementia, it seems, processes such as these are invoked again, but in a very different way. As the sense of self sustained by internal processing begins to fragment, it is the environment of others that can alone give continuity. As agency breaks down, it needs to be sustained increasingly by the facilitation which others provide. As emotional traumata continue and intensify, a greater degree of support and holding must be provided by others. Whereas in the case of an infant's development, the carer is doing 'person work' that goes along with a process of neurological matura- tion, in the case of dementia the carer is working against a process of neurological decline. Whereas, in the case of infants, the intensity of the person-work can become less as time goes on, in the case of dementia the person-work needs to become more intense. Moreover, while nature has prepared instinct-like pathways directed towards the care of infants, it is not at all clear whether this is the case with the care of those who are old and frail; it may be that it is a basically moral concern rather than a biological imperative which motivates the carer's work.

If this is the case, we may understand the course of a dementing illness in a way very different from the standard account, where dementia is seen as the inevitable consequence of an advancing neuropathology. Within a personal discourse, the prob- lem is not simply one of neurological inadequacy. It is, rather, that *the social context failed to provide those conditions that would be necessary for personhood to be retained, and that it failed increasingly as cognitive impairment advanced.* The final state of vegetation, commonly taken to be inevitable, may be reconstrued as one in which an individual has finally lost all hope of, and all means of, reaching out to others and being sustained by them. The self is irreversibly shattered. Personhood has been obliterated, never to return.

The need for a personal discourse

In this chapter we have touched on many issues related to the discourses of dementia. The crux of the matter is this. We are dealing here with one of the most bewildering and frightening conditions known to humankind: it is so both for those who are afflicted and for those who are closely involved as carers. In the dominant discourse and those which are subordinate to it the dementia sufferer – as a person – has disappeared from view, and the reasons for this are understandable. It is time for a new discourse about dementia to come to the forefront: one which puts personhood at the centre and which spells out what this means for an interpersonal psychology of caring. This discourse would not be subordinate to that produced by medical science; rather, medical science would occupy a certain space within a framework that puts the person first. Some of the key features of this personal discourse are already dis- cernible, and there have been some promising beginnings in practice; a great deal of work is needed to bring this discourse to its full strength.

The creation of a personal discourse about dementia is, then, a challenge on

two main grounds. First, it confronts an array of established material and organizational interests; for if the key problems related to the dementing process are to
be faced at an interpersonal level, then it is towards that level that the resources
need primarily to be directed. Second, it confronts a corresponding array of collusive psychological defences which prevent massive anxieties from being mobi-
lized. A discourse, then, is not simply a matter of ideas and propositions. It is also
a matter of organizational power, and of how human beings band together to deal
with realities that are often too painful to bear. The dismantling of such a structure,
and the replacement of it by something more enlightening and liberating, are a
formidable task.

References

Albert, M.S. (1982) 'Geriatric Neuropsychology', *Journal of Consulting and Clinical Psychology*
    49: 835–50.
Amster L.E. and Kraus, H.H. (1974) 'The relation between life crises and mental deterioration
    in old age', *International Journal of Aging and Human Development* 5: 51–5.
Bell, J. and McGregor, I. (1991) 'Living for the moment', *Nursing Times*, 87, 18: 45–7.
Blessed, G., Tomlinson, B.E. and Roth, M. (1968) 'The association between quantitative
    measures of dementia and of senile change in the cerebral grey matter of elderly subjects',
    British Journal of Psychiatry 114: 797–811.
Bredin, K. (1991) 'A Survey of Dementia Care Interventions', Bradford Dementia Research
    Group.
Davis, R. (1990) *My Journey into Alzheimer's Disease*, Wheaton, Illinois: Tyndale Hall
    Publishers.
De Board, G. (1978) *The Psychoanalysis of Organizations*, London: Tavistock Publications.
Feil, N. (1982) *Validation Therapy: the Feil Method*, Cleveland, Ohio: Edward Feil Productions.
Folsom, J.C. (1967) 'Reality orientation for the elderly patient', *Journal of Geriatric Psychiatry*
    1: 291–307.
Gubrium, J. (1986) *Old-timers and Alzheimer's: the Descriptive Organization of Senility*, London:
    JAI Press.
Homer, A.C., Honavar, M., Lantos, P.L., Hastie, I.R., Kollett, J.M. and Millard, P.H. (1988)
    'Diagnosing dementia: do we get it right?', *British Medical Journal* 297: 894–6.
Hope, J.A. (1986) 'When a new home "cured" the patient's dementia', *Geriatric Medicine*
    19: 8–12.
Ineichen, B. (1987) 'Measuring the rising tide. How many dementia cases will there be by
    2001?', *British Journal of Psychiatry* 150: 195–200.
Jones, G. and Miesen, B. (1991) *Caregiving in Dementia: Research and Application*, London:
    Routledge.
Kitwood, T. (1989) 'Brain, mind and dementia; with particular reference to Alzheimer's
    disease', *Ageing and Society* 9: 1–15.
Kitwood, T. (1990a) 'The dialectics of dementia: with particular reference to Alzheimer's
    disease', *Ageing and Society* 10: 177–96.
Kitwood, T. (1990b) 'Understanding senile dementia: a psychobiographical approach', *Free
    Associations* 19: 60–76.
Kitwood, T. and Bredin, K. (1992) *Person to Person: A guide to the care of those with failing mental
    powers*, Loughton: Gale Centre Publications.
McKhann, G., Drachman, D., Folstein, M., Katzman, R., Price, D. and Stadlan, E.M. (1984)
    'Clinical diagnosis of Alzheimer's Disease: report of the NINCDS – ADRDA Working

Group under the auspices of the Department of Health and Human Services Task Force on Alzheimer's Disease', *Neurology* 34: 939–44.

Menzies Lyth, I. (1988) *Containing Anxiety in Organizations*, London: Free Association Books.

Nemiroth, N.A. and Colarusso, C.A. (1985) *The Race Against Time*, New York: Plenum Press.

Norman, A. (1982) *Mental Illness in Old Age*, London: Centre for Policy on Ageing.

O'Connor, D.W., Pollitt, P.A., Brook, C.P.B. and Reiss, B.B. (1989) 'The validity of informant histories in a community study of dementia', *International Journal of Geriatric Psychiatry* 4: 203–8.

Roach, M. (1985) *Another Name for Madness*, Boston: Houghton Mifflin.

Rovner, B., Lucas-Blanstein, J., Folstein, M.F. and Smith, S.W. (1990) 'Stability over one year in patients admitted to a nursing home dementia unit', *International Journal of Geriatric Psychiatry* 5: 77–82.

Stokes, G. and Goudie, F. (1990) 'Counselling confused elderly people' in Stokes, G. and Goudie, F. (eds) *Working With Dementia*, Bicester: Winslow Press.

Winnicott, D. (1965) *The Maturational Process and the Facilitating Environment*, London: Hogarth Press.

Worden, J.W. (1983) *Grief Counselling and Grief Therapy*, London: Tavistock Publications.

1.4

Person and process in dementia (1993)

Summary

Outlines are given of an 'ethological' programme of research into the social psychology of dementia in old age. Here the manifestations and progress of a dementing illness are seen to be crucially dependent on the nature of the interpersonal context. The quality of dementia care can be evaluated, including quantitative measures. Earlier conceptualizations of the dementing process were overly deterministic and pessimistic. New challenges are created for service provision and policy.

KEY WORDS—Dementia, ethology, personhood, well-being, caregiving, evaluation.

Twenty years or so ago, the idea that there might be a social psychology of senile dementia—one which would be crucially relevant to medical and social practice—was scarcely thinkable. When psychiatry had made a probable diagnosis of a primary degenerative condition its task was virtually complete; the afflicted person was to be looked after while the disease process took its inexorable course; medication might possibly help with control of mood and behaviour. Now, however, we know much more about the dementing illnesses in their human context, and some of the gloom which pervaded that earlier understanding seems unjustified. This is especially the case for the common dementias of old age. The particular contribution which my coworkers and I have made is to develop a style of research which is 'ethological'; or, more accurately, 'ethogenic' (Harré, 1993). That is to say, the dementia sufferer is viewed as a person in the fullest possible sense: he or she is still an agent, one who can make things happen in the world, a sentient, relational and historical being. The empirical base of our work is a very detailed study of the behaviour of dementing persons in their 'natural' settings (their own homes, day centres, places of long-stay care, etc.), together with countless miniature interventions in those settings. This has led to a new way of conceptualizing a dementing condition: not in the full sense a theory, but approximating to theory and testable at many points. A further innovation by our group has been the development of a method for evaluating the care process, known as dementia care mapping.

The dementing process: towards a reconceptualization

In the traditional psychiatry of dementia, and the biomedical science that underpins it, the person has almost totally disappeared. A purely technical approach proved sufficient for many purposes (Kitwood, 1988). If, however, our concern is primarily with good caring, it is necessary to have a conceptual basis which acknowledges personhood fully. A convenient framework is to be found in the following 'equation', which suggests that the clinical manifestation of a dementia (SD) at a particular time point may be understood as arising from a complex interaction between five factors:

$$SD = P + B + H + NI + SP$$

The first, P refers to personality: that which each individual has constitutionally, overlaid with all the outcomes of social learning. Included here are such aspects as styles of coping with crisis, loss and change; defences against anxiety; and openness to help proffered by others.

B refers to biography, and in particular to the vicissitudes of later life. Some individuals embark on a dementing illness with most of the structures that formerly supported them still intact; others, however, have undergone a succession of destabilizing and demoralizing life changes, and with their personal resources already dwindling to zero.

H refers to physical health status, including the acuity of the senses. The bearing of this on mental functioning is not controversial, although many of the subtler effects still elude scientific inquiry.

The fourth factor, NI, refers to neurological impairment; according to its location, type and intensity, reducing the capacity for storing and processing information, executing 'plans', etc.

Finally, there is SP, the social psychology which makes up the fabric of everyday life; and in particular, whether it enhances or diminishes an individual's sense of safety, value and personal being.

The 'equation' given above might appear, at first sight, to be compounding neurological and psychological concepts in a barbarous way. This, however, is not the case if we accept the basic postulate that for each psychological event or state in an individual's experience there is a corresponding brain event or state (Kitwood, 1989). The 'thing as it really is' (mind–brain–body) is unknowable, but to grasp some aspects of it we find ourselves using two types of language, according to convenience; neither will ever tell us the final truth. Thus P, B, H and SP could, theoretically, be translated into one consistent set of descriptors, related to both nerve structure and neurochemistry; at present, however, we have no means for doing this.

Although the 'equation' is simplistic in some respects, it does accommodate most of the phenomena associated with the dementing conditions. For example, it accepts the great variability of symptoms, both cognitive and non-cognitive, that accompany a particular neuropathology. It can explain, in principle, the unique course of each individual's dementing illness, by combining 'structural' and 'conjunctural' means of explanation. It resolves the problem of loose correlation between intensity of neuropathology and severity of dementia, and in particular those notorious cases where relatively little pathology is found postmortem in the brain of a person who had been, apparently, severely demented. Furthermore, it can generate testable hypotheses concerning stabilization in dementia, where factors other than the damage to nerve tissue are taken into account.

The social–psychological milieu

Of the five components in the 'equation' we have examined three are already 'given'. Personality has largely been formed, and the main changes that will ensue are those of deconstruction: including, perhaps, the shattering of long-held psychological defences. The greater part of biography has now been written; nothing can change the life events that have taken place. Neurological impairments are already present, and tending to advance; biomedical interventions can do virtually nothing to arrest or reverse them. Only the other two factors still remain, crucially, as variables. Physical health may often be improved, with corresponding recoveries in mental functioning. There is also the social psychology, whose significance has, until fairly recently, passed largely unnoticed in dementia research. Psychiatry and clinical psychology have usually made the decontextualized individual their unit of analysis, and focused attention on deficits, remediable and otherwise. Studies of caregiving, moreover, have tended to prioritize caregivers, together with their problems and needs. The bizarre and troublesome behaviour of dementia sufferers was all too readily attributed to the disease process in the brain, while their real-life predicament was not taken into account.

Sustained 'ethological' inquiry, however, begins to reveal a very different picture. For example, using a form of critical incident technique it has proved possible to itemize the key aspects of the 'malignant social psychology' which often bears down on those who are dementing. (The term 'malignant' does not imply malice on the part of the caregivers; simply, that the effects are highly damaging from the recipient's point of view.) The elements of this social psychology have all been operationally defined and exemplified (Kitwood, 1990). They are:

> *Treachery:* the use of dishonest representation or deception in order to obtain compliance
>
> *Disempowerment:* doing for a dementia sufferer what he or she can in fact do, albeit clumsily or slowly
>
> *Infantilization:* implying that a dementia sufferer has the mentality or capability of a baby or young child
>
> *Condemnation:* blaming; the attribution of malicious or seditious motives, especially when the dementia sufferer is distressed
>
> *Intimidation:* the use of threats, commands or physical assault; the abuse of power
>
> *Stigmatization:* turning a dementia sufferer into an alien, a diseased object, an outcast, especially through verbal labels
>
> *Outpacing:* the delivery of information or instruction at a rate far beyond what can be processed
>
> *Invalidation:* the ignoring or discounting of a dementia sufferer's subjective states—especially feelings of distress or bewilderment

Banishment: the removal of a dementia sufferer from the human milieu, either
   physically or psychologically

Objectification: treating a person like a lump of dead matter; to be measured,
   pushed around, drained, filled, polished, dumped, etc.

The effect of this malignancy, together with the fact of continual neglect, must surely
be included in any explanation of the dementing process that aspires to scientific
truth.

  An ethological inquiry also, however, reveals a great deal about positive aspects
of dementia, and about those care practices which are conducive to the maintenance
of personhood. It has been possible, for example, to identify and operationalize 12
indicators of personal well-being in moderate or severe dementia (Kitwood and
Bredin, 1992b). These are assertion of desire, emotional ambience, initiation of social
contact, showing affection, sensitivity to others' feelings, self-respect, acceptance
of other dementia sufferers, humour, creativity, helpfulness, taking pleasure, and
physical relaxation. Some of these indicators are more robust than others, and some
are, clearly, related to enduring personality patterns. Nevertheless, each item can be
scaled 0, 1, 2, according to whether the indicator has been shown never, occasionally
or frequently day by day (to give a maximum score of 24). Our preliminary studies,
unpublished as yet, suggest that scores in the range 15–20 may be expected even from
some who have been several years in full-time care, and who score around zero on
standard cognitive tests. In such cases, so it appears, the care practice has enabled the
dementing person to retain feelings of self-worth, agency and social confidence.
Underlying that we may hypothesize a sense of hope, a basic trust that whatever ruin
and chaos there is within the psyche, the human context will still provide enough love
and stability to make life liveable. The details of the interpersonal process by which
this happens are beginning to be elucidated (Kitwood, 1993).

  There will, no doubt, be many disputes over details, but one main inference from
the ethological study of dementia is clear. It is inept to consider 'the problem' of
dementia as lying exclusively *within* the individual who carries the neurological
impairment. 'The problem' should be located, rather, in the interpersonal milieu.
'We'—professionals of all kinds, caregivers, family members, and the pattern of everyday life to which we are committed—are part of the problem too. Those who are
dementing are a problem to 'us'; they do not fit comfortably into the structures to
which we are accustomed. But conversely, 'we' are a problem to 'them', as a result of
our fears, distractions, rigidities, insensitivities, and even the professional training that
creates so deep a division between 'us' and 'them'. The evidence is growing (although
it is not thoroughly documented as yet, and a great deal of systematic research needs
to be done) that when 'we' are radically different, so also are 'they'. It begins to be
rational to doubt the idea of 'stages of dementia', if these are seen as the direct and
ineluctable consequence of advancing damage to the brain.

Mapping the care process

The social psychology which has been outlined, besides providing a rationale for good
care practice, has also given rise to a detailed method for evaluating the care process in

formal settings. The technique is known as dementia care mapping (DCM) (Kitwood and Bredin, 1992a; Kitwood, 1992). It is based on a strenuous attempt to take the standpoint of the dementia sufferer, drawing inferences from behavioural cues. As such, it provides a component that is lacking in most approaches to quality assurance in this field.

The method entails the coding of what has principally been happening to a dementia sufferer in successive time frames of 5 minutes. A letter is used to denote the general behaviour category (eg sleeping, wandering, receiving physical care). The letter is combined with a number on a six-point scale, related to the well-being or ill-being observed during each time frame. Altogether there are 110 behaviour categories. There is also a second type of coding, designed to capture those short-lived but highly significant episodes in which a dementia sufferer is subjected to some form of 'malignant social psychology'. Here there are 30 categories, representing varying degrees in the severity of personal detraction.

One trained observer can 'follow' up to five dementia sufferers with relative ease, and several more if the care process is uneventful; thus a team of three can 'map' a care environment with 15–20 dementia sufferers. The content validity of the method in use depends, clearly, on the length and typicality of the observation period(s), which might vary from 2 to 12 hours. The raw data can be processed in a variety of ways, both to summarize how individuals fared and to characterize the care environ-ment. DCM gives strong and detailed evidence concerning the social psychology of dementia, showing, at one extreme, how personhood can be continually replenished and restored and, at the other, how vegetation is actually fostered through the delivery of 'uncare'.

The course of a dementing illness

The concepts outlined in this article, together with the evidence derived from a sustained ethological inquiry, enable us to move towards a full explanation of any individual case of dementia. Also, the general course of a dementing illness may be represented in the form shown in Fig. 1. (There are analogies in the area of physical ability, particularly where the notion of a 'fitness gap' is adduced.)

Line 1 indicates the structural intactness of the brain. In principle it is measur-able, and some of its features have indeed been measured, showing the fallout of neurones, the presence of disease processes, etc. It is broadly agreed that the line slopes downwards in every adult case, but that there are great differences between persons in its gradient.

Line 2 represents the maximum possible level of psychological functioning for a given state of the brain structure. Although this is not directly measurable, it does have a close analogy in the field of computing. Here it makes logical sense to speak of a maximum computing capability for a particular configuration of the hardware.

Line 3 represents the actual level of a person's psychological functioning. Many aspects of this are directly measurable, and of course are often measured in geriatric assessments. There is very strong ground for believing that this line lies well below the second. The strongest evidence comes from examples of recovery after severe and

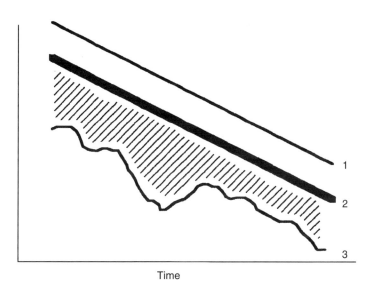

Time

Figure 1 General cause of a dementing illness.

traumatic brain damage, which, of course, is well known in persons of old age, especially in cases of stroke.

In some respects this representation is too simple, since it follows convention in ignoring the possibility of structural regeneration in the ageing brain (Roth, 1980). It does, however, show how fallacious it is to suppose that the third line—the course of the dementing illness—is a direct consequence of advancing neuropathology. The truth is, rather, that only the upper limit of psychological function is positively determined. Furthermore, this diagram points to the challenge for good dementia care. It is to work in the shaded area between lines 2 and 3: that is, to enable a person's psychological function to improve towards the upper limit. At present we have only intimations of what that limit might be, because excellent dementia care practices have not yet been widely established. This is one of the great psychogeriatric research questions of our time.

Personhood—the crucial issue

This short article has summarized only a few aspects of what is likely to be a sustained inquiry into the social psychology of dementia. Although some parts of our theoretical position are still speculative, one key point is no longer controversial. It is that far more can be done to sustain personhood than was formerly believed, even in cases where the cognitive impairments are very severe. Those highly pessimistic and deterministic accounts of the dementing process which have dominated the field for so long must be abandoned, for they are based on false logic and inadequate evidence. The diagnosis of a primary degenerative dementia should not be regarded as a sentence to 'death that leaves the body behind'. Rather, it is the requisition for a unique kind of provision. In dementia the inner sense of stability and security, held in place through memory and judgement, is vanishing to nothing. Now personhood can only be guaranteed, replenished and sustained through what others provide. And as the neuropathology advances, reducing individual capability, the need for that 'person-work' will grow more, not less. This is the fundamental challenge for good dementia care.

Acknowledgements

I would like to express my gratitude to Bradford Health Authority, the Leverhulme Trust, Charity Projects, Anchor Housing and Methodist Homes for the Aged for the funding which has enabled our work to go forward thus far. Also I acknowledge the invaluable contribution made by Kathleen Bredin, both in the conduct of research and in the development of theory.

TOM KITWOOD
Bradford Dementia Research Group,
University of Bradford, England

References

Harré, R. (1993) Rules, roles and rhetoric. *Psychologist* 16(1), 24–28.

Kitwood, T. (1988) The technical, the personal and the framing of dementia. *Soc. Behav.* 3, 161–180.

Kitwood, T. (1989) Brain, mind and dementia: With particular reference to Alzheimer's Disease. *Ageing Soc.* 9, 1–15.

Kitwood, T. (1990) The dialectics of dementia: With particular reference to Alzheimer's Disease. *Ageing Soc.* 10, 177–196.

Kitwood, T. (1992) Quality assurance in dementia care. *Geriatr. Med.* 22(9), 34–38.

Kitwood, T. (1993) Towards a theory of dementia care: The interpersonal process. *Ageing Soc.* 13, (in press).

Kitwood, T. and Bredin, K. (1992a) A new approach to the evaluation of dementia care. *J. Adv. Health Nursing Care* 1(5), 41–60.

Kitwood, T. and Bredin, K. (1992b) Towards a theory of dementia care: Personhood and well-being. *Ageing Soc.* 12, 269–287.

Roth, M. (1980) Senile dementia and its borderlands. In *Psychopathology in the Aged* (J. O. Cole and J. E. Barrett, Eds). Raven Press, New York.

1.5

A dialectical framework for dementia (1996)

Introduction

If we follow any person's dementing illness carefully, observing its course in the realities of everyday life, it is extremely difficult to conclude that we are simply witnessing the inexorable consequences of a process of degeneration in nervous tissue. Anyone who has dementia exists in a human context, for good or ill, and is powerfully affected by the behaviour of others. Those who are being cared for by their spouse or a family member are the inheritors of deeply rooted patterns, now changed because of the new situation; although there is often an almost superhuman love and self-sacrifice, it is also the case that fears, resentment and failures of communication that were already present may now be intensified. Those who are in "formal" care are liable to some degree of institutionalization, accompanied by various forms of misperception and misunderstanding; at worst their social life becomes that of a collectivity of strangers. The situation of those with dementia is often made more insecure because they are subjected to many changes and disruptions at the very point when they need greater safety and stability.

Although social and personal aspects of dementing illness such as these are widely recognized, for a long time there were only a very few attempts to incorporate them into a consistent body of theory. Psychiatry, with its underpinning of biomedical science, was largely impotent in this respect; however humane its practice, there was no corresponding body of theory (see, for example, Roth, 1980), Clinical psychology, too, offered very little; it tended to make the individual the unit of analysis, and its focus was often on the detailed description of deficits (see, for example, Hanley & Hodge, 1984). Some help was provided from the theory, such as it was, that accompanied certain dementia care interventions, for example reality orientation, reminiscence and validation (Holden & Woods, 1995), but here there was virtually no reference to research in neuroscience. There were also some moves to put dementia into a biographical and social-psychological context. Perhaps the most notable was that of Barnes, Sack & Shore (1973), who postulated an involutional spiral of personal deterioration, in which interpersonal factors had a major place.

In a series of papers dating from 1986 (see Kitwood, 1993a), I have attempted to develop an account of the dementing process and of dementia care that attempts to remedy this situation. It has three particular features, when compared to earlier work. First, the theoretical framework aims to remain close to the findings of biomedical research, even if not to the mythical penumbra that surrounds it. Second, it attempts to bring together both structural and conjunctural factors. (An analogy would be explaining the collapse of a bridge, where one might draw both on the general theory of statics and on the specific combination of traffic density, wind speed and direction, subsidence and corrosion.) Third, it grasps a nettle that has generally been avoided in the theory of dementia: the relationship between mind and brain. From this, as we shall see, arises the idea of a dialectic.

The "standard paradigm" and its problems

Underpinning a very large body of research into dementia—neuropathological and neurochemical investigations, brain scanning, drug trials, genetic research—there is an assumptive framework which can be expressed in very simple terms. In fact it is only rarely made explicit, but its subliminal presence is very easy to discover. The origins of the framework lie in developments in psychiatry around a century ago, when organic correlates for certain serious mental disorders were being discovered (Berrios, 1990). A major reason for its persistence is the innovation of many highly successful techniques for examining the structure and function of nervous tissue. The framework is not a theory as such, but rather the "generative grammar" from which specific theories may be derived as a field is opened up for investigation. It is, in Kuhn's terms, a paradigm: a disciplinary matrix backed by notable exemplars (Suppe, 1976).

This "standard paradigm" may be expressed as follows:

$$X \rightarrow \text{neuropathic change} \rightarrow \text{dementia}$$

The paradigm of course, allows many variants, and there is controversy among investigators about the details of the process they postulate. In pure research the aim is to identify X as a set of necessary conditions, together with the precise causal mechanism; in drug research the aim is to prevent or retard the efficacy of X, ideally with the causal process sufficiently elucidated; and in genetic research, the ultimate aim is to remove X altogether. In all of this the basic linear sequence remains largely unchallenged.

This paradigm has been taken to apply to all dementing conditions, whether cortical or subcortical. Within the former category the nature of X is now fairly clear in the so-called multi-infarct conditions. However, for those pathologies now commonly clustered together as Alzheimer's disease, the nature of X remains unknown; there are several promising lines of inquiry, accompanied by a great deal of speculation. The part played by genetic factors, whether as direct causes or as determinants of predispositions, has received particular attention of late (Roses et al., 1994).

Although the "standard paradigm" has provided an orientation for biomedical research, it has certain fundamental flaws as a basis for explaining the dementing process. At a purely conceptual level it is far too individualistic, ignoring the fact that human beings are not monads, but parts of complex systems. Also, the paradigm completely evades the question of how mind and brain are related. Neuropathology is a brain category, whereas dementia is "mental" in the broad sense of being clinically identified (McKhann et al., 1984). In virtually all biomedical research into dementia the slide from neurological to mental categories is not charted in any way.

Empirically, too, the paradigm runs into serious difficulties, three of which are particularly significant here. The first is the now notorious problem of the weak correlations between measures of dementia and indices of the extent of neuropathology. Some of the facts have been plain in the research literature for a long time (Kitwood, 1988), but they have been glossed over in secondary sources. And for those well documented instances in which a person had, apparently, gone through the whole course of a dementing illness as classically described, but whose brain showed no neuropathology beyond what would be typical for a person with no impairments, the common move was to suggest that the original diagnosis was incorrect (e.g. Homer et al., 1988). Evasions such as this, however, do not overcome the difficulties, which are so great as to lead one leading neuroscientist to the following conclusions:

> Over the years, investigators have fought assiduously for lesions or tissue alterations in the Alzheimer's brain which ... might at least correlate with clinical determinants of the disease severity. Plaque and tangle densities have been measured, specific neuroanatomic locations have been sought, neurons have been counted, and neurotransmitter deficiencies have been quantified. Despite 30 years of such efforts, clinico-pathologic correlations have been so weak or entirely lacking that determination of the proximate, let alone the ultimate, cause of Alzheimer's disease (AD) has not been possible. (Terry, 1992)

Elucidation of this enigma proceeds slowly. Recent work, for example, has confirmed the probable irrelevance of amyloid plaques, while pointing more strongly to neurofibrillary tangles in the frontal and parietal lobes (Nagy et al., 1995). The relation of correlation to causation, however, remains obscure.

The second empirical problem with the paradigm is the well attested observation that some people with dementia, under certain conditions, deteriorate in their functioning very much faster than can be attributed to the consequence of progressive degeneration of nervous tissue. A person may, for example, move rapidly from moderate to very severe dementia (in terms of some stage theory) following entry into a residential or nursing home, or show clear stepwise decline after each successive period of respite care, or emerge from hospital after a small operation in a state of drastic and apparently irreversible confusion. Changes such as these occur over a period of months, whereas the time-course of typical neurodegeneration, even in instances where it is fairly rapid, is a matter of years. There is an order of magnitude in the difference.

The third difficulty for the standard paradigm is less well known, but is highly significant for our understanding of the dementing process. This is the phenomenon of stabilization—the virtual arrest of deterioration—under certain conditions (e.g. Bell

& McGregor, 1991). Even more striking is the process which I have termed "rementing" (Kitwood, 1989), that is, the partial recovery of some powers which were, apparently, lost for ever. Research into rementing is only in its very early stages, but it is now documented in at least one major study (Sixsmith, Stilwell & Copeland, 1993).

The standard paradigm, then, is deficient on both conceptual and empirical grounds, and a more adequate way of framing the dementing process is required. No doubt the paradigm will persist for a long time yet, because it is supported by such great organizational power and so many material interests. It is in a position rather similar to that of pre-Copernican astronomy: empirically well grounded in a limited way, but continually having to "save appearances" as anomalies emerge. The alternative is to look for another paradigmatic framework, one with greater explanatory power.

On the problem of brain and mind

In much of the research on dementia two discourses tend to be conflated: one related to a person's behavioural and cognitive impairments, and the other related to processes occurring in the nervous system. A relationship between the neurological and the psychological is evidently assumed, but it is hardly ever made explicit. Perhaps there is an assumption that the relationship is a simple one. In fact, however, this is far from being the case; a long-standing debate within philosophy, going back at least to the 17th century, bears witness to the fact. This debate is far from being resolved, and it has taken on a new intensity with the arrival of computers and artificial intelligence. Both psychiatry and clinical psychology might benefit through a clarification.

The position which I shall outline here rejects the Cartesian idea of two fundamentally different "substances": matter and mind. Instead, it is monistic, in that it assumes the existence of one (exceedingly complex) reality. We can call it a material reality, but we must at once bracket commonsensical ideas of materialism. As human beings we act upon and within this reality, and in reflection upon our experience we create sets of categories. Our capacity for receiving, processing and storing information is extremely elaborate; it is excellent for securing our survival as a social species, but it could never provide a complete understanding of what is "really" there. Thus every discourse which human beings create in order to give coherence to their experience is limited in its scope.

In relation to the so-called mind–brain problem, Western civilization has developed two distinct types of discourse. One uses such language as "I feel hungry", "I regret having had that quarrel," "I plan to go to the theatre tomorrow", "I believe that you are telling the truth", and so on. This is an intentional discourse, and in using it we generally experience a sense of freedom. In contrast to this there is the language of natural science, based on critical and systematic observation. Within this discourse regularities are observed and corroborated, and causal relationships established. When we use it there often arises a sense of absolute determinism.

Each discourse has its function and its appropriate domain. It is a great error to mistake the categories of any one discourse for the reality itself, and a whole set of pseudo-problems arises as a consequence: for example, whether or not we have free will, whether the mind is inside the brain, whether the emotions are merely biochemical, and so on. The reality, whatever it is, is much greater and more complex than any of our conceptual frames.

We can apply these ideas usefully to the conceptualization of dementia, in the following way. An event or state within a person that is experienced psychologically (ψ) is also a brain event or state (b). (In this discussion the term "brain" may be taken as a shorthand for the whole neurophysiological system of which it is the core.) The happening is being described in two different ways. Hence:

$$\psi \equiv b$$

The brain events or states occur within an "apparatus" that has a structure, an architecture; and the nature of that architecture (especially, so neuroscience tells us, the number and type of synaptic connections) sets limits to what the brain can do. Now there are two crucial aspects to brain structure. The first relates to how this has developed as a result of learning and experience; hence B^d. The articulation of the nervous system proceeds rapidly during the first few years and it continues throughout life, right into old age. The other aspect of brain structure relates to the loss of neurones, interneuronal connections, etc., through such processes as the thermodynamic accumulation of disorder and specific disease processes. We might call this pathology, in its broadest sense; hence B_p

So, very crudely, the general representation will be:

$$\frac{\psi \equiv b}{B^d, B_p}$$

(Any mental state is also a brain event or state, instantiated in a brain with such-and-such a structure, which is the consequence of both developmental and pathological factors.)

If this account is correct in principle, even if grossly simplified, it helps us to order many observations related to dementia. Rapid decline (and depressive pseudodementia) involve changes in $\psi \equiv b$, but without, initially, significant enhancement of B_p. However, since the brain (unlike a computer) is a plastic organ, changes in function may, in the longer term, be translated into changes of structure. The weakness of correlations between dementia and neuropathology is now what would be expected; so also is the great heterogeneity of clinical presentation, even when the pathology is very similar (Boller et al., 1992). A person's condition is very inadequately represented by B_p alone.

This conceptualization raises a very serious issue for both psychiatry and clinical psychology. It is that B^d has been almost totally neglected in theories of dementia. There may be very great differences between human beings in the degree to which nerve architecture has developed through learning and experience, and hence in their resilience to dementogenic tendencies in the brain. Even psychodynamic processes such as repression or denial may have their counterparts at a neurological level. A rementing process may be attributable to the enhancement of B^d within a more restricted supply of neurones. At present, in human beings, the direct evidence to support these hypotheses in not available. There is, however, abundant data concerning brain development in animals near to the end of their life span (e.g. Diamond, 1978) and concerning the recovery of the nervous system after such a catastrophic event as a stroke (Kidd, 1992; Kandel, 1993).

The conceptualization that I have proposed here (a single reality, with pluralism of descriptions) is but one of several possible resolutions of the mind–brain problem, and its full explication is a matter for technical philosophy (see, for example, Davidson, 1970). It will suffice, however, for our more modest and pragmatic purposes.

Understanding dementia

Having set out a basis for relating the categories "brain" and "mind", we can now return to familiar ground, closer to everyday practice. In order to understand the manifestation of dementia (D) in any particular individual, what, principally, do we need to bear in mind? There are five key factors, as shown in the "equation" below:

$$D = P + B + H + NI + SP$$

The first factor (P) is personality. For our purposes here, descriptive concepts of personality in terms of traits are too bland and superficial. It is more helpful, following theorists such as Mischel (1977) or Burkitt (1993), to consider personality as resources for action. Each person develops his or her own repertoire in a unique way (beginning with tendencies which are given constitutionally) according to the opportunities that life provides; these opportunities are interpersonal, but can be related to broader factors such as locality, culture and position within the class structure of society. Resources are consolidated through experiences of success, and become deeply habituated. Each person also carries a repertoire of avoidances and blocks (in popular jargon, "hang-ups") acquired through experiences of failure, fear or powerlessness; accompanying these are various defences against anxiety. As life progresses, the content of the two repertoires may change to some degree; personality patterns do, however, show a remarkable endurance over time. Thus each individual brings a unique structure of action tendencies into his or her dementing illness. Many of the apparent changes in personality that then occur can be understood either as the losing of resources or the enhancement of "hang-ups", together with a stripping away of some of the psychological defences.

The second factor (B) is biography, which is clearly related to personality as it has been characterized here. It is self-evident that we cannot understand a person in later life unless we have some sense of his or her life story: childhood, family, occupation, interests, great adventures, and so on (although often records in formal care settings are remarkably deficient even in these essentials). Among all aspects of biography, perhaps it is that of loss that we need to be particularly aware of in understanding those who have dementia (Burnside, 1971): multiple bereavements, changes in health, mobility, economic power, and so on. Even if there were no failing of mental powers, with its accompanying anxiety and sense of disintegration, there is enough loss in the lives of many older people to render the sense of efficacy and self-esteem exceedingly fragile.

The third factor (H) is physical health. The main point here is that some degree of confusion is directly induced by problems at a metabolic level. There may be toxins in the system as a consequence of infections, kidney failure (or, ironically, the build-up of certain drugs), hormonal imbalance, or severe vitamin deficiency. Other health problems, particularly loss of mobility, sight or hearing, affect the opportunities for interaction and maintaining competence.

Fourth, there is neurological impairment (NI), according to its type, intensity and location, setting limits to the data-processing capacities of the nervous system.

The fifth factor is the social psychology (SP) that surrounds the person with dementia from day to day. Here, as with the theorization of personality, it is helpful to have an "ethogenic" model, rather than one which is derived in some way from behaviourism. From this standpoint each individual is viewed as a creative agent: one who attempts to define situations, to make sense of what others are doing, and to put out appropriate actions in a context of meaning. Social psychology of this kind has a long ancestry and has had a notable exposition during the last 20 years or so (see, for example, Harré, 1993). To work through its implications in the case of those who have dementia is complex, but at least some of the foundations of such a social psychology have been laid (Kitwood, 1993b).

To see dementia in terms of these five factors is very helpful for practical purposes, both for forming relationships that are rich in human contact and enablement, and for routine purposes such as assessment. More theoretically, it might appear at first sight that neurological, physiological and psychological categories have been compounded in a barbarous way. The point, however, is that all five factors can, in principle, be translated into a consistent set of neurological descriptors related to structure and biochemistry: it is simply that the practical means for so doing are not available, and probably never will be because the subject matter is so complex.

Of the five factors three are, in some sense, fixed or given. Personality has been consolidated over a long period (presumably with its counterpart in nerve architecture). Biography, by definition, is what has happened. The neurological impairments are already present, and at the current state of biomedical science there is no way of reversing them. The two factors which are clearly open to positive change are H and SP. In relation to the first of these everything possible should, of course, be done to ensure the highest level of physical health and to reduce the toxic burden on the system; no more will be said on this important issue here. This leaves us with the second, to which remarkably little attention has been given; ten years ago the phrase "the social psychology of dementia" was absent from the literature. It is clear, even on the basis of naive observation, that the social psychology surrounding those who have dementia has enormous variability, from that which is highly enlivening and reassuring to that which takes away from people their last remaining traces of competence and self-respect. In a very general way, then, the symptomatic presentation of dementia in any individual arises from a complex interaction between all five factors, while the progression of the illness depends primarily on the interplay between NI and SP, and this interplay, as we shall see, may properly be characterized as dialectical.

The social psychology of dementia

The full explication of social psychological processes in dementia is a task beyond the scope of this chapter. Here we shall focus simply on certain kinds of interaction that promote either the destruction or the maintenance of personhood. All of us are, of course, affected by interactions of these two kinds. If our cognitions are intact, we do have certain inner stabilizers: primarily defences against invasion by anxiety, and our capacity for rational understanding. So, for example, if an extremely hurtful and disparaging remark is made to us, we may be able to offset the feeling of being devalued and undermined through the knowledge that the remark was untrue factually, and that it arose from the other's state of stress. Generally those who have dementia do not have strong inner stabilizers, with the consequence that they are extremely susceptible to social-psychological processes. Also, while their capacities for assimilating cognitive content are weakened, their sensitivity to non-verbal information often seems to be increased. Thus the social psychology that surrounds them is extremely significant, whether for their well- or ill-being.

I have researched this social psychology in considerable detail, through the study of critical incidents (Kitwood, 1990), through the observational technique of dementia care mapping (DCM) (Kitwood & Bredin, 1992), and in a less structured way simply through involvement in the care process. There can be no doubt that we have inherited from the past some ways of interacting that are extremely damaging to those who have dementia, amounting to a "malignant social psychology". This strong term refers to the effects upon those who have dementia; it does not imply malice on the part of careworkers, who generally carry out their tasks with good intentions. Some of the principal components of this malignancy are treachery, disempowerment, infantilization, condemnation, intimidation, stigmatization, outpacing, invalidation, banishment and objectification. These are operationalized in detail in the DCM method, as 46 types of "personal detraction", graded into five different levels of severity. Our experience with DCM suggests that it is extremely difficult to eliminate these episodes, even in care setting that might be judged of generally high quality (Fox, 1995).

In contrast to this, it is possible to identify elements of a social psychology that make for well-being; we have often observed that when this has consistently been in operation for, say, half an hour, a person gains enough confidence and security to cope well for the two or three hours that follow, as if personhood has temporarily been restored. Here are five examples of such processes.

Holding

This term is used in the sense that Winnicott used it in his accounts of parenting (Davis & Wallbridge, 1981). Holding is a metaphor for providing a safe and steady place where powerful and frightening emotions can be experienced, without the person being overwhelmed by the terror of disintegration or annihilation. As in the case of children, the psychological holding of those who have dementia may well involve a physical holding too.

Validation

This term has a long history in psychotherapeutic work. It means to accept the reality and "personal truth" of another's experience, often in contrast to those who would dismiss it as unreal or of no account. Validation has now been shown to be of crucial importance in dementia care, largely through the work of Feil (1993).

Facilitation

At its simplest, this refers to enabling people to do what they otherwise might not be able to do, by providing those parts of the action schemata that are missing—and no more. Less obviously, and again drawing on Winnicott, facilitation entails responding to a gesture in such a way as to evoke a further response, and providing the interaction with structure and meaning. In true facilitation, nothing is taken away from the person who makes the gesture—there is no overriding or impingement; yet a solitary gesture is transformed into a complete action in the social world.

Celebration

Processes of this type involve the person with dementia and the carer being together and doing something which they both sincerely enjoy: singing, dancing, laughing, having a good meal, walking at the seaside. In the terms of Berne's transactional analysis, both participants are in the ego state of the "free child" (Stewart & Joines, 1987). In contrast to this, the majority of dementia care interactions are of the parent–child type, whether that parent is controlling and critical or primarily nurturing.

Timulation

This term is a neologism, coined during the development of dementia care mapping. It means the direct and pleasurable stimulation of the senses, in a way that accords with the values and scruples of the person with dementia. This might include those forms of massage whose prime aim is to provide bodily contact and comfort, the use of aromatic oils, the exploration of materials and the creation of a personal conversation through music. The direct involvement of the senses is, in its own way, a form of orientation to reality.

These five processes are far more than techniques, although technical competence is required. Each one demands something profound from the caregiver, something that may entail personal change on his or her part. To be able to "hold" another means having overcome the fear of powerful emotion, the dread of annihilation; to validate the experience of another involves the ability to give free attention and use one's own feeling states; to facilitate requires imaginative sensitivity and creative power; to celebrate means having ready access to one's own spontaneity, one's own "free child"; to provide timulation requires that one should be free of puritanical inhibitions, comfortable with one's own sensuality. The setting up and maintaining of processes such as the five mentioned here may be considered as "positive person-work".

The dialectics of dementia

In its original sense dialectics was a form of argumentation in which thesis and counter-thesis were brought together and explored; the argument "moved on" as each conclusion was then subjected to a new counter-thesis. When the idea of dialectic is applied to a process, it means an interaction between a state and one or more causal tendencies, to provide a new state; this then comes under the influence of new tendencies, and so on. So, simplistically, for a succession of states S1, S2, etc., and tendencies T1, T2, etc., this is shown in Figure 14.1.

If we apply this to the dementing process the states refer to the whole person; or, with some reduction, to the nervous system; and hence, if we adopt a monistic view of the mind–brain relationship as we have seen, to $\dfrac{\psi \equiv b}{B^d, B_p}$. The tendencies are social psychological, whether malignant or benign, and although we commonly represent these in psychological categories, they have their neurological counterparts.

So the central thesis in the dialectical framework is that the dementing process arises from an interaction between neurological impairment and social psychological processes. The biographical events are accounted for better in this way than through looking at neuropathology alone. In reality, or course, an individual is likely to experience a mixture of both malignant and benign social psychologies. We might, however, consider two ideal types, by way of clarification.

In the first, the social psychology tends to undermine and discourage those who already carry neurologically based disabilities. So, for example, a person who is criticized and blamed for a lack of competence that is genuinely present will find the sense of efficacy and self-esteem dwindling, and come to believe that the disability is greater than is in fact the case; a person whose attempts to reach out to others are disregarded will sooner or later lose heart, and sink into apathy and despair; a person whose experience is not treated as valid may come to doubt the reality of that experience, and even the reality of his or her own being. In this kind of way, then, a vicious circle is set up, where genuine disability is enhanced at a social-psychological level, and where each negative outcome tends to recruit more of the malignant social psychology. Thus an involutional process goes forward, each of its stages appearing to be part of an inexorable programme of decline. The microstructure of this process becomes clearly visible in the course of dementia care mapping. The long-term consequence is a radical depersonalization, and perhaps a vegetative state, as shown in Figure 14.2.

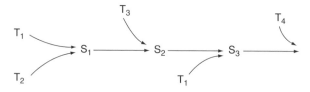

Figure 14.1 A diagrammatic representation of a dialectic process.

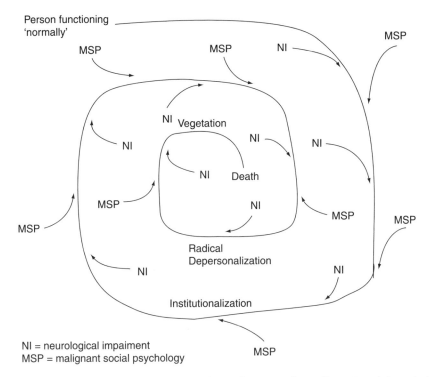

Figure 14.2 Interaction between neurological impairment and a malignant social psychology.

Within this dialectic, then, we may find the dementing process as classically described, including the various stage-schemes of deterioration; the explanation, however, is very different from that offered by the "standard paradigm".

The second ideal type is one in which the neurological impairments and their direct consequences are offset or mitigated by the social psychology: by the positive person-work caried out by carers. The "holding" is sufficient to enable the person with dementia to tolerate powerful feelings of anxiety or grief; the facilitation is such that many competences are retained; there is enough celebration for life to have joy and meaning; and so on. In this kind of way a person is able to "relax into" his or her dementia; although there is anguish and devastating loss, there is an underlying security and well-being. So a different kind of interaction is set up; in a sense the process is more truly dialectical than the first, because it is derived from contradictory rather than mutually reinforcing tendencies. The person with dementia is, of course, diminished in certain respects, and the situation may truly be described as tragic. There is, however, no radical loss of personhood. In a few instances personal qualities may even become apparent that were not in evidence before the dementing illness began; some of these pertain to the "free child," who perhaps was hidden away for years behind layer and layer of repression (Kitwood, 1995). The form of this second dialectic is shown in Figure 14.3.

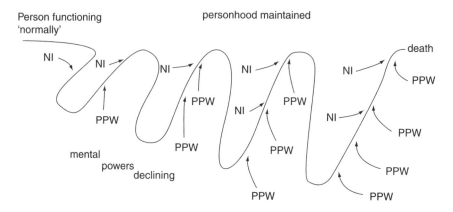

Figure 14.3 NI = neurological impairment; PPW = positive person-work.

Advantages of a dialectical approach

We do not know, of course, what is happening from moment to moment in the brains of those who have dementia, whether the dialectic approximates more to the first type or the second. Scanning methods, even of the most powerful kind, give very incomplete information, and they inevitably involve taking people away from those environments in which they feel most secure and supported, where their brain function is likely to be optimal. Much, then, remains speculative at the present time. The great merit of the framework that I have proposed here is that it begins to accommodate a far greater range of information, both clinical and neurological, than the standard paradigm of biomedical science. Much that was, so to speak, noise—contributing to a vast amount of error variance in research—begins to be converted into clear signals. Moreover, by bringing social psychology into the same picture as neurology we are not reverting to dualism, but retaining a high degree of theoretical coherence.

More controversially, the door is opened for considering the possibility that a prolonged and pervasive malignant social psychology might actually cause damage to the brain, and even that there might be, in some instances, psychological antecedents to dementia (for example, the massive uses of such defences as denial and displacement). On the positive side there is the possibility that a benign social psychology might, over a period, even provoke some structural regeneration among the neurones that remain. Evidence related to dementia, albeit of a rather indirect kind, is just beginning to appear in the literature (e.g. Brane, Karlsson, Kihlgren & Norberg, 1989). It is a general principle of epigenetics that function becomes structure in the phenotype.

Finally, on a directly practical level, a dialectical framework such as I have proposed points clearly to what we should and should not be doing in care practice. There is no need to wait in fantasy for some golden future when biomedical science has at last delivered magic bullets, or genetic intervention has removed even the propensity to develop dementia. There is much that can be done now that makes sound neurological sense, provided that we relinquish all utopian expectations and simply retain confidence in our human powers.

References

Barnes, T., Sack, J. & Shore, J. (1973). The cycle of dementia. *Gerontologist*, **13**, 513–527.

Bell, J. & McGregor, I. (1991). Living for the moment. *Nursing Times*, **87**, 18, 45–47.

Berrios, G.E. (1990). Alzheimer's disease: a conceptual history. *International Journal of Geriatric Psychiatry*, **5**, 355–365.

Boller, F., Forette, F., Khachaturian, Z., Pancet, M. & Christen, Y. (eds) (1992). *Heterogeneity of Alzheimer's Disease*. Springer Verlag, Berlin.

Brane, G., Karlsson, I., Kihlgren, M. & Norberg, A. (1989). Integrity-promoting care of demented nursing home patients: psychological and biochemical changes. *International Journal of Geriatric Psychiatry*, **4**, 165–172.

Burkitt, I. (1993). *Social Selves*. Sage, London.

Burnside, I.M. (1971). Loss: a constant theme in group work with the aged. In S.H. Zarit (ed.), *Ageing and Death: Contemporary Perspectives*. Harper and Row, New York.

Davidson, D. (1970). Mental events. In L. Foster & J.W. Swanson (eds), *Experience and Theory*. University of Massachusetts Press, Boston.

Davis, M. & Wallbridge, D. (1981). *Boundary and Space*. Penguin, Harmondsworth.

Diamond, M.C. (1978). The ageing brain: some enlightening and optimistic results, *American Scientist*, **66**, 66–71.

Feil, N. (1993). *The Validation Breakthrough*. Health Professionals Press, Baltimore.

Fox, L. (1995). Mapping the advance of the new culture in dementia care. In T. Kitwood & S. Benson (eds), *The New Culture of Dementia Care*. Hawker Publications, London.

Hanley, I.G. & Hodge, J. (eds) (1984). *Psychological Approaches to the Care of the Elderly*. Croom Helm, London.

Harré, R. (1993). Rules, roles and rhetoric. *Psychologist*, **16**(1), 24–28.

Holden, U. & Woods, R. (1995). *Positive Approaches to Dementia Care*. Churchill Livingstone, New York.

Homer, A.C., Honavar, M., Lantos, P.L., Hastie, I.R., Kellett, J.M. & Millard, P.H. (1988). Diagnosing dementia: do we get it right? *British Medical Journal*, **297**, 894–896.

Kandel, E.R. (1993). Synapse formation, trophic interactions between neurons, and the development of behaviour. In E.R. Kandel & J.H. Schwartz (eds), *Principles of Neural Science*. Elsevier, New York.

Kidd, G. (1992). *Understanding Neuromuscular Plasticity: A Basis for Clinical Rehabilitation*. Arnold, Sevenoaks.

Kitwood, T. (1988). The technical, the personal and the framing of dementia. *Social Behaviour*, **3**, 161–179.

Kitwood, T. (1989). Brain, mind and dementia: with particular reference to Alzheimer's disease. *Ageing and Society*, **9**, 1–15.

Kitwood, T. (1990). The dialetics of dementia: with particular reference to Alzheimer's disease. *Ageing and Society*, **10**, 177–196.

Kitwood, T. (1993a). Person and process in dementia. *International Journal of Geriatric Psychiatry*, **8**, 541–545.

Kitwood, T. (1993b). Towards a theory of dementia care: the interpersonal process, *Ageing and Society*, **13**, 51–67.

Kitwood, T. (1995). Positive long term changes in dementia: some preliminary observations. *Journal of Mental Health*, **4**, 133–144.

Kitwood, T. & Bredin, K. (1992). A new approach to the evaluation of dementia care. *Journal of Advances in Health and Nursing Care*, 1(5), 41–60.

McKhann, G., Drachman, D., Folstein, M., Kulzman, N., Price, D. & Stadlan, E.M. (1984). Clinical diagnosis of Alzheimer's disease: report of the NINCDS-ADRDA Working Group. *Neurology*, 34, 939–944.

Mischel, W. (1977). The interaction of person and situation. In D. Magnusson & N.S. Endler (eds), *Personality at the Crossorads*. Erlbaum, Hillsdale, NJ.

Nagy, S.Z., Esiric, M.M., Jobst, K.A., Morris, J.H., King, E.M.-F., McDonald, B., Litchfield, S., Smith, A., Barnetson, L. & Smith, A.D. (1995). Relative roles of plaques and tangles in the dementia of Alzheimer's disease: correlations using three sets of neuropathological criteria. *Dementia*, 6, 21–31.

Roses, A.D., Strittmatter, W.J., Pericak-Vance, M.A., Corcher, E.H., Saunders, A.W. & Schmedchel, D.E. (1994). Clinical application of apolipoprotein E genotyping to Alzheimer's disease, *Lancet*, 343(8912), 1564–1565.

Roth, M. (1980). Senile dementia and its borderlands. In J.O. Cole & J.E. Barrett (eds), *Psychopathology in the Aged*. Raven Press, New York.

Sixsmith, A., Stilwell, J. & Copeland, J. (1993). Rementia: challenging the limits of dementia care. *International Journal of Geriatric Psychiatry*, 8, 993–1000.

Stewart, I. & Joines, V. (1987). *TA Today*. Addison-Wesley, Reading, Mass.

Suppe, F. (ed.) (1976). *The Structure of Scientific Theories*. Unviersity of Illinois Press, Urbana.

Terry, R.D. (1992). The pathogenesis of Alzheimer's disease: what causes dementia? In Y. Christen & P. Churchland (eds), *Neurophilosophy and Alzheimer's Disease*. Springer Verlag, Berlin.

Part 2

ILL-BEING, WELL-BEING AND PSYCHOLOGICAL NEED

Ill-being, well-being and psychological need

Readings

Kitwood, T. (1988) The contribution of psychology to the understanding of senile dementia. In Gearing, B., Johnson, M. and Heller, T. (eds) *Mental Health Problems in Old Age: A reader*. Chichester: John Wiley & Sons.

Kitwood, T. (1990) Understanding senile dementia: a psychobiographical approach, *Free Associations*, 19: 60–76.

Kitwood, T. and Bredin, K. (1992) Towards a theory of dementia care: personhood and well-being, *Ageing and Society*, 12(3): 269–287.

Kitwood, T., Buckland, S. and Petre, T. (1995) Findings relating to well-being, and findings related to ill-being, in *Brighter Futures: A report into provision for persons with dementia in residential homes, nursing homes and sheltered housing*. London: Anchor Housing Association 19–28.

Kitwood, T. (1998) Toward a theory of dementia care: ethics and interaction, *Journal of Clinical Ethics*, 9(1): 23–34.

Critical commentary

At the heart of Kitwood's approach to person-centred care lies a conviction that in dementia, no matter how severe the cognitive losses, there is a 'core self', which remains recognizable and fundamentally intact. The person with dementia may be confused, distressed, adrift, but she or he is still 'there', still able to be reached by the lifebelt of human contact. Moreover, at least some of the confusion, distress and loss of identity experienced by people who have dementia are of our own and society's making. Psychological ill-being in dementia is not, in Kitwood's view, solely the result of pathological changes to the brain, as has so often been implied. It is also the result of failures of human communication, social support and service provision. If we accept this reflectively, rather than at a merely superficial level, we also have to consider the potential for maintaining or enhancing the well-being of people with dementia if the quality of care and human interaction are very high. In order to provide person-centred care it is vital to recognize that each person with dementia is unique; to draw on a detailed knowledge and understanding of his or her life history, and to value individual tastes, preferences and beliefs.

Kitwood made a significant distinction between cognition (or mental acuity), which he acknowledged was always compromised in dementia, and other aspects of personhood or identity that can remain relatively intact if the quality of care and support are high. Kitwood's overall position on the relationship between quality of care, ill-being and well-being, is one that will already be familiar to many readers. Like other aspects of his thinking, however, Kitwood's work on this subject developed and changed over time, and the emphases within it often differ depending on the intended audience. The practice-oriented publications have, in general, a more didactic and instructional tone than the more discursive and exploratory theoretical papers. In this section we will set practice interventions such as Dementia Care Mapping (DCM) alongside Kitwood's theoretical publications related to ill-being and well-being. We will also consider some of the methodological issues arising from related empirical research.

Kitwood's work on ill-being and well-being in dementia appears to have unfolded in three main phases. In the earliest of these (from around 1987–1990) the emphasis is almost entirely on ill-being, which is considered to be an inevitable consequence of dementia and is frequently suggested by him as a precondition for its onset. In the mid-phase (1991–1995) the emphasis shifts to both ill-being and well-being in the context of interpersonal interaction with the person with dementia, largely in formal care settings. In the latest phase of Kitwood's published work (1995–1998), the focus moves again from a binary distinction between ill-being and well-being to a more detailed consideration of the psychological needs of people with dementia and the challenges of equipping caregivers to meet these needs.

In this chapter we will first summarize the key elements of Kitwood's thinking on well-being and ill-being in dementia, as these had come to be formalized at the time of his death. We will then briefly consider the nature of well-being as a philosophical concept. Finally, we will go on to chart the development of Kitwood's thinking on what might broadly be termed 'the psychology of dementia' within the three-phase framework just outlined, with reference to the five articles reproduced in this section of the Reader, which span a 10-year period from 1988 to 1998. What can be seen here is that Kitwood advanced a series of conjectures about the impact of ill- and well-being on the onset, progression and experience of dementia, which over time were tempered by the evidence that was then available and adapted accordingly.

Key concepts related to ill-being and well-being in Kitwood's work

The most accessible account of Kitwood's position on well-being and ill-being at the time of his death was the, then current, seventh edition of the *Dementia Care Mapping Manual* (Bradford Dementia Group 1997). See Box 2.1 for a fuller explanation of Dementia Care Mapping (DCM). Here, Kitwood noted that although the nature of dementia means that 'it cannot ever be considered a state of well-being ... it is possible for many people to fare relatively well even though they have a dementing condition' (p. 4).[1] Kitwood argued that because cognition is only one aspect of our personhood, the problems with memory, understanding, judgement and so on which accompany dementia still leave many other aspects of personhood intact (for example, feelings, attachments, a sense of identity). Kitwood proposed a range of states of

---

Box 2.1   Dementia Care Mapping (DCM)

As many readers will already know, DCM is an observational method designed to assess the quality of care for people with dementia in formal care settings (e.g. residential and nursing homes, assessment units and day care centres). The DCM method was developed by Tom Kitwood and Kathleen Bredin in the late 1980s and has since been taught to many hundreds of people working in the field of dementia care both in the UK and internationally. Following its formal introduction in 1991, DCM was constantly revised and updated on the basis of feedback from users of the method and in line with developments in Kitwood's own thinking. The 7th edition of the DCM manual was introduced in 1997 (the year before Kitwood's death), following a very thorough consultation with experienced users of the method.

When carrying out Dementia Care Mapping, qualified users (or 'mappers') sit unobtrusively in a communal area of the care setting and observe several people with dementia (typically around six) over a number of hours. At the end of each five minute time frame each mapper makes codings based on his or her subjective assessment of the experience of each of the people being observed during that five-minute period. The aim of this process is to gain a detailed picture of what life is like in the care setting in question from the perspective of the people with dementia themselves.

The 7th edition of the DCM manual, current at the time of Kitwood's death, had three main coding frames. The first, the behaviour category code (BCC) related to the main kind of activity that the person had been engaged in during the previous five minutes, e.g. F = food (eating or drinking); G = games; P = receiving physical care and so on. The second coding frame related to 'well- or ill-being value' (WIB value) and was based on an assessment of the quality of care the person was receiving during the activity in question as demonstrated by his or her apparent well-being or ill-being. Coding ranged from a maximum of +5 for 'exceptional well-being – it is hard to envisage anything better: very high levels of engagement, self-expression, social interaction' through moderate and mild well-being (+3, +1), to mild and moderate ill-being (−1, −3) and extreme ill-being, a state in which 'extremes of apathy, withdrawal, rage, grief or despair' are observed (coded as −5). The third coding frame was the recording of any incidents of personal detraction (PD) – see Box 2.3. The data generated by DCM observations can then be used to calculate individual and group measures of well-being and behaviour category profiles.

The introduction of the coding frame known as the 'WIB value' in the 7th edition of the DCM manual was a significant departure from all previous versions of the DCM manual in which this coding frame had been known as the 'care value' (CV). Introduction of the WIB value coding effectively broke the link between care practice and well-being which had been implicit in the previous CV coding.

---

relative well-being and ill-being in dementia which for DCM purposes were divided into six bands (Bradford Dementia Group 1997: 24).

Because, Kitwood suggested, people with dementia have a reduced ability to 'buffer' themselves against external events, they will tend to move from one state of well-being or ill-being to another relatively quickly. This is where quality of care is very important, since care which does not meet the person's psychological needs will lead to a state of enduring ill-being. Kitwood went on to identify 12 key indicators of well-being and seven indicators of ill-being which are shown in Box 2.2.

Kitwood recognized that being able to identify signs of well-being or ill-being in a person with dementia requires more than simple observation: 'It requires the faculty known as empathy: being able to put oneself, imaginatively, into the place of another person, and sense what life might be like from within that person's frame of reference' (Bradford Dementia Group 1997: 5).

A strong claim Kitwood made in the context of DCM is that relative well-being corresponds to good-quality care, while the converse is also applicable: relative ill-being corresponds to poor-quality care. Kitwood's stance on well-being and ill-being in dementia can thus be presented as three specific propositions:

1   It is possible for a person with dementia to remain in a relatively high state of well-being provided his or her psychological needs are met. Kitwood challenges

---

Box 2.2   Indicators of well-being and ill-being

Indicators of well-being

Assertiveness, or being able to express wishes in an acceptable way
Bodily relaxation
Sensitivity to the emotional needs of others
Humour
Creative self-expression (such as singing, dancing or painting)
Taking pleasure in some aspects of daily life
Helpfulness
Initiation of social contact
Affection
Self-respect (such as being concerned about hygiene, tidiness and appearance)
Expressing a full range of range of emotions, both 'positive' and 'negative'
Acceptance of others who also have dementia

Indicators of ill-being

Unattended sadness or grief
Sustained anger
Anxiety
Boredom
Apathy and withdrawal
Despair
Physical discomfort or pain

Source: Bradford Dementia Group 1997: 5

what Post (1995) has identified as 'hypercognitivity', i.e. the view that equates a person's worth with his or her intellectual prowess or intelligence.

2   Ill-being in dementia is not solely the result of neuropathology (i.e. of a progressive disease process in the brain), it is also influenced by other factors, particularly the quality of care and support provided. In this Kitwood counters 'therapeutic nihilism' (Burns et al. 1995) by suggesting that there is much we can do to help people with dementia simply through human care and kindness.

3   Actions on the part of the person with dementia which would be described within the 'standard paradigm' as problem behaviours can better be understood as indicators of ill-being. Ill-being itself arises largely from unmet needs. The neuro-logical or neurogenetic determinism (Rose 1997: 272) of the biomedical model are questioned and we are encouraged to see the behaviour of people with dementia as purposeful and as similar to our own response to frustrating, un-familiar or anxiety-provoking situations. In this view, for example, the behavioural label 'wandering' is replaced by an interpretation of the person's action as walking with a purpose, i.e. in order to go somewhere or to find something that will meet a need.

It is these claims related to well-being and ill-being that followers of Kitwood's work are most likely to find familiar. In the discussion that follows, we will attempt to outline the process by which Kitwood's thinking arrived at this point and also to demonstrate that this was still 'work in progress' at the point of Kitwood's death, by referring to the concept of psychological need in dementia which was outlined in his last major work, *Dementia Reconsidered: The person comes first* (Kitwood 1997a).

Well-being as a philosophical concept

Beyond identifying outward signs that would indicate its presence, Kitwood did not enter into a discussion of what well-being means; the nature of well-being tends to be taken as given in his work. In moral philosophy, however, a number of definitions of well-being have been proposed. From the perspective of *utilitarianism*, for example, well-being is defined as what is 'good for' a person, how well the person's life is going. Against this, ill-being is defined as a lack of the 'goods' which are generally considered to lead to well-being (e.g. prosperity, happiness, health).

Early utilitarians, such as Bentham (1789), who equated well-being with pleasure and argued that we should act in order to maximize our pleasure and to avoid pain as far as possible. This, however, raises questions about the relationship between the pursuit of what is 'good for' ourselves and our moral commitment to others. Often, for example, the things which give us short-term pleasure or well-being (e.g. eating chocolate or drinking alcohol) may be bad for us in the longer term and pursuit of our own aims may make us selfish or ungenerous to other people. In dementia, of course, the right to pursue short-term personal satisfaction becomes far more complex because the per-son may lack the ability to make an informed decision about what is in his or her best interests. The utilitarian concept of well-being is, thus, certainly not irrelevant to dementia. It could aptly be applied to a discussion of the actions of people with dementia who become sexually disinhibited, who prefer to eat only sweet food or who gain pleasure from singing the same song over and over again very loudly (for a fuller discussion of utilitarianism, see Beauchamp and Childress 2001).

Kitwood's notion of well-being and the way that this has been operationalized (e.g. in terms of the indicators of well-being he identified) are rather different. What we seem to have here is a set of indicators that someone is, although cognitively impaired, still capable of displaying 'appropriate' (albeit somewhat compliant) emotional responses. Indeed, Harding and Palfrey (1997: 64) note that Kitwood's signs of well-being are 'remarkable for their neutrality or attractiveness'.

So rather than adopting the hedonistic view of well-being favoured by some utilitarians Kitwood's approach to well-being seems closer to the *objective list theory* (Griffin 1986). In this view it is possible to generate a list of things that people ought to want (for example, knowledge, friendship, status in society), even if they do not in fact want them or pursue them. What is good for people is what works to improve (or even to perfect) human nature. The aim is not immediate personal fulfilment and physical pleasure, but the development of higher goals related to spiritual and emotional fulfilment. Indeed, the central claim in Kitwood's work – that the main aim of dementia care practice is to successively increase the extent to which these indicators of well-being are expressed and to eradicate indicators of ill-being – fits most closely the *perfectionist* model of well-being (Hurka 1993). Here the roots of Kitwood's thinking on dementia in his earlier Christian faith are clearly evident. The transition from ill-being to well-being is very reminiscent of the 'new birth' of becoming Christian, as he had described it in his early book *What is Human?:* 'The dishonest becomes truthful; the idle, hardworking; the fearful, bold; the sullen, sweet-tempered; the shiftless, reliable; the selfish, concerned for others . . . God . . . recreates from within, until the qualities of the life of Christ, love, joy, peace, patience, kindness, goodness, faithfulness, humility, self-control are produced' (Kitwood 1970: 114–115/200).

Happiness, or 'the good life' in the context of dementia care, is thus viewed by Kitwood not as the pursuit of personal gratification or immediate pleasure, but as the expression of more spiritual indicators of inner peace, humility and acceptance of cognitive losses. While this view of 'the best that can be achieved' through person-centred care has many attractions, it might also be contested for a number of reasons:

1   It reinforces stereotypical ideas of the 'well-adapted' older person as one who is, or ought to be, without embodied passion, desire or legitimate hostility in the face of authority (i.e. it depoliticizes ageing).
2   It 'sells' person-centred care as a means of making life easier for caregivers; if the quality of care is good the person with dementia will become more tractable, compliant and pleasant to work with. There seems little room within Kitwood's conception of well-being for the person who expresses him or herself with 'rage against the dying of the light' (Thomas 1951).
3   It does not consider that – in a secular context – and with little time left to them to enjoy life, those with dementia might benefit from short-term immediate gratification of their wishes, even if what they prefer to do is bad for them in the longer term.

Development of Kitwood's thinking on the psychology of dementia: three conjectures

As already mentioned, Kitwood advanced three rather different propositions on the psychology of dementia during his career. These can broadly be summarized as follows:

> *Phase 1*: Ill-being as a precondition for the onset of dementia.
> *Phase 2*: Ill-being and well-being as indicators of quality of care.
> *Phase 3*: Positive person-work as a way of meeting psychological need.

The term conjecture is used advisedly here; it means 'an opinion based on incomplete information' (*Oxford Paperback Dictionary* 2001: 179). As we will go on to argue, Kitwood put forward each of these conjectures before empirical support was available and then modified his position in the face of the emerging evidence.

Ill-being as a precondition for the onset of dementia

In Kitwood's early work a key concern is the reframing of the prevailing technical–rational model of dementia in such a way that psychological factors are also taken into consideration (see Part 1 on 'Kitwood's critique of the standard paradigm'): 'We may make a distinction, then, between two possible ways of framing human ill-being, whether of body or of mind: the *technical* and the *personal*' (Kitwood 1988a: 123/109).

Kitwood's work during this period was to challenge the prevailing explanatory framework offered by biomedical science with its taken-for-granted view that dementia could be understood entirely in terms of neuropathology. Here, however, Kitwood puts forward the strong claim that the social and psychological (personal) factors he refers to *predispose* certain people to develop dementia. This is not a theme that has been much recognized or critiqued in Kitwood's work, but it is a strikingly tenacious one over time, particularly where particular personality traits are concerned.

What we might term Kitwood's first and most ambitious conjecture suggested, then, that experiential ill-being predisposes a person to the onset of dementia. The causes of psychological and emotional ill-being he cited ranged from the macro-social, global and economic, such as the inhumanity of city life: 'the social environment of modern urban America might be regarded as highly dementogenic for those in later life' (Kitwood 1988a: 129/117) to the individual incident (e.g. redundancy), to failures in interpersonal communication within families. Kitwood recognized that this model of explanation would not be popular. For family members in particular the technical framework, he noted, 'provides a small consolation, insulating people from certain deeply disturbing truths which, at some level, they do not wish to know' (Kitwood 1988a: 128/115).

Drawing on the work of Phillipson (1982) Kitwood describes the experience of retirement, and the fear of loss of income, social roles, and increased dependency as a basis for collective, collusive denial which favour the unthinking acceptance of dementia as a problem of biochemical engineering, rather than one set at the heart of our forms of social organization and their correspondingly deformed modes of personal relationship. From a psychological point of view, he argues, dementia can be regarded as a progressive 'loss of self', in which both the 'experiencing self' and the 'adapted self' are seriously compromised (see also, Part 3, on 'Personhood'): 'In short we might hypothesize that the psychological *precondition* for dementia is an underdeveloped experiencing self, while the adapted self is seriously undermined. The secret hope of being really understood and validated by another is finally abandoned' (Kitwood, 1988a: 129/117, emphasis added).

As with much of Kitwood's work, there is a tension in this article between the macro- and micro-social, the political and the personal, the distal and the proximal. (For a fuller discussion of distal and proximal sources of human unhappiness, see Smail 1993.) While Smail's work was an unacknowledged influence on Kitwood during this period, there is an interesting inversion in the way he interpreted and applied Smail's thinking. A key strand in Smail's work is the suggestion that people habitually assume that the causes of their unhappiness are proximal – i.e. close at hand, in personal relationships and day-to-day life – and are thus the result of their own personal failings and inadequacies. In actuality, Smail argues, the true causes are always distal – political or socio-economic – and thus outside the person's own sphere of influence. Smail thus criticizes the tendency to 'psychologize' political and economic sources of human distress. Kitwood, it might be argued, attempts a more subtle synthesis by providing an account of how lived experience deforms the individual psyche – via personality formation – so that an attenuated sense of identity predisposes the person to mental ill-health. In doing so, however, Kitwood runs the risk of returning to the very psychologization that Smail counsels against.

Moreover, the suggestion of psychological predisposition begs a difficult question: given that fear, unhappiness, and lack of personal fulfilment are so prevalent in modern Western societies and that their effects become more pronounced with advancing age, we should expect that the prevalence of dementia would be much higher than it actually is. As Woods points out: 'The lack of dementia pathology in many who have been subject to just such a dehumanizing social environment through institutionalization suggests that this is not the case' (1999: 6). Kitwood was, however, careful not to propose the psychological framework he puts forward as an *alternative* to the technical framework. Instead he argued that they must be seen as complementary to each other; the medical–scientific model of dementia must still be part of the picture. In this, Kitwood did not go so far as other opponents of the medical model (see Harding and Palfrey 1997) who have argued that dementia is merely a term for labelling socially constructed 'deviancy' in later life.

Kitwood did, however, relegate neurological impairment to a marginal role in the aetiology of dementia. Dementia is, he says, 'an existential crisis of a person, of an embodied, social and sentient being, and indeed a crisis of an interpersonal milieu; neuropathology, of whatever degree of severity becomes a part of a whole range of peripheral considerations' (Kitwood 1990b: 60/119). Kitwood went on to liken dementia to 'senile psychosis': 'It is as if the self, together with its defences, has been subjected to extreme attenuation; then the threats which relate specifically to death and dying fasten onto *psychotic elements that are already present from earlier life*, and their invasion is a relatively easy matter' (Kitwood 1990b: 74/129, emphasis added).

It is clear, then, that at this stage, Kitwood viewed the person with dementia as one who was marked out for this fate because of psychopathology due to earlier life experience. In his subsequent empirical work Kitwood attempted to find evidence for this by conducting a number of psychobiographical interviews with the relatives of people with dementia.

Kitwood's psychobiographical method

As Adams (1996) has pointed out, the article *Understanding Senile Dementia: A psychobiographical approach* (Kitwood 1990b) has some significant methodological flaws. Here a great deal is claimed on the basis of a single case study – albeit one drawn from a larger body of unpublished work – on the role of life events in the aetiology of dementia and in which data from the key informant (the daughter of the person in question) will inevitably be biased to some extent. Further, in putting forward what are some quite bold claims (for example, that there is evidence that a propensity to dementia may be related to personality), Kitwood does not cite any sources beyond his own earlier publications. Although conventions in citation have changed significantly in the years since this article was published, this is, as Adams points out, wholly inadequate in order to establish an evidence base. His suggestion in a later publication (Adams and Bartlett 2003: 11) that this was the only empirical work Kitwood ever published is, however, seriously misleading. As we shall see later, though, when attempts were made to present empirical data based on a much larger study, the methodological problems associated with this kind of work, and often flagged up by Kitwood himself, became increasingly apparent.

The article *Understanding Senile Dementia: A psychobiographical approach* is based on the case history of a woman, Rose, whose account of her life story was given by her daughter, Sarah (not their real names). It is not clear whether Rose was present during the interview with Sarah, or, indeed, whether she was still alive at the time. The method Kitwood used was to take a detailed life history from the relative he was interviewing and then split this into seven periods of 14 years each (in Rose's case only six periods are reported on, since the life history ends when she is in the 70–84 period). The key life events for each 14-year period are then summarized (see Reading 2.2 for a full account). So, for example – in Rose's case:

Period 1 (0–14)
The family was large; material and psychological impoverishment were intertwined, Rose was the fifth child. *Probably she lacked attention and care.* Her success at school came to nothing. She suffered a major bereavement. Her first job was one in which she adapted to others' needs. There is little to suggest a strong beginning to an experiencing self. (Kitwood 1990b: 70/126, emphasis added)

Then later:

Period 5 (56–70)
No fundamental change in her way of living and experiencing took place. *Her work with the theatre and her paid employment came to an end.* She found a valid way of being as a member of her daughter's household. Four of her siblings died. (Kitwood 1990b: 70/126, emphasis added)

It is noticeable that the events recorded are almost entirely negative, but it is unclear whether this is because Rose's life was particularly unhappy or whether it is a result of the psychobiographical method itself and the kinds of question her daughter was asked. One suspects that there was a tendency to select data that supported Kitwood's hypothesis that traumatic life events influence personality development, which then becomes a precondition for dementia. Evidence of this can be seen in two ways in the extracts just given. First, Kitwood hypothesizes that Rose probably lacked care and attention as a child. Belonging to a large family is seen as a disadvantage when it might equally be considered to increase the potential for forming close relationships and having access to a wider social support network. Second, Kitwood records the deleterious effects of paid employment coming to an end, without ever having recorded meaningful employment as a 'good' in earlier periods. As mentioned later in the article, Rose had been a theatrical costumier – presumably a skilled, rewarding and creative career – and had raised thousands of pounds for local charities. These positive aspects of Rose's life and personality are not mentioned in the summarized data. Even so, these data do not suggest someone who had a particularly traumatic life. Although it certainly carries its share of deprivation and disappointment, it is, perhaps, a typical history for a woman of Rose's generation and upbringing.

On the basis of this case study, Kitwood goes on to say:

> In the light of psychobiographical evidence such as we have discussed here, it seems overwhelmingly probable that the states of being that are clinically known as senile dementia arise from an interaction between psychological factors and the declining functional capacity of the brain . . . In other words, the demented person is one who suffers a *psychological* affliction that is 'carried' by a brain whose processes are, to some degree, impaired. (Kitwood 1990b: 74/128, emphasis in original)

The basis of Kitwood's argument in these early papers is that the ill-being he saw, at this stage, as inevitable in dementia was not solely the result of a disease process in the brain. Rather, it was as though a lifelong state of existential unhappiness was then compounded by neuropathology to the extent that the person's sense of identity and ability to cope were entirely eroded. The person is not so much a victim of dementia, as a lifelong victim of society who now experiences the additional assault of neurological impairment. While this is a strikingly original argument for its time, it does not help to explain why so many women whose lived experience has been very similar to Rose's never develop dementia, while others who have had – on the face of things, at least – much happier and more affluent lives, do.

Kitwood's psychobiographical approach to investigating traumatic life events suspected of predisposing people to dementia did not yield the empirical results that he had hoped for and his first conjecture was gradually abandoned. In a later article he notes that in 27 out of 44 cases the psychobiography revealed 'critical life events as precipitants' (1993a). While this number is, in itself, inconclusive, Kitwood must also have come to suspect that the biographical data taken from relatives was unreliable for various reasons. For example, Gubrium (1986) had drawn attention to the very tendency of relatives to construct an explanation for the onset of dementia which was based on a single precipitating cause, whether or not this was plausible. So when Kitwood quotes, for example, the case of the man whose wife asserted that his dementia began on the precise day that he sold a musical instrument he had enjoyed playing after neighbours complained about the noise (1993a) this is exactly the kind of post hoc attribution that would be expected in terms of Gubrium's theory. Whether or not Kitwood was perman-ently dissuaded from the view that life events play a critical role in the onset of dementia by these discoveries is a moot point. It may well have been that he simply became more aware of the methodological problems researching this presented. Whatever the reason, Kitwood now began to turn his attention increasingly towards the quality of interpersonal relationships *during or after* the diagnosis of dementia, and their impact on ill-being and well-being in dementia.

Ill-being and well-being as indicators of quality of care

In what we have termed the mid-phase of Kitwood's work on ill-being and well-being, a noticeably different perspective began to emerge. The new conjecture was that much of the deterioration seen in people with dementia following diagnosis was due to 'malig-nant social psychology' (Kitwood and Bredin 1992a) rather than, as was commonly believed, to neurodegenerative disease. In order to explore this Kitwood was particularly concerned to investigate 'evidence . . . concerning relative well-being even in those who are, from a cognitive standpoint, severely demented' (Kitwood and Bredin 1992a: 269/ 131). In addition, where Kitwood's previous emphasis had tended to be on family psychodynamics, there was now a move towards the experience of people with dementia in formal care settings. This is explained at least in part by the preliminary work that had been done just prior to this time to develop Dementia Care Mapping (DCM). The DCM method was piloted and developed in formal care settings, thus, no doubt, focusing Kitwood's thinking on the issues that arise in residential, nursing and day care contexts. Kitwood and Bredin (1992a) pointed out that there was then no current theory of dementia care practice and that 'thousands upon thousands of hours of dementia care work pass by, in which the people involved generally do not understand what they are doing. This applies, moreover, even to some who are doing excellent work' (Kitwood and Bredin 1992a: 270/132).

Now, the ill-being that often accompanies dementia is seen not as a manifestation of lifelong maladaptation, as tended to be suggested in the earlier work, but as a result of inept or insensitive care practice *following* a diagnosis of dementia. Kitwood and Bredin refer here to the insidious effects of 'malignant social psychology' on the person with dementia. Poor care is, they suggest, characterized by high levels of malignant social psychology while good care is 'singularly free of this, and is highly respectful of personhood' (Kitwood and Bredin 1992a: 271/132). See Box 2.3 for the 17 indicators of malignant social psychology/personal detractions.

In a noticeable departure from the earlier work, those with dementia are now valor-ized as generally more authentic, less hypocritical, more accepting of dependence on others and more able to live in the present than those who are unaffected by dementia. For both those with dementia, and those who care for them, the goal is to move towards a life in which there is more joy, fluidity, growth and change. Clearly discernible here is the influence of humanistic psychology with its emphasis on human potential and

---

Box 2.3   Indicators of malignant social psychology/personal detractions

---

1 *Treachery* – using forms of deception in order to distract or manipulate a person with dementia, or force them into compliance.

2 *Disempowerment* – not allowing a person to use the abilities they do have; failing to help them to complete actions they have initiated.

3 *Infantilization* – treating a person very condescendingly, as someone lacking sensitivity might treat a very young child.

4 *Intimidation* – inducing fear in a person, through use of threats or physical power.

5 *Labelling* – using a category such as dementia, or 'organic mental disorder', as the main basis for interacting with a person and for explaining their behaviour.

6 *Stigmatization* – treating a person as if they were a diseased object, an alien or an outcast.

7 *Outpacing* – providing information, presenting choices, etc., at a rate too fast for a person to understand; putting them under pressure to do things more rapidly than they can bear.

8 *Invalidation* – failing to acknowledge the subjective reality of a person's experience, and especially what they are feeling.

9 *Banishment* – sending a person away, or excluding them, physically or psychologically.

10 *Objectification* – treating a person as if they were a lump of dead matter; to be pushed, lifted, filled, pumped or drained, without proper reference to the fact that they are sentient beings.

11 *Ignoring* – carrying on (in conversation or action) in the presence of a person as if they were not there.

12 *Imposition* – forcing a person to do something, overriding desire or denying the possibility of choice on their part.

13 *Withholding* – refusing to give asked for attention, or to meet an evident need; for example, for affectionate contact.

14 *Accusation* – blaming a person for actions or failures of action that arise from their lack of ability, or their misunderstanding of the situation.

15 *Disruption* – disturbing a person's action or inaction; crudely breaking their 'frame of reference'.

16 *Mockery* – making fun of a person's 'strange' actions or remarks; teasing, ridiculing, humiliating, making jokes at their expense.

17 *Disparagement* – telling a person that they are incompetent, useless, worthless etc.; giving them messages that are damaging to their self-esteem.

Source: Adapted from Kitwood 1997a: 46–47

---

self-actualization (cf. Rogers 1951; Rogers et al. 1967). The role of negative personality traits in the onset and progression of dementia appears to have receded from Kitwood's explanatory framework during this period.

It is at this point that we begin to see the emergence of the concept of well-being as it later became known to followers of Kitwood's work. The preservation of personhood *is* fundamentally, in this view, the preservation of well-being. It is suggested that good care and support may often enable a person with dementia to stabilize, to experience little or no further deterioration in their condition. Further, it is implied that when the quality of care is very high, a degree of 'rementia' may occur. In this respect, care intervention is clearly viewed as 'therapeutic' in the strictest sense; that is, it is not just intended to make the person feel happier, it is also suggested as a means of reversing the process of dementia itself. 'As social being is recovered, so "mind" (in some of its aspects) is restored' (Kitwood and Bredin 1992a: 278/138). Flicker (1999: 880) writing in the *British Medical Journal* challenged the evidence base for claims related to rementia, commenting that: 'The main concern about these hypotheses is the lack of evidence to support them and the author's assertion that there is no requirement for rigorous testing . . . The major basis for Kitwood's hypothesis is some sketchy case histories and allusion to some small case series in which some individuals with dementia are said not to have deteriorated as quickly as others.'

Here again we have an example of the rather frequent criticism that Kitwood did not provide a sound empirical evidence base to support his claims (see Part 1) – in this case on the postulated link between well-being and 'rementia'. It is, of course, difficult to provide evidence in a new field, and particularly in a context where existing standards of care are sufficiently poor to make the identification of likely 'test beds' problematic. Comments such as those put forward by Flicker also, however, help to demonstrate the dismissive and defensive responses with which Kitwood's work tended to be greeted by members of the medical profession.

Kitwood and Bredin (1992a) use a series of vignettes to demonstrate the 12 signs of well-being identified during their observational work in care settings. While these small case study examples are helpful in exemplifying the ways that well-being might be identified, there are also significant philosophical and methodological problems in attempting to infer a state of well-being (or, to an even greater extent, ill-being) from a set of external behavioural indicators. This is particularly difficult when the examples provided have been, one suspects, subjected to some simplification and 'narrative smoothing' (Spence 1986) in order to make them demonstrate what the authors wish to show. Such examples are always capable of alternative interpretation. For example, 'helpfulness', a suggested well-being indicator, may, in some cases, be shown by a person who is acting out of an anxious desire to comply with the regime of the home, and some forms of 'humour' may be obscene, racist or self-denigrating. Expressions of anger have proved particularly difficult to classify in practice in terms of Kitwood's taxonomy since although being able to express justifiable frustration or indignation can clearly be a sign of assertiveness and ability to display a range of emotions, we cannot infer from this that the person expressing those feelings is in a state of well-being at the time.

In 1995 Kitwood was the lead author of *Brighter Futures*, a report on a significant empirical research project with joint funding from Methodist Homes for the Aged and Anchor Housing Trust (Kitwood et al. 1995). The full report presents findings from two parallel studies, one set in residential and nursing homes, the other in sheltered housing. In all, 224 people with dementia in 77 care settings were observed using DCM. Residents without dementia and care staff were also involved in the study. The authors claim this as the most thorough study in this field that has ever been undertaken in

Britain. While it has not been widely cited or discussed, it is of interest in that it presents a large body of empirical data, thus going some way to contest the criticism that Kitwood did not provide empirical support for his claims. The methodological problems arising from this study are significant. The findings reported are, in one sense, entirely non-controversial. For example, it is found that well-being is higher when there are high levels of engagement and plenty of things to do; when people have meaningful relationships and regular contact with other residents, and when the physical amenities of the home are good. On the other hand, some aspects of the report gloss over the means of production of its findings. Or to put it another way, the methodological standpoint that has led to the choice of research methods and the construction of certain measures and operational rules is not made explicit and it is clear that some of the findings are actually artefacts of the methods used. For example, the findings related to ill-being, report that:

> One of the most important factors which led to increased ill-being was for people to be left unattended, showing signs of ill-being, for long periods of time. This lack of attention, *once over thirty minutes*, very significantly contributed toward a high state of ill-being. Apathy and loneliness were the most common forms of ill-being observable in those who were left unattended. (Kitwood et al. 1995: 25/151)

It is not in question that leaving people with dementia on their own for long periods of time is undesirable. Nevertheless, this statement raises specific methodological questions. First, can we in fact observe that a person 'feels' apathetic or lonely simply from observing outward expression and demeanour? We can certainly see that someone is sitting alone, doing nothing, but whether we can make a judgement about an inner psychological state on this basis is much more difficult to say. Older people in general may prefer to spend considerable amounts of time in quiet contemplation, or day dreaming, and some religions would see a state of transcendence through withdrawal from the world as being the highest state of existence it is possible to reach. Indeed Kitwood himself, refers to the benefits of meditation (for example, 1997a: 131).

In addition, the operational rules for DCM itself stipulated that after 30 minutes of unattended ill-being, the coding level would drop automatically even if the signs of ill-being themselves did not become worse. If a person had been coded socially withdrawn −1 (mild ill-being) for 30 minutes and was still unattended to at the end of that time the coding would drop to −3 (moderate ill-being) even though the *observed* signs of ill-being remained mild. Further, in presenting the statistical data – for some reason that is not made explicit – the usual six-point interval scale of well-being has been converted into a dichotomous one with only 'high' or 'low' measures. It is perhaps with this kind of consideration in mind that Murphy (1997: 104), in his review of the *Brighter Futures* report, commented: 'The reader should be prepared to distinguish those conclusions in the report which represent the authors' (considerable) experience in the field, and those which derive directly from the data.'

It is also noticeable in this article that the concept of personality has regained ascendance. For example, it is reported that 'well-being is specifically related to two dimensions of personality, openness and conscientiousness' (Kitwood et al. 1995: 21/ 148) and that:

> Neuroticism, agreeableness and conscientiousness were three dimensions of personality which discriminated between high and low ill-being . . . Neuroticism is a tendency to view things in a negative way . . . Agreeableness is basically how easy to get on with, and easy going a person is . . . People seen as 'disagreeable' are in fact those who are likely to manage and implement their own ideas. In the residential setting such people may find themselves in conflict with organisational rigidity with respect to staff and resident role. (Kitwood et al. 1995: 26–27/152)

The identification of personality traits such as these, which are then presented selectively either as the way people actually 'are' or as a way that they are constructed by others is theoretically unsatisfactory. If one person's 'disagreeableness' can be seen as a construction of care staff who dislike residents taking independent action, then another person's 'neuroticism' can equally be seen as a construction of care staff who dislike those who complain about things. Similarly, in relation to 'conscientiousness' (defined as 'a person's "get up and go", their commitment and sense of responsibility') it is claimed that 'few people have high levels of conscientiousness, and those who do are sometimes viewed by staff as interfering and troublesome' (Kitwood et al. 1995: 21/148). One has to question here whether these are actually distinct personality traits or whether they are merely ways of labelling people who challenge the system in one way or another (see Harding and Palfrey 1997). Sloan (1997) makes a similar point in relation to theories of personality in a more general context:

> It would be fairly simple to show that although two people have identical profiles on a trait inventory, the meanings or intentions typically fulfilled by the actions related to those trait dimensions would be ridiculous. The 'aggressiveness' of the first person, for example, might be directed towards finding houses for the homeless, while the same trait in the second leads him to get into fights in bars . . . The objectivism of trait theory turns out to be yet another ideological trap. (p. 100)

From the mid-1990s onwards it is clear that Kitwood became increasingly dissatisfied with the concepts of ill-being and well-being when used in relation to individuals. It may be considered surprising, given the ascendancy they had achieved in the DCM field, that the terms well-being and ill-being are not indexed – and indeed are barely referred to – in Kitwood's major work *Dementia Reconsidered*. This is particularly striking when we note that the 7th edition of the DCM manual and *Dementia Reconsidered* were both published in 1997. It seems evident that another major shift in Kitwood's thinking was taking place at this point.

There appear to be a number of reasons for Kitwood's growing discontent with the notions of well-being and ill-being and we may relate these in part back to his initial conjecture about the connection between malignant social psychology and ill-being in dementia. Particularly significant were the findings from DCM data available at the time, which did not appear to be showing that attempts to improve care practice led consistently to improved measures of well-being. Some experienced users of the DCM method had become concerned by the implications of feeding back, to hard-pressed staff, negative findings from DCM evaluations carried out in contexts where their efforts did not appear to be leading to improvements in clients' well-being.

To some extent it seems likely that this was a feature of the DCM method itself, in which well-being and ill-being values were effectively averaged out over a period of time, so that individual improvements tended to get lost in the overall data (Capstick 2003). Moreover, individual scores indicating that an individual was in an overall state of mild well-being could easily mask significant episodes of distress or poor care practice. Kitwood was genuinely concerned that measures derived from DCM data should not be used to draw unjustified inferences about the quality of care provided to individuals, but there must also have been some disappointment that the approach he had pioneered and implemented did not appear to be producing evidence of enhanced well-being.

Pointing to the limits of the general validity of his equation 'relative well-being corresponds to good quality care', Kitwood (Bradford Dementia Group 1997: 11) now acknowledged that 'good care (the social psychology) may not necessarily be successful in generating relative well-being in some people with dementia' among whom he included:

- those whose neurological impairments were particularly damaging
- those with longstanding depression
- those whose lived experience had been particularly traumatic
- those whose physical health problems might be exacerbating their confusion.

In one sense, this appears to be evidence of a significant 'backing down' on Kitwood's part, not least because these four categories would exclude from his general equation such significant numbers of people with dementia living in formal care settings. On the other hand, Kitwood's reluctance to make these concessions at all is manifest in the fact that they are immediately followed by the following 'note of caution':

> It is all too easy to explain low DCM aggregate scores by reference to attributes of the people receiving care, and so to deflect attention from the social psychology of the care environment . . . The fact that the staff are at their limits – or that the mappers can envisage no better form of care – does not mean that nothing further can, in fact, be done. (Bradford Dementia Group 1997: 11)

Perhaps in recognition of the need to raise the consciousness of practitioners, Kitwood now started to turn to a more detailed consideration of the experience of dementia, the psychological needs of people with dementia, and the skills and values that were needed by caregivers in order to provide a *benign* rather than malignant social psychology.

Positive person-work as a way of meeting psychological need

Unlike Kitwood's earlier two conjectures related to well-being and ill-being in dementia, this last phase of his work is characterized by the more modest suggestion that the personhood of people with dementia will be maintained if their core psychological needs are met. Kitwood's work on the five core psychological needs was published for the first time in *Dementia Reconsidered*, where it is elaborated in the context of the subjective experience of the person with dementia and his or her acceptance of death.

Kitwood begins by considering the reasons why each person's experience of dementia will be unique. It is interesting here, that rather than considering aspects of life experience, culture, social diversity or state of general health, Kitwood discusses only the effects of individual personality. Drawing on the work of Jacques (1988) he identifies five main personality types, described respectively as: dependent; independent; paranoid; hysterical and psychopathic. Here Kitwood does not appear to abide by his own 'dementia equation' (D = P + B + H + NI + SP) in characterizing the unique individual experience of dementia, instead he focuses on the single component of personality. The personality types, moreover, are ones which have the potential to pathologize the person with dementia and it is difficult to understand why Kitwood considers them 'helpful' to the project of person-centred care (Kitwood 1997a: 71). As Richards (1996: 81) points out, there has been a long tradition within psychiatry of using personality types to identify those who are 'especially prone to different types of insanity . . . as in Eysenck's model where schizophrenia and hysteria constitute extreme introvert and extravert modes of high neuroticism', but such methods have been widely criticized for their determinism and divisiveness.

Kitwood goes on to suggest that there are a cluster of needs in dementia that are common to each person and that centre on an all-encompassing need for love – 'a generous, forgiving and unconditional acceptance, a wholehearted emotional giving, without any expectation of direct reward' (Kitwood 1997a: 81). The five needs Kitwood identified as clustering around the central need for love are comfort; attachment; inclusion; occupation and identity.[2] This choice seems a fairly arbitrary one and does not include needs that Kitwood had stressed in earlier work, such as agency and hope, for example.

While accepting that this is still work that was in its infancy, it is, however, noticeable that Kitwood's suggestions on how these needs might be met – by improving communication and by developing awareness of the impact that psychological factors have on physical health – seem more grounded, achievable and less world-changing than Kitwood's earlier suggestions about the role of ill-being in the aetiology of dementia or the dementogenic effects of malignant social psychology.

In *Towards a Theory of Dementia Care: Ethics and interaction*, one of Kitwood's last papers, published in 1998, he goes on to elaborate in detail 10 kinds of 'positive person work' that he believed could do much to 'mitigate the disablement that so often accompanies the process of dementia'. These are: recognition, negotiation, collaboration, play, timalation (a neologism combining sensory stimulation with an 'honouring' of the person), celebration, relaxation, validation, holding and facilitation (1998b: 27–29/ 160–162).

These forms of positive interaction are presented within an ethical framework derived from hermeneutics, in which 'actions and utterances are assumed to be meaningful, and an attempt is made to understand them in their historical and concurrent context' (1998b: 27/160). In other words, the essential qualities of good person-centred care are interpretation, reflection and informed response, in order to meet the psychological need that is being expressed by the person with dementia. There is no suggestion here, however, that positive person work might lead to rementia.

Indeed, Kitwood acknowledges that in the kind of non-repressive social order that emerges when people with dementia are recognized and validated in this way, suffering and conflict may actually be more in evidence than in the over-controlled regimes dependent on chemical and physical restraint. The difference, he suggests, is that when 'pains and problems are dealt with openly . . . they can be faced and the necessary help provided' (1998b: 33/167).

In a sense, perhaps, Kitwood's theory had begun to come home. Ultimately, we should care for and respond to the psychological needs of people with dementia because this is the only decent way to treat our fellow human beings. We may hope that it makes a difference, although often we will have no consistent or abiding evidence for this. Those who work with people who have dementia are always contending with the realistic likelihood that the person they are caring for and supporting will deteriorate, cease to recognize them and will, ultimately, die.

Kitwood's earlier conjectures that dementia might be eradicated under different forms of social organization, or that it might be cured by more benign care practice, could be argued in themselves to contribute to the denial and defensive avoidance that he saw as so damaging to the cause of people with dementia. For some, Kitwood's work undoubtedly carried with it, if only for a while, a hope similar to that of the 'magic bullets' or manipulated genes promised by biomedical research – a hope that this need never happen to us or those we love. There is little glamour in accepting that old age, dependency and physical and mental frailty are not going to go away. There is, however, a great deal of courage in facing this realistically and doing what we can to make what is left of life enjoyable.

Conclusion

We have argued that in Kitwood's overall body of work related to ill-being, well-being and psychological need, a series of conjectures are put forward. The first, and earliest, was that ill-being or traumatic experience earlier in life – particularly in its impact on personality formation – predisposes the person to develop dementia in old age. The second was that malignant social psychology accounts for – or at least exacerbates – mental decline in those with dementia, while good-quality care can lead to a process of rementing. The final conjecture, still under development at the time of Kitwood's death was that positive person work (or a benign social psychology) could enable the person with dementia to live out his or her remaining years in a climate of respect, understanding and fundamental equality with others, but without illusions of cure or a reversal in cognitive decline.

There are some dangers in putting forward such a framework for understanding the development of Kitwood's thinking. The conjectures identified here are not necessarily mutually exclusive and while the earlier themes became marginalized over time they can often be seen to re-emerge in the later work. The idea that lived experience in a more macro-social and political context might be dementogenic was sidelined in Kitwood's later work, for example, while his fascination with personality traits and their role in the onset, progression and experience of dementia frequently re-emerged. The overall picture is thus perhaps less neat and chronologically ordered than we have suggested. What remains interesting, however, is that Kitwood put forward the first two conjectures in advance of empirical evidence to support them. When such empirical evidence did not quickly emerge, Kitwood allowed them to fade from view rather than publicly disavowing them.

In putting increasing emphasis on what could be achieved to maintain or increase well-being at the micro-social level it seems likely that Kitwood made a conscious and pragmatic decision to avoid the more contentious political and socioeconomic critique of late capitalism and its disregard for the old and needy that had characterized his earlier, more challenging and certainly less popular work. This should not mean, however, that this work is overlooked or forgotten or that we should cease to ask difficult questions about the aetiology of dementia. The work of materialist psychologists such as Sève (1978) and Leonard (1984) proposes a model of the process by which forms of social organization – particularly labour relations – under late capitalism lead to an alienation of the individual. This work has fallen from favour in recent years. It may still, however, have much to offer our understanding of the psychology of dementia. Against the dismal anti-humanism of, for example, Smail (1993; discussed earlier) these writers are not pessimistic; instead they view resistance through informed collective action as the route to both personal and social transformation. Or, as Walker (1993: 270) has put it, in a rather different context: 'the secret of joy is resistance'.

Notes

1   Although this is referenced as Bradford Dementia Group 1997, it is clear that the text is attributable to Kitwood. This applies equally to quotes attributed to Kitwood but cited as Bradford Dementia Group later in the chapter.

2   These five psychological needs have now been incorporated into the 8th edition of the *Dementia Care Mapping Manual* introduced since Kitwood's death, in 2005.

2.1

The contribution of psychology to the understanding of senile dementia (1988)

I would like to begin this article with two vignettes from my own recent experience. Both relate to a symposium organized by the Alzheimer's Disease Society in Britain, of which I am a member. After a presentation on the aetiology of dementia a discussion developed about one of the most puzzling, yet well-established findings of recent research: that there is a higher prevalence of dementia, in all degrees of severity and throughout the whole age range, in New York than in London (Gurland *et al.*, 1983). Various hypotheses were aired: there might be differences in the metallic content of the water, in atmospheric pollution, in diet, in ethnic (and hence genetic) mix, and so on. No one suggested the possibility that New York might be a more stressful environment than London for those in later life. Had our discussion been about cardiac disorder or diabetes mellitus, this surely would have been raised at least as a possibility. I was reminded of the memorial service for a member of my family, who had practised for many years as a doctor and psychoanalyst in New York, but who had returned to an English village for the last months of her life. Her best friend, herself a New Yorker, had said in her short speech of remembrance: 'New York is a wonderful place in which to live: but it is a terrible place in which to die'.

The other vignette concerns disclosures made to me by a woman to whom I was a total stranger. Her husband had developed a dementing illness. He had been employed for over thirty years in industry; then, when his company began to contract its operations, his job became threatened, and eventually he took early retirement. Apparently he showed no emotional reaction to this, either at the time or later. He then had a year at university, attempting to gain a teaching qualification. Here he found the work very difficult, although he would not admit it, and eventually he failed. After this he took on some part-time teaching in further education, but in due course he was told he was no longer required. Around this time the older daughter qualified as a doctor, and was preparing for marriage. One day, so my acquaintance told me, she arrived home to find her husband in a totally confused state, which lasted about 24 hours. Soon afterwards he was diagnosed as a case of Alzheimer's disease. It seems that none of the medical professionals gave even the faintest hint that the affliction might be related in some way to his life-experiences; Alzheimer's disease was simply a mysterious and tragic 'bolt from the blue'. My acquaintance, however, had wondered whether there were connections. As she told me the story, I felt that I had heard something like this a number of times before (Kitwood, 1987a).

In certain respects our understanding of dementia is in a state resembling that of cancer some twenty or thirty years ago. At that time the main emphases in research were upon identifying environmental carcinogens, examining the details of cellular change, and so on. Since then the emphasis has changed to some degree, as it has become clear that cancer-formation is linked to a weakening or breakdown of the immune system; the key problem is not so much why cancer cells are produced, as why they are not rejected. Moreover some cancers, at least, appear to be linked both to personality type and to psychosocial stress (Cooper, ed., 1984). In other words, the way is gradually being opened up for viewing cancer as an illness of the person.

We may make distinction, then, between two possible ways of framing human ill-being, whether of body or of mind: the *technical* and the *personal*. Those who adopt a technical approach see illness very much in the way that a mechanic might look at the breakdown of an automobile, or an electronics engineer the malfunction of a computer. Medical science in the West is strongly committed to this approach, which has indeed yielded some remarkable victories. In the case of dementia in old age it holds sway virtually to the exclusion of all other possibilities. The brain is failing: discover, then, precisely what is going wrong, using such natural-scientific disciplines as neurology, biochemistry, virology, pathology and genetics, with the hope of eventually uncovering and controlling the causal process. The point about my two vignettes, of course, is this. It is not that the framing of dementia in personal terms has been 'weighed in the balance and found wanting'; on the contrary, it is not on the official agenda at all. And yet, as we shall see, the findings of neuropathological research themselves point to the need for a complementary psychological understanding. Moreover, the literature shows that promising beginnings were made some years ago; but as research from a technical standpoint gained in momentum, these were either forgotten or ignored.

The technical frame

According to geriatric medical science there are several fairly well defined organic diseases which cause dementia in old age, of which two are especially significant. The first (AD) is a condition in which the cerebral grey matter shows clear degenerative changes, including the plaques first identified by Simchowicz and the neurofibrillary tangles identified by Alzheimer early in this century. The second (MID) is associated with the destruction of tissue that follows some form of circulatory failure in the brain (multiple infarction). The two conditions are sometimes, but not always, distinguishable at a clinical level. Authorities vary considerably in their accounts of the relative prevalence. According to a typical report (Albert, 1982), over 50% of senile dementias are of the first type; 10–15% are of the second; another 10–15% are a mixture of both; and the remainder belong to a number of minor categories, relating to metabolic dysfunction, alcoholism, hydrocephalus, tumours, etc. There are also several 'pseudodementias', in which the symptoms are reversible; these are associated with such factors as depression, metabolic imbalance, or the side effects of drugs. In sound clinical practice, of course, the possibility of pseudodementia must be eliminated before the final diagnosis of an organic dementia can be sustained. MID can often be diagnosed positively. AD tends to be diagnosed by default; it is something of a residual category.

So far as aetiology is concerned, the core of the technical research consists of 50 or so papers, dating from the late 1960s, which deal with the relationship between the state of the brain and the degree of dementia as assessed by clinical judgement and/or psychological testing. These papers are not read by many doctors, let alone those involved in the day-to-day business of geriatric care; indeed, it is likely that they have been scrutinized, closely by only a very few persons. Somehow it has come to be assumed widely that they have established beyond all reasonable doubt the case for exclusive neuropathological causation in the 'true' dementias. This, however, is some way from the truth, although of course this work has made an absolutely fundamental contribution to our understanding of the organic basis to these disorders.

Research on the neuropathological correlates of dementia may be divided into several main categories. The 'classical' work consists of observations made on the brains of old people after death, using either macroscopic or histopathological techniques. Another corpus of research is based on computed tomography. This is a sophisticated development from photography using X-rays, where data from successive sections of the brain are reconstructed by a computer. In recent developments the technique has been extended beyond its original use, to include nuclear magnetic resonance and positron emission. The latter looks as if it may prove to be a very powerful tool in due course, since it can give many indications of brain metabolism (Hawkins and Phelps, 1986).

Among the other categories of technical research particular mention must be made of biochemical studies, particularly of neurotransmitter levels; of regional blood flow; and of nerve conduction velocity outside the brain. Only the first two categories will be discussed here. They are complementary, in that they provide evidence about the state of the dead and of the living brain. In their fine detail the findings reported here may not, in the end, prove to be definitive, and some may have been superseded already. The most important point for our purposes, however, is the type of research, and the general approach to the problem of dementia, that they exemplify. For a more detailed discussion, see Kitwood (1987b).

1. Evidence from post-mortem studies

The first major quantitative study of a neuropathological correlate of dementia was that of Blessed, Tomlinson and Roth (1968). Using the very reliable, although not very sensitive, technique of plaque counting, they examined the brains of 60 subjects, 26 of whom had been diagnosed clinically as demented. Very strikingly, they found 'no one kind of pathological change peculiar to the severely demented individuals . . . the differences between the "senile dements" and other subjects reflect a quantitative gradation of a pathological process common in old age, rather than qualitative differences' (p.805). For the whole group there was a highly significant correlation between the plaque count and degree of dementia as assessed by two tests. This, however, was much reduced for the 'senile dements' alone; only about 16% of the variance could be accounted for. Moreover, if the data are examined in detail, it is apparent that those with a high dementia score are randomly distributed according to plaque count. A parallel set of data for MID are presented by Roth (1980), with correlations and scatter rather similar to those found with dementia of the Alzheimer type. Thus although, in general, dementia is associated with neuropathic change, a very considerable part of the variance remains unexplained.

In two further papers (Tomlinson, Blessed and Roth, 1968, 1970), the same authors report a more detailed examination of the brains of 50 old people who had become demented and of 28 who had remained mentally intact. One of the most remarkable features here, too, was the degree of overlap between the state of the brains of the dements and of the controls. For example, 40% of the dements showed no cerebral atrophy (controls 46%); 28% showed no neurofibrillary change (controls 39%). The most severe neuropathology, however, both Alzheimer type and multi-infarct, was shown only in the brains of the demented persons. Among the dements, two brains were highly anomalous, in that they showed no significant damage of either type.

These are among the foundational studies that have set the tone for many other more detailed investigations. To give but one example, Ball *et al.* (1985) report their observations on the hippocampal region of the brain and claim that neuropathology here, and here alone, is specific to AD. This hypothesis, however, runs into difficulties. There is considerable variation in the amount of neuropathic change that is associated with dementia; dementia has been shown in some cases without hippocampal damage as detectable by current methods; and most crucially, as Collerton and Fairbairn (1985) have pointed out, the total non-function of the hippocampus results not in dementia but amnesia. In work such as this the loose fit between dementia and neuropathology still remains.

Findings from post-mortem studies certainly suggest that when the degeneration of grey matter has passed beyond certain limits, dementia is the inevitable outcome. To assert this, however, is a very different matter from assigning causation uniquely to neuropathology. The data have shown consistently that the state of the brains of some dements are well within the range of those of the mentally well preserved, and that a psychological condition of dementia can accompany varying degrees and kinds of neuropathic change. This point was emphasized repeatedly in the earlier work of Rothschild. In one paper (Rothschild and Sharpe, 1941), for example, detailed case studies were presented of three persons who were severely demented, but whose brains appeared to be virtually 'normal', and of two who had remained mentally intact despite severe brain damage.

2. Evidence from computerized tomography

Here we will look at a small body of research, based on the scanning of the brains of 50 well-preserved old people, 40 who were assessed clinically as probably demented and 41 who were suffering from an affective disorder, principally depression (Jacoby, Levy and Dawson, 1980; Jacoby and Levy, 1980a, 1980b). The data indicated a slow, age-related process of atrophy in the grey matter of the cortex among all three groups. Although this was significantly greater for the dements, there was considerable overlap with the other two groups. No clear point could be established where the CT measures would unequivocally indicate dementia; depending on the measure, the authors estimated that up to 40% of the subjects might be misclassified. Thus although CT is very useful in screening out other conditions (for example tumours), it is limited value in the positive diagnosis of dementia. A similar point was made by Wells and Duncan (1977), who report on the way CT has been implicated in the misdiagnosis of this condition.

A reexamination of 27 survivors was carried out after an interval of about 4 years (Bird, Levy and Jacoby, 1986). Taking the group as a whole, no significant changes were found either in the CT measures or in cognitive function. When CT was used to identify a putative dementing subgroup, no significant cognitive differences emerged between these persons and the rest. The authors conclude:

> It is important not to place undue significance on cut-off points of dementia; it is now clear that those determined in our earlier studies cannot be used to define a dementing group. . . . Atrophy does not necessarily indicate dementia; the diagnosis must still be made by means of a global clinical assessment (p.83).

Thus if these studies are typical, CT certainly indicates an association between dementia and a degenerative process in the brain, but not the conclusion that dementia is caused exclusively by neuropathic change. The research group whose work we have examined estimates that about 20% of normal old people have enlarged ventricles, and that about 25% of demented persons have ventricles within the normal range. In giving these figures, they point out candidly that workers such as Earnest *et al.* (1979) find an even greater degree of overlap. In general, then, these findings corroborate those obtained from post-mortem studies, although of course they are far less precise.

Looking at the whole body of work carried out within the technical frame, the key facts relevant to our discussion are as follows:

1. In clinical terms the dementias fall into a small number of overlapping syndromes, only loosely correlated to recognizable neuropathology as identified *post mortem.*

2. The neuropathology can roughly be classified into two main types, Alzheimerian and multi-infarct, although many brains show a mixture of both.

3. The neuropathic changes found in the demented are present, to some degree, in many well-preserved old people.

4. 'Alzheimer's disease' is a very loose category, almost certainly covering several different conditions.

5. A form of neuropathology clearly specific to AD, or to one of its types, has not yet been discovered.

6. Some people become demented with very little accompanying neuropathology. The correlation between degree of dementia and severity of neuropathology for both AD and MID falls far short of a basis for sufficient explanation.

7. There is probably a neuropathological threshold beyond which a demented state is inevitable, although this may vary from person to person.

A certain determinism does seem to be built into the technical frame. For example, the assertion 'the true dementias of old age are irreversible (and hence incurable)' is now immune to falsification. If any condition is found to be reversible it is simply not held to be one of the genuine conditions, organic in the old-fashioned sense. The 'saving of the appearances' is aided by another device, quite commonly used in clinical work. Suppose an old person suffers an accident, or undergoes an operation, or has an extended period away from home, and that thenceforward a process of senile impairment clearly ensues. This is often explained by saying that he or she already 'had' a dementing illness, but that it was 'unmasked' by the critical life events. In ways such as this the possible contribution of psychology to the genesis of dementia tends to be excluded from consideration; as also the existence of a hinterland where dementia might be reversible, that lies en route to the terminal condition.

Brain and mind in dementia

At this point we must face a question that has never been prominent in the work of those who have framed dementia in a technical way: it is the relationship between states of the brain and states of the mind—a relationship that is as important in 'mental sickness' as in 'mental health' (cf. Rose, 1984). If we reject dualism and assume that mental and neurophysiological descriptions refer to the same reality, to talk in psychological terms is never to be dealing with a domain that is mysteriously independent of brain function. To propose that some part might be played by psychological factors in the aetiology of dementia is thus to talk about exceedingly subtle events and states in a way that is readily accessible to experience and investigation, although with less precision than that to which natural science aspires. Moreover, and most crucially, the human being who is the subject of the inquiry can still be regarded a person, even for the purpose of research.

Let us suppose, for a moment, that the correlation between the most powerful neuropathological indices and the most robust measures of dementia approached 1.0; in other words, that all the variance was accounted for. If so, the proximal causation of dementia might be entirely attributable to neuropathology; this, however, would still have to be clearly demonstrated, because correlation does not in itself prove causation. Even then, psychology might be involved in more distal aspects of causation, by analogy with diseases such as cancer (see p. 123). In the case of the senile dementias, however, matters are more complex. The present state of research indicates that some 50% of the variance might be accounted for; although as we have seen, if cases of low dementia and small neuropathic change are excluded, the amount is much smaller. It seems highly improbable that this falling short of 100% is solely due to error variance. Thus psychology seems to be implicated proximally in the causation of dementia, even if it contributes to the distal causation as well. Putting matters in a way that does not do justice to the subtlety of the mind–brain problem, but which accords with a technical mentality, dementia in old age is not only caused by malfunction of the hardware but by faulty software as well.

Perhaps the most crucial question posed by neuropathological research, and which at present it seems unable to answer, is what brings about the change from normal to demented functioning in an individual, granted a certain degree of degeneration of grey matter. It may, of course, be the case that there are obscure pathogens yet to be discovered, or biochemical disturbances too subtle to be monitored by today's techniques, and so on. There seems to be a strong case, however, for the inquiry to include factors of a personal kind. It is irrational to rule them out a *priori*.

The technical frame and the taken-for-granted world

Why, then, has one particular type of approach to dementia achieved such prominence during the last 20 or so years, virtually to the exclusion of all others? Very speculatively, it may be suggested that there has been a convergence of interests in adopting a purely technical frame, and that as research within it has gathered momentum, clearly achieving results, other approaches have come to appear irrelevant or absurd.

Most significantly, perhaps, medicine in the West has increasingly tended to view human illness by analogy with problems in engineering. Moreover, as high technology has become available to medical science, those carrying out research have often been lured by what is 'technically sweet'. Their good faith is not in question here. The point is that their milieu, the world with which they are familiar by training and experience, is one deeply impregnated by technology and natural science, and the objectifying mode that accompanies them. The skills of interpersonal understanding, on the other hand, belong to another milieu, which only a minority of health professionals have entered. The technical framing of dementia, it need hardly be added, has had powerful support from some drug companies, which could then produce specific sedatives and palliatives; and even, in certain instances, complete schedules for the assessment and management of the dementing illnesses. Within the medical profession there are, however, some indications of dissent; for example recently a group of doctors openly rejected the 'medicalization of dementia' at a symposium of the American Gerontological Society (Klass, 1985).

The technical frame is generally adopted, too, by nurses and others who are employed in geriatric care—even if there are times when it conflicts with their more direct intuitions. The majority of carers will have absorbed the standard view without subjecting it to critical appraisal. Also, since their professional life-position is one of subservience and deference to medical authority (Salvage, 1983), there is a very strong pressure on them to continue with taken-for-granted views. But there is a further point. Under the current provision for medical and social services for old people it is virtually impossible for them to engage in a fully personal way with their confused, fearful and sometimes despairing patients. It is often merely a matter of 'managing' their behaviour. The professional carers are not sufficiently resourced themselves, either at an organizational or an individual level, to do more. Thus the technical frame provides a kind of distancing; it helps to make their working life more bearable, and rationalizes the woes that they encounter day by day.

But we must consider also the predicament of relatives and, in some cases, friends. For them, too, the technical frame is helpful, for it enables them to cope with the feelings of grief, anger, fear, guilt and inadequacy in which they are often enveloped. Also, it can give grounds for an apologia, since it is far easier to describe the afflicted person as 'having' Alzheimer's disease or some other condition than to express matters in everyday terms. Moreover, by adopting the technical frame the caretakers are relieved of having to face the immensely threatening possibility that there might have been, and might still be, psychologically malignant processes going on within the family, including even their own relationship to the dementing person. Perhaps this is why the associations of carers contain people for whom the technical frame virtually provides a mythology, and why some of their own written contributions express a touching yet tragic combination of sentiment and subservience to the technical view.

If we move even further onto speculative ground, we come upon another possible reason why the technical frame has come to be accepted so widely. Does it aid a widespread and collusive denial of what is involved in ageing and dying in the modern world, and even perhaps the denial of death itself? The disintegration of the embodied person that we witness as a slow process during a dementing illness is something that will happen to us all. It is liable to activate our deepest forms of *angst*, attached to the ultimate facts of isolation and mortality. In a society such as ours the age of retirement involves, for many people, a disastrous disempowerment through lack of income, work role and mobility; great personal insecurity; a progressive loss of social connections; and possibly an entry into a world where there is little genuine love and understanding. Some of the burdens and losses bear especially heavily on women, who may have spent much of their lives attending to the needs of others, while their own needs were unrecognized or unfulfilled. Many of these problems arise from the structural position of old people; they are not the necessary accompaniment of the ageing process (Phillipson, 1984).

These are hard truths to face existentially, when the culture makes so great a fetish of youth and beauty, and when social structures are so firmly embedded. To view dementia as a problem in neurological or biochemical engineering provides a small consolation, insulating people from certain deeply disturbing truths which, at some level, they do not wish to know. The technical framing of dementia is a paradigm of the technical framing of the universal facts of ageing and death. There are only very few settings, perhaps most notably some of the hospices for the dying, where the technical frame is genuinely transcended.

Towards a psychological understanding of dementia

To consider dementia as an illness of the whole person, rather than merely a disease of the brain is, of course, not a new idea. Some of the relevant literature is reviewed by Gilhooly (1984), who comes to the very proper conclusion that while there may be something of significance here, it is clearly an instance of 'case not proven'. Her discussion, however, is somewhat unsympathetic. In some of this earlier work there is a richness that is lacking in the more precise research carried out within the purely technical frame. It has, however, remained as little more than a collection of fragments, and never been coordinated into a coherent research programme. One reason for this, undoubtedly, is the power, prestige and success of work in medical science such as we have examined. But it is also arguable that the more psychologically oriented research never had a theoretical basis adequate to the task. It required, but lacked, a well-founded concept of the person as an embodied being in a social setting. Thus systematic psychological work in this field has yet to be carried out.

Of course, all that is said from a psychological standpoint must, ultimately, be compatible with the established findings of neurophysiology and neuropathology. But the key to a psychological approach that is genuinely personal is that it does not 'stand outside', taking the position of a detached, unaffected observer. Its aim is to work interpretively and empathically, going far beyond the measurement of indices or the codification of behaviour. This involves personal risk for the researcher, for his or her own self-hood becomes involved, engaged, and thereby subjected to all manner of psychodynamic processes such as identification, projection and counter-transference. These are not to be guarded against, but to be used as data. It is on the ground of our own experience in relationship that we can gain some inkling of what is happening to another. Yet when we encounter deep distress we often defend ourselves against it, lest we too should be engulfed.

From a psychological standpoint the more obvious symptoms of dementia, such as impairment of short-term memory, emotional disinhibition, paranoid reactions, and the failure to complete schemata of action, might be understood as aspects of a slow and progressive 'loss of self'. The continuing thread of 'I am' experience, which was first spun together from tiny strands during infancy, becomes disturbed, fades from view, or is fragmented. This is often compounded by fear and bewilderment, because the person lacks sufficient insight to recognize what is happening. If he or she did, this meta-level understanding might itself be a sufficient basis for continuing identity, as in Luria's famous case of the 'man with a shattered world', whose brain had suffered massive damage from a bullet wound (Luria, 1972). Our task, then, is to give a psychological account of this loss of self, and this requires a theory or model of the self that is lost.

Here we need a distinction, conceptualized in various ways in the theories that have arisen from psychoanalysis and psychotherapy. It is between the experiencing, sentient centre (sometimes, but ineptly, called the 'true self') and the self that is formed in everyday interaction, as a person adapts, often without awareness, to existing social reality. Modern social psychology, with its strongly cognitive emphasis, tells us mainly about the latter, showing how a self-concept arises out of processes such as social feedback and social comparison. The experiential self is what many forms of psychotherapy seek to recover, by enabling the person to be more in touch with his or her own organismic life, less subject to the distortions of experience that are imposed by others. The experiencing self, so depth psychology suggests, develops mainly in contexts where a person is valued, where he or she is attended to with respect, where discourse is available in which sentient experience is accepted, named and shared. To be in touch with this self is to be psychologically healthy, and this would be highly conducive also to physical well-being. The experiencing self is often impaired, obscured, malnourished; how could it be otherwise, when that which would enrich and validate it is largely absent? In some people this self is hidden away, put into cold storage and then forgotten, in the secret hope that one day it will be allowed to grow and flourish. Meanwhile, living in the taken-for-granted world, they exist on the ground of their adapted selves, mistaking this for the true psychic reality. They have a certain kind of stability, but only so long as that world remains intact.

If we view self-hood in this kind of way, a problem area comes into focus. Dementia might be understood, psychologically, as the consequence of the removal of the main cognitive supports that had preserved a person's sense of ontological continuity, even if in an alienated state, through loss of roles, impoverishment of social life, and so on. But not only this; these losses are likely to be far more damaging in those whose experiential self is poorly developed; who cannot genuinely assimilate them, and ward them off by such defences as denial. In short, we might hypothesize that the psychological precondition for dementia is an underdeveloped experiencing self, while the adapted self is seriously undermined. The secret hope of being really understood and validated by another is finally abandoned. All this, of course, has its neurophysiological correlates, and it is not inconceivable that it might have neuropathological consequences as well. These ideas could certainly be related to the two vignettes with which this paper began. The social environment of modern urban America might be regarded as highly 'dementogenic' for those in later life. The case of the man who developed dementia soon after being made redundant seems to be a paradigmatic example of what we have been discussing.

Thus, from what has been found in the more technical research, and from directly psychological considerations, there is a strong case for viewing dementia in personal terms. The technical frame is not likely to deliver anything like the full aetiological picture, despite the power of its research methods and the precision of some, at least, of its results. There are other kinds of inquiry to be made into dementia, grounded in that intersubjective sensitivity that lies at the heart of psychotherapeutic work. Dementia is an existential plight of persons—not simply a problem to be investigated and managed through technical skill.

Author's note

I wish to thank the editors of *Free Associations* for their permission to draw on papers of mine which they have already published. These are listed in the references.

References

Albert, M.S. (1982). 'Geriatric neuropsychology', *Journal of Consulting and Clinical Psychology*, **49**, 835–50.

Ball, M.J., Blume, W., Fisman, M., Fox, A., Fox, H., Hachinski, V., Kral, V.A., Kirsher, A.J., and Merskey, H. (1985). 'A new definition of Alzheimer's disease: A hippocampal dementia', *Lancet*, 5 January, 14–16.

Bird, J.M., Levy, R., and Jacoby, R.J. (1986). 'Computed tomography in the elderly: changes over time in a normal population', *British Journal of Psychiatry*, **148**, 80–5.

Blessed, G., Tomlinson, B.E., and Roth, M. (1968). 'The association between quantitative measures of dementia and of senile change in the cerebral grey matter of elderly subjects', *British Journal of Psychiatry*, **114**, 797–811.

Collerton, D., and Fairbairn, A. (1985). 'Alzheimer's disease and the hippocampus', *Lancet*, 2 February, 278–9.

Cooper, C.L. (ed.) (1984). *Psychosocial Stress and Cancer*, Wiley, Chichester.

Earnest, M.P., Heaton, R.K., Wilkinson, W.E., and Manke, W.F. (1979). 'Cortical atrophy, ventricular enlargement and intellectual impairment in the aged', *Neurology*, **29**, 1138–43.

Gilhooly, M. (1984). 'The social dimensions of senile dementia'. In I. Hanley and J. Hodge (eds.), *Psychological Approaches to the Care of the Elderly*, Croom Helm, London.

Gurland, B., Copeland, J., Kuriansky, J., Kellever, M., Sharpe, L., and Dean, L.L. (1983). *The Mind and Mood of Ageing*, Croom Helm, Beckenham.

Hawkins, R.A., and Phelps, M.E. (1986). 'Positron emission tomography for evaluation of cerebral function', *Current Concepts in Diagnostic Nuclear Medicine*, **3**, 1–13.

Jacoby, R.J., and Levy, R. (1980a). 'Computed tomography in the elderly: 2. Senile dementia: diagnosis and functional impairment', *British Journal of Psychiatry*, **136**, 270–5.

Jacoby, R.J., and Levy, R. (1980b). 'Computed tomography in the elderly: 3. Affective disorder', *British Journal of Psychiatry*, **136**, 270–5.

Jacoby, R.J., Levy, R., and Dawson, J.M. (1980). 'Computed tomography in the elderly: 1. The normal population', *British Journal of Psychiatry*, **136**, 249–55.

Kitwood, T.M. (1987a). 'Dementia and its pathology: in brain, mind or society?', *Free Associations*, **8**, 81–93.

Kitwood, T.M. (1987b). 'Explaining senile dementia: the limits of neuropathological research', *Free Associations*, **10**, 117–40.

Klass, D. (1985). 'Medicalization of dementia: gain or loss?', Gerontological Society of America (unpublished).

Luria, A.R. (1972). *The Man with Shattered World*, Basic Books, New York.

Phillipson, C. (1984). *Capitalism and the Construction of Old Age*, Pluto Press, London.

Rose, S.P.R. (1984). 'Disordered molecules and diseased minds', *Journal of Psychiatric Research*, **18**, 351–60.

Roth, M. (1980). 'Senile dementia and its borderlands'. In J.O. Cole and J.E. Barrett (eds.), *Psychopathology in the Aged*, Raven Press, New York.

Rothschild, D., and Sharpe, M.L. (1941). 'The origin of senile psychoses: neuropathologic factors and factors of a more personal nature', *Diseases of the Nervous System*, **2**, 49–54.

Salvage, J. (1983). *The Politics of Nursing*, Heinemann, London.

Tomlinson, B.E., Blessed, G., and Roth, M. (1968). 'Observations on the brains of non-demented old people', *Journal of Neurological Science*, **7**, 331–6.

Tomlinson, B.E., Blessed, G., and Roth, M. (1970). 'Observations on the brains of demented old people', *Journal of Neurological Science*, **11**, 205–42.

Wells, C.E., and Duncan, G.W. (1977). 'Danger of over-reliance on computerised cranial tomography', *American Journal of Psychiatry*, **134**, 811–13.

2.2

Understanding senile dementia: a psychobiographical approach (1990)

What is happening, and what has happened, when a person becomes demented in later life? In one gestalt configuration – perhaps the prevailing one at present – the central figure is a process of degeneration, or some other physical impairment, in the grey matter of the brain; psychological and social factors fade into the background, at least for the purposes of research. Another gestalt, however, equally valid, can emerge; in this the figure becomes an existential crisis of a person, of an embodied, social and sentient being, and indeed a crisis of an interpersonal milieu; neuropathology, of whatever degree of severity, becomes part of a whole range of peripheral considerations.

The main thesis of this paper is that if the dementias of old age are to be understood and responded to in a way that does justice to our humanity, the second gestalt must have a central place; not to the exclusion of the first, but in a dialectical tension with it. This is acknowledged, if tacitly and common-sensically, by many people who are involved in practical care-giving, whether as family members or professionals. Geriatric care is not easy, at the best of times; it is doubly difficult when resources are cut to the bone and there is a prevailing climate of resentment and demoralization. Nevertheless, a respect for demented persons continually emerges: a belief in their capacity to feel, relate and respond – and even to recover to some degree. Among care-givers there is often a deep reluctance to accept that the demented are merely the victims of a crippling neurological affliction: and there is a reaching out – expressed in praxis rather than in theory – towards a fuller understanding of their predicament.

Curiously, however, this humanism is far less evident in formal research. On the one hand there is now a very strong tradition of inquiry orientated around the first gestalt, looking at the nature of the neuropathic and biochemical changes that accompany dementia, and searching for causes at levels ranging from the molecular to the cellular (Kitwood, 1987b). On the other hand, there is a small and far less coherent body of research concerned with social and personal factors; but this generally lacks either the breadth or depth to generate an adequately personal understanding. For example, there is some evidence that a propensity to dementia may be related to personality, to critical life events and, more broadly, to an imperfectly avowed awareness of the powerless and often hopeless predicament of advanced old age in contemporary industrial societies, together with the prospect of impending death. The literature on dementia, however, contains few if any examples of attempts to relate dementia in old age to the larger pattern of life history, and to the nature of a person's social relations and experience. To do this is difficult conceptually, and involves slow and careful empirical work; also, it places a heavy responsibility on the researcher as interpreter, as compared to methods that rely centrally on the quantification of supposedly objective data.

If we are to have an adequate and humane understanding of dementia, it is crucially important to be aware of the personal dimension; and this not from the standpoint of a narrow individualism, but from a genuinely social perspective. One approach is to think in terms of an experiential and an adapted self, both of which coexist 'within' any individual, and both of which are socially formed (Kitwood, 1987a). The experimential self is grounded in a kind of feeling-knowing or affectivity. It develops as experience is accepted, named and validated by others, and to the extent that a person can apprehend the self as an agent, one who creatively brings new things into being in the world. The adapted self has its basis in conformity to others' expectations, whether informally or in clearly structured roles. In industrial capitalist society at least (and almost certainly in all societies where there are severe inequalities and impositions of power) there is a disjuncture between the two selves. The project of psychotherapy, then, may be regarded as that of enabling a person to recover contact with – and to live more clearly on the basis of – the experiential self, since this is the vital source of well-being and relatedness.

We can take these fairly simplistic ideas in order to make psychological sense of a person's biography, by asking about the vicissitudes of the two types of self. For the majority of people the adapted self grows steadily from early childhood, as a greater number and variety of roles are taken on; it continues strongly until the seventh decade of life, and then declines as roles are withdrawn and opportunity for a range of social contacts diminishes. The progress of the experiential self shows, perhaps, much greater variability. Some people develop psychic defences very early in life and maintain them through its whole span: others grow up with relatively few defences and remain extraordinarily open to experience; others, perhaps as a result of major life changes, intense love or suffering or perhaps with the aid of psychotherapy, allow their defences to be lowered, and become more integrated and self-accepting. Psychoanalytic theory indicates that the first basic patterns are formed in infancy. Whether a person can develop an experiential self depends in part on whether certain crucial thresholds are crossed successfully, and in particular on how the basic problem of primary ambivalence is dealt with. Adaptation in later life is in some respects the successor to infantile compliance.

In this paper we shall use this framework to examine the psychobiography of one person who was diagnosed as suffering from senile dementia of the Alzheimer type (SDAT). The aim here is primarily to illustrate a method, and to exhibit the second type of gestalt. This points towards a type of research into senile dementia that is, arguably, much in need of development.

Constructing a psychobiography

In our method for grasping something of the social and psychological context of a dementing illness, two researchers jointly carry out one or more fairly lengthy interviews (typically around two hours) with the main care-giver(s) and any other family members who are available. One person carries out the greater part of the interviewing, while the other makes detailed notes. The aim is to acquire a basic outline of the person's whole life, and to focus specifically on any events or developments that pertain to the vicissitudes of the experiential and the adapted selves; for example, life crises and how they were dealt with. Part of this involves a modified form of existing life-events methodology. We also build up a portrait of the person at different stages by collecting up any remarks made about his or her typical reactions, ways of relating to others, and so on. The interview has an atmosphere rather like that of non-directive counselling, and indeed in some cases it seems to have a therapeutic effect; the care-giver may be able to bring into the open a range of hidden feelings and tentative understandings – possibly it is the first time the fragments have ever been put together into a total picture. As researchers, however, we do have an agenda whose aim has been made explicit to the person we are meeting. We maintain the therapeutic informality throughout the greater part of the interview, but towards the end, or at a subsequent meeting, there is a 'mopping-up' operation: that is, the note-taker brings forward in a more systematic way any points on our agenda that have not been covered. Through this combination of freedom and structure much of the threat of the situation seems to be removed, and the threshold for personal disclosure is lowered.

This research method is close to psychotherapy in another respect. As interviewers we are not detached observers, coolly collecting objective data. We are involved sharing with the care-giver in a joint venture of intersubjectivity, allowing our intuitions and feelings into the experiential field. Without this a genuinely personal understanding would be impossible, and the 'truth' generated by the research would be of an exceedingly shallow kind. Our own reactions to the narrative, and our own experience of being with the care-giver, are highly relevant as evidence. In some cases we have been left with difficult feelings of pain, frustration or oppression, which it has been necessary to deal with for ourselves in a later, private 'de-briefing'.

The psychobiographical material is ordered into successive periods of fourteen years. (The choice is convenient, but has no theoretical justification; only a few lives extend beyond the seventh period, which ends at ninety-eight.) We apply this schematization also to our version of life-events methodology. Thus we do not follow the usual practice of covering a period backdated from the supposed onset of an illness; for in the case of the senile dementias this is usually impossible to discern – and, indeed, the question of the point of onset may well turn out to be meaningless. During the first three periods, up to age forty-two, it may be supposed that various patterns of relating and problem-solving are generally being established, according to whatever resources a person brings from infancy and early childhood. The fourth period, from forty-two to fifty-six, covers many typical midlife crises: children are growing up and leaving home, a person gains some inkling of what his or her career will amount to, and for most women this is the time of the menopause. The fifth period, from fifty-six to seventy, is one in which for many people retirement and several other major role losses occur, and old age comes clearly into sight. The sixth and seventh periods (seventy to eighty-four and eighty-four to ninety-eight) are, in Western society, those of old age proper. Statistics show that the incidence of dementia rises sharply; the figures are notoriously unreliable due to the lack of clear criteria for defining dementia, but suggest that about 10 per cent in the first of these two age brackets, and about 20 per cent in the second, may be seriously afflicted. In studying psychobiography, we look here particularly for factors that might stabilize or undermine the self, perhaps already rendered fragile through earlier losses.

Through ordering the data in this kind of way, and through collating the descriptive material concerning the one who has become demented, it becomes possible to build up some kind of picture of psychological life history. In this process the researchers' empathy and imagination are necessarily – and unashamedly – involved; it is a creative act, a search after meaning, which can be undertaken only by fellow-human beings. Gradually it becomes possible to compare cases of dementia, and also to bring these into juxtaposition with the psychobiographics of others who remain psychologically well preserved in old age. When this is done it becomes extremely difficult to see Alzheimer's disease as a purely neurological affliction. More, perhaps, than any other 'disease', it is intimately bound up with the vicissitudes of personal and social life.

All this might seem highly subjective and undisciplined, and therefore open to many of the objections that have been levelled against qualitative research. We have ourselves taken note of a dozen or so serious methodological problems. Our method of research does, in fact, allow the operationalization and quantification of certain key variables, and hence the collection also of data according to the canons of more positivistic social inquiry. This, however, is not the subject here. Suffice it to say that such a tactic is valuable at the very least as a check against certain gross distortions such as researchers' projections or special pleading case by case, even if it cannot in itself lead to a particularly creative understanding.

Rose: a case history

In 1986 Rose H. was found to be seriously demented and was taken into institutional care. Physically she was very active and in fairly good health, but she was clearly quite unable to look after herself. The extent of her dementia had come to light after her brother Thomas, with whom she had been living for about ten years, died. What follows is a brief account of her life story, as given by her daughter Sarah. For purposes of confidentiality, all names have been changed.

Rose was born in 1904, the fifth child of a family of nine, to which was added the 'illegitimate' son of one of her older sisters. They lived in one of those streets of small terraced houses that are typical of the North of England, with a factory nearby. The family was poor but 'respectable'. Rose's father was killed in the First World War. The war indeed left many marks upon the street: among the neighbours were three widows, two men who had lost a leg, and another whose lungs were permanently damaged through gas attacks. Rose was, apparently, a very intelligent girl who might have gone some way further with her education. Her widowed mother, however, could not afford to keep her at school. Her first job was helping to look after the babies of women who were doing war work, which suggests that she must have been about thirteen or fourteen at the time. Soon afterwards she went, with her older sister Anna, to work in a clothing factory, and this continued for many years. The work was monotonous, but she enjoyed her Saturday nights out with the girls from the factory, and was even known to get 'merry' on occasions – rather out of keeping with her sober upbringing. Rose married in 1930 at the age of twenty-six, after a very long engagement. She would have married earlier, but times were hard and the fear of unemployment pervasive; Jim, her fiancé, was working about a hundred miles away and was sending money home to his widowed mother, as well as trying to save for the wedding.

After the marriage Rose and her husband rented a house three doors away from the family home. She continued to go to work with her sister Anna. Each day the two sisters, together with another sister and brother, would all go home to a midday meal prepared by their mother. In 1936, when Rose was thirty-two, her daughter Sarah was born; she was the only child. Within a few weeks Rose was back at work, leaving the baby in her own mother's care. During her thirties and forties Rose was quiet, 'lady-like', undemonstrative and reserved: a small woman with long black hair, attractive to men. Her husband was an extrovert with a strong sense of humour, perhaps tending to cast his wife into the shade. In addition to his attempts to breed an all-white canary, he took a leading part in local entertainment. At that time many Northern streets and factories had their own troupe of dancers; he trained some of these, and was often called upon to be the Master of Ceremonies at local functions. Around 1946 he began to produce an annual pantomime; Rose designed and made many theatrical costumes, at which she was very skilful and assured. The marriage was a sound one by the standards of the day, although somewhat lacking in physical closeness and real intimacy. Typically, Jim would go out with 'the boys' on a Friday night; there would be a ritual row in which Rose complained that she was being left to do the cleaning, after which he slammed the door and left. On Saturdays, however, Jim would 'take her out'.

In 1952, when Rose was forty-eight, Jim died suddenly. At the funeral she was, untypically, very distraught, and afterwards she found it very difficult to reassemble her life. She spent a few weeks at the home of her sister Anna, who was now married. Around this time, apparently, Anna's husband was heard to complain: 'I have lost my wife', so great were Rose's demands on her sister's time and attention. When Rose took up the threads of her life again her daughter Sarah had succeeded her father in running the theatrical productions. She continued as wardrobe mistress, accompanying her daughter to rehearsals and committee meetings. Rose sometimes seemed to be extremely dependent, and even wanted to sleep in Sarah's bed. Sarah at times felt 'almost suffocated' by her mother's presence. In 1957 Sarah got married. Rose showed some ambivalence to her daughter's husband-to-be; he was not local, and she 'knew he would take her away'. Perhaps significantly, Rose did not arrange her daughter's wedding, although she did make the dresses. Sarah and her husband set up home five miles away; she was working full-time, running a large dancing school. After a fairly short period Rose moved into her daughter's home, keeping her own house for storing the theatrical costumes. Sarah and her husband moved south in 1962, and the theatrical productions in which she and her mother had been so closely involved for ten years came to an end. Rose stayed on in her own home, and continued to work with her sister Anna, until they both retired in 1968.

At this point Rose sold her house, and came again to live with Sarah and her husband, who now had a son. She was very helpful as a grandmother, and showed the child a lot of affection. However, she seemed to be extremely dependent and clinging; she made no friends in her own right, and would not go shopping alone. Sarah and her husband had a bed-sitting room built for her, hoping she would create a life of her own and give them a little more space. She never took this up, preferring to live and eat with them all the time. Sarah did, however, succeed in introducing her to art classes, and these she seemed to enjoy. Around this time four of Rose's siblings died. Anna had become a widow and went to live with her younger brother Thomas, who had never married. Every Christmas and summer Anna and Thomas would come to stay at Sarah's house.

In 1971 Sarah had another child, a daughter, and they moved house yet again, together with Rose. There was no change in her general reluctance to create a more independent life; also, although she would take the new baby out in her pram, she would go nowhere else unless accompanied. Sarah was very much taken up with her work, being out three nights each week and most weekends; her husband also was extremely occupied with his business. Thus Rose had a valued place in the household, and the granddaughter recalls that she felt more cared for by her than by her own mother. This state of affairs continued until 1976, when Rose was seventy-two years old.

Then Anna, the sister with whom she had gone to work for so many years and who was undoubtedly her favourite, died. Rose moved back to the area from which she had originally come, in order to keep house for Thomas. She was, in fact, the third sister to have this role. At first she seemed to take on a new lease of life. She took control of the home and bought new carpets and curtains. Also, she found a way of coping with Thomas, who was a difficult man: a 'bit of a bully', rather inconsiderate, unable to listen or share in any mode beyond extreme formality. Rose found that she was able to go out shopping alone, and met up with some of her old friends. Around this time another brother and sister died; now only Rose and Thomas were left, out of the original family of ten. Sarah, her husband and the two children moved yet again, a hundred miles or so away. Rose and Thomas continued to visit them for about two weeks each Christmas, and again in the summer; also Sarah would go to visit them each year. Rose was coping fairly well, although she was becoming more forgetful.

By 1980 Rose was beginning to show signs of serious impairment. She might go to the shops and then forget what she wanted to buy, or return having bought large quantities of what was not needed. Her conversation had become voluble and repetitive, and sometimes she seemed agitated. Thomas was often irritated by her, and reacted aggressively. Sarah had an illness which lasted for about three years, making contact more difficult. Then in 1983 Rose was found to have cancer of the bladder. There was an operation, after which she and Thomas came to stay with Sarah, remaining there while Rose received a course of radiotherapy. She was now exceedingly confused; she was unable to find the different rooms in her daughter's house, and sometimes she would wander off and get totally lost. Also, she began to urinate and defecate on chairs, or in corners of the room. Thomas went back home, and it was thought that Rose would die.

Remarkably, however, she began to recover, both in physical health and in mental facility. She worried about Thomas, and fretted to return to her own home. Following the doctor's advice, Rose was taken back to her familiar surroundings, there to resume her life with Thomas. Her condition continued to improve; she recovered her continence, and clearly enjoyed gardening again. During this period a curious symbiosis developed between brother and sister. He was now so afflicted by arthritis that he could (or would) do very little about the house; her memory was so impaired that she could carry very few tasks through to completion on her own. Together, however, they were able to do the cooking and the housework, maintaining a shared existence with a little outside help. In 1984 Sarah's husband died, at almost the same age as Rose's husband Jim had done. Rose and Thomas continued to visit her, but the situation was evidently deteriorating. There would be occasional urgent calls to Sarah to come and visit her mother when events got out of hand.

In 1986 Thomas died. Rose found him in his chair. She would not, apparently, accept that he was dead, and it seems that all acknowledgement of his existence was blanked out; Sarah has never heard Rose mention him since, even though she has often spoken of her sister Anna. It was after this crisis that the diagnosis of senile dementia of the Alzheimer type was made, and Rose was taken into full-time care. Since then her physical health has remained generally good, but her confusion has slowly deepened. Sometimes she seems to believe that she works at the home, making attempts to take care of the others. She has been slowly losing the capacity to recognize her daughter, and all contacts with her former social world have gone.

These are the bare bones of a long life history, as filtered through the experience of Rose's daughter Sarah. Many impressions were conveyed about the kind of person Rose was in middle life, and here are a few examples. She was, in her own way, 'very outgoing and friendly', and affectionate to her grandchildren. She was very skilled at making costumes and dresses, shrewd and resourceful in shopping around for materials. When she learned to paint during her sixties she enjoyed it, and became quite competent in technique. On the other hand, as Sarah put it. 'You organized Rose; you told her what to do'. Rose found it difficult to live an independent life. She 'liked to be where the action was' – but it was other people's action. She hardly ever showed emotion; she 'seemed to shut things out'; or, in her granddaughter's words, 'she had a lot of barriers'. She generally avoided conflict, tending to 'take it on herself' – for example in the way she excused her brother Thomas's rude and insensitive behaviour. She seemed to be frightened and disturbed by Sarah's ventures into philosophy and meditation, as if this were a kind of forbidden territory. 'When you hugged her, it didn't feel like hugging another human being.' She 'was never really a mother', although she was wardrobe mistress, helper, cleaner. 'It was difficult to love her', said her granddaughter. 'I don't think anyone ever got really close to my mother', was Sarah's own appraisal.

The self and its vicissitudes

When data are collected after a person has become demented, and through the mediation of a family member, there is not sufficient for a detailed psychoanalytic interpretation. It is certainly possible, however, to go some way in that direction, using the rather loose categories of the experiential and the adapted self. First let us look briefly at Rose's life, considered as a succession of fourteen-year periods.

Period 1 (0–14) The family was large; material and psychological impoverishment were intertwined. Rose was the fifth child. Probably she lacked attention and care. Her success at school came to nothing. She suffered a major bereavement. Her first job was one in which she adapted to others' needs. There is little to suggest a strong beginning to an experiencing self.

Period 2 (14–28) She was involved in monotonous manual work. Her family life was intact and supportive, although not conducive to 'personal growth'. With 'the girls' at work she experienced a modicum of playfulness and spontaneity. She made a 'sound' marriage, but without real intimacy.

Period 3 (28–42) This was a period of relative stability and fulfilment; but without obvious development. Rose had a child, but was not closely involved as a mother. She was a dutiful wife. She continued to be close to her own family, and to do the same work as before.

Period 4 (42–56) With the death of her mother and her husband, life was temporarily destabilized. She showed marked signs of defence and dependency, and moved even further into a pattern of adaptation (primarily now to her daughter).

Period 5 (56–70) No fundamental change in her way of living and experiencing took place. Her work with the theatre and her paid employment came to an end. She found a valid way of being as a member of her daughter's household. Four of her siblings died.

Period 6 (70–84) After Anna's death she moved from the relatively secure position in her daughter's home to the much more demanding task of looking after her brother Thomas. She gained in confidence, improved her social life. However, her mode of being was still primarily one of adaptation, and she herself received little affirmation. Another brother and sister died. Her life became much more precarious with her cancer and the subsequent radiotherapy. After her return to Thomas, adaptation had become transmuted into symbiosis. At Thomas's death she was found to be 'demented'.

Psychobiographically, what we see here is surely the history of someone whose personal resources were only poorly developed for the living of a long life within the social relations of an evolving and then declining industrial capitalist nation, disrupted by two major wars. There is much more than the relatively late encroachment of an 'organic mental disorder' leading to severe cognitive impairment in an individual; although a neuropathological process is surely part of the whole picture.

The material provided by Sarah is rich in evidence pertaining to her mother's experiential self. As with many people of her generation, it had little opportunity for development. This is apparent in some of the general characterizations of Rose, such as her lack of affect and her inability to create new bonds with others. It is also manifested in some specific accounts, most notably of her way of dealing with bereavement. In the case of her husband's death, it seems, there was one fairly brief and catastrophic irruption of chaos and desolation into consciousness; but here, and with the other bereavements, there is no indication of the 'working through' of a grief process. On the death of her favourite sister Anna she showed no emotional reaction; and later, on the death of her brother and companion Thomas, she was not even able to make a cognitive acknowledgement of her loss. Her attitude to sentient experience is also shown in her view of Sarah's attempt to enrich her own subjective life through meditation and philosophy. Rose saw this as some kind of threat: 'You shouldn't meddle with what you don't know'. More circumstantially, it seems unlikely either that Rose's hard-pressed and bereft family or her work would have given much opportunity for the development of her experiential self. Her marriage lacked warmth and intimacy, and having a child, which for some people provides a breakthrough into affectivity and sensitive awareness of others, did relatively little for Rose; for her baby was mainly looked after by her mother.

It appears, then, that Rose's life was lived primarily on the basis of the adapted self. During the first three fourteen-year periods of her life she was, in this respect, intact and developing; she had clear roles in her own family, her marriage, her paid employment, and later as a helper in the theatrical activities. After her husband's death, although she was profoundly disorientated for a short while, she soon reconstructed her adaptive mode – now focusing primarily on her daughter and her family life. During the later periods the progress of the adapted self seems to have been through a succession of plateaux, each one lower than its predecessor. There was one while she and Anna were still going out to work together, and another longer one when she was fully established as a grandmother, living in her daughter's house. A further plateau was maintained when she was looking after Thomas. The last, after she had recovered from her cancer operation, was one of extreme adaptation; and when that came to an end with Thomas's death, her personal resources were exhausted. In one crucial sense, her selfhood ceased to exist.

The story of Rose has, of course, its unique features, but it is certainly not out of the ordinary: also, the dementia was clearly not a consequence of institutionalization. In her case the experiential self, which might have sustained her sense of ontological security, her sense of agency, and her capacity for relatedness despite some degree of brain failure, was only poorly developed; and her adapted self, as with the great majority of people who survive into their seventies and eighties, underwent progressive decline; in her case, to vanishing point. Psychologically, it would seem that dementia was the inevitable consequence.

To do justice to Rose's psychobiography, we must place it in the broader context of life under industrial capitalism. The exceedingly poor provision which societies of this kind make for old age is certainly part of the story; but we need to look also at the psychological consequences of inequality on the whole pattern of a life: most crucially here the depredations brought about by the extraction of surplus value from wage labour, and the exigencies of war. Rose was one of a large family, struggling to make ends meet and remain respectable; throughout her early life the threat of unemployment was never far away. Under such conditions survival is the top priority; tenderness and sensitivity are often in short supply – perhaps even considered a weakness – while loyalty is strong. The interpersonal life of Rose's family was never well developed; there was no milieu for the growth and enhancement of the experiential self, while there were very strong pressures to lay down long-term patterns of adaptation. The premature death of Rose's husband was probably a consequence, at least in part, of the stress of working life and the struggle to remain employed; that of her son-in-law seems to be related to his striving to develop a career that would make him secure against the trap of poverty. A widow at the age of forty-eight, Rose then moved from place to place at the behest of others, without ever putting down roots for herself.

In part also Rose's predicament can be seen as a consequence of the social construction of gender, for women of her generation, even more than generally today, were viewed as those who respond to others' needs, fulfil others' expectations. As Sarah expressed it in a letter to the geriatrician who was in charge of Rose's case, protesting about the conditions to which her mother had (temporarily) been subjected when in institutional care:

> This lady has suffered the bereavement of all her nine brothers and sisters; she has lived a life devoted to others – from caring for the babies of working women during the First World War when only a child herself, to raising thousands of pounds for local charities and making hundreds of costumes for the children of her local Theatrical Society. On retirement even a horse would be given a field of grass and daisies.

When a person is required so strongly and persistently to attend to others, while her own needs are disastrously unmet, is it any wonder that her own self disappears?

In Rose's case it is impossible to say when the 'Alzheimer's disease' began, as indeed with most people who become demented in this kind of way. In a strictly medical framing of the problem, what we have here is a neurological disease of insidious origin – nothing more. But when we look closely at the afflicted person's psychobiography we are bound to see matters in a different light. The story of Rose is also that of a person in whom selfhood and the sense of agency were not well established, and yet who had to face difficulties in old age such as would tax to the limit even the most resourceful. She was required to do it, moreover, without the kind of support that would, in some other societies, at least have kept the mode of adaptation in good repair. For it is a feature of contemporary industrial capitalist societies (and to some extent also of those with centrally planned economics) that they have no clear place for those in later life; at the very point where high-quality social support is required, often very little is forthcoming. Concomitant with an increasingly difficult existential predicament. Rose's brain function was declining, thus giving her even less flexibility. Her 'senile dementia of the Alzheimer type' is the outcome of the confluence of these two processes.

Towards a theory of SDAT

In the light of psychobiographical evidence such as we have discussed here, it seems overwhelmingly probable that the states of being that are clinically known as senile dementia arise from an interaction between psychological factors and the declining functional capacity of the brain. This is especially the case with SDAT, where the correlations with neuropathology are not particularly strong (Kitwood, 1987b). In other words, the demented person is one who suffers a *psychological* affliction that is 'carried' by a brain whose processes are, to some degree, impaired. In some of the older literature that affliction was termed senile psychosis, and similarities were demonstrated with; certain forms of schizophrenia. This point is worth taking seriously; at the very least, a psychosis may be understood as a profound disturbance in the self process, as if the continuing thread of 'I-ness' has been broken. Psychosis in earlier life often seems to be associated with a violent perturbation or disruption of the self, a bursting through the defences, an invasion by material so powerful and damaging that it cannot be assimilated into conscious experience. The psychotic aspect of senile dementia, however, seems to have a rather different dynamic. It is as if the self, together with its defences, has been subjected to extreme attenuation: then the threats which relate specifically to death and dying fasten on to psychotic elements that are already present from earlier life, and their invasion is a relatively easy matter. Presumably everyone has some degree of psychotic tendency; but whereas for the great majority this does not feature to any marked degree in the normal run of adult life, it is more readily activated in the extremities of old age and particularly where a person encounters again, in helplessness, the archaic terror of abandonment.

To talk about a senile psychosis as well as a process of degeneration in the grey matter of the brain is not to fall into a naive dualism, as might at first appear. Within a monistic interpretation we may suppose that for every mental event or state there is, in any individual, a corresponding neurophysiological event or state; and in general the relation between the two may be characterized as one in which mental descriptions supervene upon the neurophysiological.[1] In senile dementia, however, matters are more complex. As the neuropathological process sets in, a severe limitation is imposed upon what can occur at the psychological level; it is reasonable to suppose that beyond a certain threshold the brain can only 'carry' a demented state, and supervenience breaks down.

Thus tentatively, and a shade simplistically, we may express matters as shown below:

(i)   Benign senescence: $\dfrac{\psi}{B_{(f)}}$

(ii)   Reversible psychosis: $\dfrac{\psi'}{B}$

(iii) SDAT: $\dfrac{\psi'_2}{B_{(f)}}$

Here ψ indicates normal psychological functioning, and ψ' indicates psychosis. (Admittedly, there are grave difficulties in clearly demarcating the two.) ψ'_2 indicates that special kind of psychosis which relate to attenuation of selfhood in old age. B indicates the brain without significant neuropathic change, and $B_{(f)}$ the brain in some degree of irreversible failure. Clearly the affective pseudodementias of old age (so called because they can be reversed) can be related to category (ii). Perhaps they might be characterized as

$$\frac{\psi'_2}{B}$$

Much now can, in principle, be explained. The diverse manifestations of the same dementia (as defined by neurological criteria) are attributable to variability in the proportions of ψ'_2 and $B_{(f)}$ The clinical resemblance that is sometimes observed between different dementias is attributable to similarities in ψ'_2 despite different types of brain failure. Some cases of dementia show more evident psychotic features than others; the limiting case would be one in which there was severe brain failure with virtually no psychosis.

If these points are basically correct, it becomes clear why a programme of research that focues exclusively on the causes of $B_{(f)}$, with the aim of bringing about a 'technical' cure or prevention, cannot fully encompass the problem of senile dementia. With SDAT at least, and probably in all cases, it is necessary also to develop an account of psychotic tendencies in later life. This can be done only through an act of personal understanding; and here psychobiography has a central place.

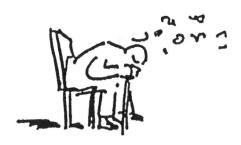

Note

1   In the philosophy of mind, the relation of supervenience is often expressed as follows: states of type X supervene on states of type Y if there is no difference among X states unless there is a corresponding difference among Y states. Thus, crudely, whenever minds differ, brains differ; but when minds are identical, brains may still differ.

Acknowledgement

I would like to thank Joan Carter for her invaluable help in the preparation of this paper.

References

Kitwood, T. (1987a) 'Dementia and its pathology: in mind, brain or society.' *Free Assns* 8: 81–93.
— (1987b) 'Explaining senile dementia: the limits of neuropathological research', *Free Assns* 10: 117–40.

Address for correspondence: Interdisciplinary Human Studies, University of Bradford, West Yorks BD7 1DP, UK

2.3

Towards a theory of dementia care: personhood and well-being (1992)

ABSTRACT

Some foundations are laid for a social-psychological theory of dementia care. Central to this is a conceptualisation of personhood, in which both subjectivity and intersubjectivity are fully recognised. Evidence is brought forward concerning relative well-being even in those who are, from a cognitive standpoint, severely demented. In the light of this it is argued that the key psychological task in dementia care is that of keeping the sufferer's personhood in being. This requires us to see personhood in social rather than individual terms.

Introduction

At present there is no coherent theory of the process of care for those who have a dementing illness in old age. Neither psychiatry, clinical psychology, nor any of the related disciplines has provided what is needed in this respect. In place of theory there is a considerable body of folklore and an abundance of tacit knowledge, the latter embodied often in the work of outstanding practitioners. Also there is a substantial portfolio of practical approaches, some adorned with the term 'therapy', which provide good advice drawn from everyday experience; in some of these there are the beginnings of a theory, but little more. Often it is a fairly crude pragmatism that leads to the decision to adopt one of these approaches rather than another.

Considering its great significance for gerontology, and indeed for the whole pattern of contemporary life, the absence of a theory of dementia care is remarkable. Why should there be such a gap? One can attempt to answer this question at various levels, where each proposed explanation requires another. Most obviously, there is the fact that the psychiatry of old age has had an overwhelming tendency to make the brain rather than the personhood of the dementia sufferer its central focus of attention; the inquiry has been technical rather than personal.[1] This has been very useful for medical-scientific research, but it has delivered almost no valuable theoretical insight into the practicalities of care. Behind this lies the fact that both psychiatry and clinical psychology have been extremely reluctant to articulate and implement a clear concept of the human subject, preferring to work even at a clinical level with regularities among fairly simple observables. It might be argued that this feature has run as a great fault-line through work on mental distress ever since the days of Kraepelin, despite a succession of attempts to set matters to rights.[2] So, pressing the question further, one might ask, 'Why this flight from personhood and subjectivity?' In an obvious sense this avoidance enabled psychiatry and psychology to conform to a notion of natural science, although a rather narrow and stilted one. Less obviously and much more controversially, a stance that is mainly technical keeps distress at bay. Professionals and informal carers are vulnerable people too, bearing their own anxiety and dread concerning frailty, dependence, madness, ageing, dying and death. A supposed objectivity in a context that is, in fact, interpersonal is one way of maintaining psychological defences, and so making involvement with conditions such as dementia bearable.[3]

Whatever may be the weight of truth in these and other possible reasons, the fact is that thousands upon thousands of hours of dementia care work pass by, in which the people involved generally do not understand what they are doing. This applies, moreover, even to some who are doing excellent work. The need for a theory can hardly be doubted. A care practice, however good it might be judged to be, is relatively ineffective without a coherent theory; it is powerless at the clinical, pedagogical, and political levels. A thorough theoretisation – or, as the followers of Paulo Freire might say, a conscientisation[4] – provides awareness, a sense of value, and the basis for concerted action.

In this paper we attempt to set out the grounding for such a theory, focusing on the concept of personhood, and drawing on an observation that is gradually being recognised as crucially significant: that a dementing illness, although it often does involve a dismantling of the person, need not necessarily do so; and that a dementia sufferer can be in a state of at least relative well-being. In a subsequent paper the actual process of caregiving will be examined. Behind the view of care that we are putting forward lies a theory of dementia that has already been outlined in this journal.[5] Briefly, it suggests that the clinical presentation of dementia is far from being a direct consequence of a degenerative process in nervous tissue. Rather, the dementing process should be viewed as the outcome of a dialectical interplay between two tendencies. The first is neurological impairment, which does indeed set upper limits to how a person can perform. The second is the personal psychology an individual has accrued, together with the social psychology with which he or she is surrounded. Such a dialectical account can, in principle, rationalize the whole range of phenomena associated with dementia better than one derived simply from medical science. This does not yield a comprehensive general theory of the dementing process: that, it may be argued, is impossible. Here, however, are the conceptual tools through which to construct, at least in outline, the unique course of dementia in any particular individual. Crucial to this account is a recognition of the 'malignant social psychology' which often bears down powerfully on those who are aged and confused: a psychology in which the others involved are usually well-intentioned but lacking in insight. One implication is that 'bad care' involves this malignancy to a high degree. 'Good care', conversely, is singularly free of this, and is highly respectful of personhood.

There is a problem: where is the problem?

At the very beginning of that disruption of social life which is later identified as a particular individual's dementia, a problem is developing. A person is starting to forget the shopping, or gets lost in town, or puts the electric kettle on the gas cooker. Something new and disturbing is happening in the interpersonal field. On this single point every theorist of dementia is agreed. For those who are actually involved, the problem is usually first clearly identified by others; the individual whose behaviour appears to be strange may be extremely reluctant to acknowledge that a problem exists at all.

Beyond this extremely general description – 'there is a problem' – no clear agreement exists.

How is the growing problem in the interpersonal field going to be rationalized? At the extremes, there are two main possibilities. The first is by far the most common, since it underpins the greater part of medical, nursing and social work practice, as well as the taken-for-granted world of residential care. It can be illustrated diagrammatically as shown below.

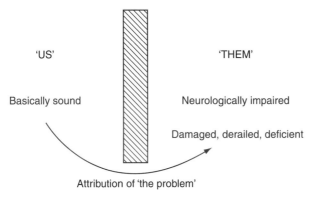

Figure 1

Here there is a clear division between *us* (members of the 'normal' population) and *them* (the dementia sufferers). *We* are basically sound, undamaged, competent, kind. *They* are in a bad way, for they are afflicted with a primary degenerative disease in the grey matter. *They* are thus damaged, de-railed, deficient. *We* may not always be the most effective carers. So there is a need for training to give us knowledge about *their* illness; and to develop skills, especially in managing *their* 'challenging behaviours'. In the long run *they* will have to learn to accommodate themselves to the provision that *we* make for them.

This may be something of a caricature, but in one crucial respect there is certainly no exaggeration. The focus of attention is overwhelmingly on *them* as the problem, while *we* are not problematized at all. A detailed survey of all the main approaches to dementia care, for example Reality Orientation, Behaviour Modification, Reminiscence Therapy, Validation Therapy, makes this point abundantly clear.[6] The problem is to be located with *them*, while *we* bring nothing seriously problematic to the situation. Putting matters in a different way, and rather less contentiously: there is here no clear view either of relationship or of intersubjectivity. Although the subject-matter is that of caregiving, there is still an infection from the detached and supposedly objective stance that pervades psychiatry and clinical psychology.

There is, however, a different view, as illustrated below.

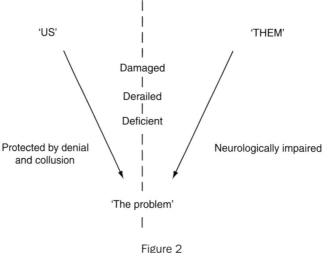

Figure 2

According to this, *we* are also contributors to the problem, for both *we* and *they* are human beings with our failures, limitations and suffering. In some respects, indeed, *we* might be considered more problematic than *they*. *They* are obviously damaged, derailed, deficient: a neurological process has interfered with their everyday functioning. But *we*, in our very varied ways, are damaged, derailed, deficient too. What is particularly dangerous here is that generally *we* do not acknowledge these facts. Indeed, much of our professional socialization involves a systematic training in how to avoid such a painful insight; we learn to live with very high defences against any recognition.[7] What is more, it is arguable that the general pattern of everyday life, with its hypocrisy, competitiveness and pursuit of crass materialism is, from a human standpoint, deeply pathological; those whose way of being dovetails smoothly into this pattern are the most 'normal' and well-adjusted. The truth, from this other standpoint, is that such people simply participate in an unacknowledged 'pathology of normality'.[8] Thus when the interpersonal field surrounding the beginnings of 'dementia' is looked at in this way, the problem is by no means focused on a single person whose brain is failing. Those others who have face-to-face contact are also involved; and, in the background, so also is the prevailing pattern of social relations.

This view can be taken further. For one might even suggest that in some respects *they* are rather less of a problem than *we*. *They* are generally more authentic about what they are feeling and doing; many of the polite veneers of earlier life have been stripped away. *They* are clearly dependent on others, and usually come to accept that dependence; whereas many 'normal' people, living under an ideology of extreme individualism, strenuously deny their dependency needs. *They* live very largely in the present, because certain parts of their memory function have failed. *We* often find it very difficult to live in the present, suffering constant distraction; the sense of the present is often contaminated by regrets about the past and fears concerning the future.

The view that is represented in figure 2 has never (so far as we are aware) been fully articulated in the literature on dementia and dementia care, although some of the ideas expressed in recent work do point in that direction.[9] It is in a different field – that of psychotherapy and counselling – that is it clearly recognized that *we* are, or may be, or may become part of the problem. Here it is axiomatic that any person who would help others to deal with their distress and self-defeating patterns must first get acquainted with his or her own personal difficulties, and understand his or her familiar ways of being with others. There must always be awareness, and where there are serious drawbacks growth must be allowed to take place. Without this vital preparation the would-be helper or healer may become caught up in any number of noxious interactive patterns, or get continually seduced into unproductive 'games'. We would argue strongly that a 'therapeutic' awareness of this kind could and should be a central part of caring for those who suffer from dementia. The dementing illness of one person brings to the surface a much larger problematic which challenges our commonsense and customary ways of being.

Personhood: the central issue

The presence of dementia on a large scale in contemporary society, and the dire process which it often entails, raises very deep questions about what it means to be a person. The encounter with dementia is deeply paradoxical. On the one hand, people involved in caregiving often have a strong intuitive sense that even an individual who is disastrously impaired is still recognizably a person: on the other hand the progress of a dementing illness, especially if it involves a long stay in residential or nursing care, seems to be taking personhood away.

Contradictory impressions such as these invite us to enquire closely into the nature of personhood. What is that state which we might properly call being a person? If we can engage accurately with this question, so tragically neglected in psychiatry and clinical psychology, we may come to find the proper basis for developing a theory of dementia care. Like Gilleard,[10] who has already made some very valuable suggestions on this topic, the core of our position is that personhood should be viewed as essentially social: it refers to the human being in relation to others. But also, it carries essentially ethical connotations: to be a person is to have a certain status, to be worthy of respect. In developing this view briefly here we draw on a large body of theory, much of it derived from work in counselling and psychotherapy.[11] It must be acknowledged that in this field theory often rests on rather fragmentary data, although it is a rich resource for understanding. This is somewhat in contrast to experimental psychology, where theory is often impoverished, but the fit between theory and data is relatively tight.

In the main traditions of the western world, which date from the break-up of feudalism and the theories of the Enlightenment, the term *person* has often come to be taken as having virtually the same meaning as *individual*. This idea is certainly not a cross-cultural universal. Also, it is evident that personhood is not so closely allied to individualism in the development of a single human life. The transformation of a neonate into a being who has the full range of human attributes is very clearly a social process, and not one of simple maturation. An infant exists in a kind of psychological symbiosis with the mother or other main caregiver, and comes to form definite attachments. Out of interaction, and particularly out of those occasions when the infant's gestures meet a sensitive response, selfhood emerges; the infant acquires a sense of agency and an 'inner' subjective world, progressively enriched through the acquisition of language. The greater part of infant and early child development requires the involvement of others, providing subtle support and safety, while giving the 'space' for exploration of both the interpersonal and the physical world. In an ethical sense, personhood is attributed even to the newborn infant. In an empirical sense, personhood emerges in a social context. Thus personhood is not, at first, a property of the individual; rather, it is provided or guaranteed by the presence of others. Putting it another way, relationship comes first, and with it intersubjectivity; the subjectivity of the individual is like a distillate that is collected later.

Sometime in late childhood, perhaps around the age of 8, 9 or 10, and associated with a general concretization of cognition, the basic structure of personality tends to become set. The individual has acquired by this time a set of strategies for dealing with people and situations, a view of the self, a particular array of psychological defences. There is some evidence that this structure tends to persist, being elaborated rather than radically changed as the individual moves into adolescence and adulthood.[12] What was, in the early part of life, fluid, 'held' on the individual's behalf by others, now becomes relatively fixed; or – to use a less favourable image – frozen.

So we have here one crucial parameter of personal being: the construct fluid-frozen. In adult life many people remain, more or less, in the frozen state, maintaining their defences and simply developing resources upon the same basic personality structure. Their subjectivity receives little further nourishment. The frozen state is maintained by various forms of collusion, particularly in organizations, where individuals unwittingly consent to work together in certain very restricted ways, and avoiding any deep intersubjectivity. The frozen state is fostered by extreme individualism, because this both forces a person away from the support of others and requires a reinforcement of defences against anxiety. It is ameliorated just a little by such approaches as 'humanistic management'. When a person remains frozen and unsupported but with heavy demands to deal with, he or she is liable to depression or burn-out. There is some return to fluidity, even if only very partial, in intimate friendship and in sexual love. This is also the case in counselling and psychotherapy. Jung, with his sense of an analogy between alchemy and psychology, took the term analysis in an almost literal sense. It meant a dissolving of the personality, a return to fluidity, so that new ways of being might be developed: a synthesis. Despite the variety of schools of therapy, there seems to be agreement regarding the therapist's own state of being. Those who themselves remain fixed or frozen, their subjectivity limited by highly elaborated defences, will not enable others to become fluid. It is when one person in the dyad is fluid and resourceful that the condition is provided for the other to begin to melt and change. All this may be summed up, as shown below.

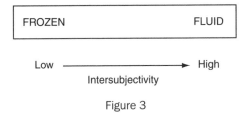

Figure 3

This, however, is not the whole story, for there is another main state of personal being to be included. If we retain the fluid-frozen image, the third state could be described as 'shattered'. It is as if the ice block has been broken up into fragments, but without the melting that could enable a new synthesis. This approximately describes a severe psychotic breakdown. The remarkable fact here, as some of the investigators of psychosis have shown, is that an individual might be desperately alone in the sense of lacking intersubjectivity, and yet be surrounded by others. Their presence, and their contradictory meanings, are a major part of the problem.

So, condensing and simplifying a vast amount of psychological theory, the full contruct has the form shown below.

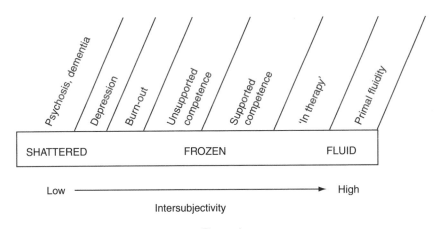

Figure 4

Using this, severe and unattended dementia can be understood as a particular form of the 'shattered' state. With many individuals the neurological insult is resisted for a while, and some of the defences remain intact. Gradually these break down, leaving subjectivity fragmented. Here the dementia sufferer is often dreadfully isolated and unsupported. Maybe it is at this point that many of the more alarming behaviour disturbances are manifested.

Tentatively, also, a general social inference may be drawn. Everyday life continues by maintaining individuals in a relatively frozen state; its way of being positively requires it, even though the cost to personal well-being is immense. A more desirable form of life would be one in which there was vastly more intersubjectivity, and where there would be a continuing opportunity for people to be fluid; or, to alter the image, to grow and change. Our taken-for-granted world, however, is so permeated with the ideology of extreme individualism that this possibility, and the fundamental notion of personhood that underpins it are almost totally obscured.[13]

The preservation of personhood in dementia

In the foregoing brief excursion into the nature of personhood we have, in a sense, brought the dementia sufferer and the 'other' into a single frame. This opens the way for exploring the basis for good caring; or, more broadly, for a way of meeting, of creating an intersubjectivity. Now, however, it is necessary to return specifically to the dementia sufferer, and to make a separation between personhood and cognitive ability. The two have been bound up too closely in western psychological theory, especially of late; its 'hypercognitivism' is something of a disadvantage for a humane understanding of dementia, and needs to be resisted.

Dementia is often presented as a dire condition, a terrible and progressive loss. It is easy to characterise it as a state of continuing and ever-deepening ill-being. This can hardly be disputed if attention is focused on highly developed cognitive powers to the exclusion of other human faculties. There are, however, certain lines of evidence that begin to point in more hopeful directions. Three are particularly significant for our purposes here.

The first comes directly from the care context. It is that some individuals who had seriously deteriorated in all their functioning, including some who had been written off as hopelessly demented, show considerable reversal or 'rementia' when their conditions of life, and especially their social relationships, are changed. The positive changes that are most notable are in the areas of social skill, independence and continence. As social being is recovered, so 'mind' (in some of its aspects) is restored.[14] In our own research on the evaluation of dementia care we have been given many examples of this phenomenon, and in some cases actually met the individuals concerned. There seems to be no reason to doubt the basic truthfulness of care workers' accounts, even when some allowance is made for their humanistic hopes, and their desire to convey a good impression about their work. However, it must be acknowledged that virtually all the evidence that we have on this topic is anecdotal; clearly it is very important for the understanding of dementia that this be put to the test of systematic inquiry.

The second line of evidence concerns the stabilization of some individuals who have been clearly diagnosed as suffering from one of the main degenerative dementias. We ourselves know individuals who are 5–8 years on from the first recognition of their dementia; but, who, in their present care context, are showing no signs of further deterioration, and certainly not moving towards that vegetative condition which is often held out as the inevitable end-point. Again here much of the evidence is anecdotal, but there is now one piece of research in the literature that corroborates this point with systematic data.[15] This is a study comparing two groups, each of 14 dementia sufferers, in residential care. The two groups were comparable in the degree of their dementia, and received roughly the same amount of basic nursing care.

The first group, which occupied a special dementia unit, was given a programme of activities covering about 40 hours per week, whereas the second group was in a traditional form of care, with activities taking up around 3–5 hours per week. Also the first group received a medical and psychiatric check-up weekly, leading, where appropriate, to changes in the programme of care; the second group received only a monthly medical check-up. After one year only 2 of the first group showed signs of further deterioration, whereas 9 from the other group did so. This finding is strengthened by the fact that those in the first group were slightly younger, and the conventional wisdom is that personal decline proceeds more quickly with those for whom the onset of dementia is relatively early. Of course this is only a single study, the time span was short, and the numbers involved are small. The most that can be said at present is that it accords with what many experienced workers in the field of dementia care believe they have observed.

The third line of evidence comes from those experiments with 'geriatric' rats which are occasionally reported, but very rarely interpreted, in the context of writings on dementia. Diamond and her colleagues, in one such study,[16] examined a group of rats, a few right into very old age. Of these, some were put at maturity into exceedingly impoverished and solitary environments. As the rats aged, so did their brains deteriorate (as indicated by conventional post-mortem study). Some of the rats that had been subjected to the impoverished conditions were then transferred to new environments, where there were plenty of activities, and the company of other rats. After a period, their brains appeared to have undergone considerable neurological development. Putting it crudely, then, these experiments show that the brain of a declining geriatric rat can be revived solely through a change in environmental conditions. The rat, of course, is not a human being, and does not (so far as we know) have comparable problems with intersubjectivity. Yet there are great similarities in the nature of the grey matter of rats and humans. It is curious that research of this kind, which provides highly relevant direct evidence about brain structure, is almost totally ignored in the literature on dementia. There can be little doubt that comparable neurological development can occur in the ageing human brain, possibly offsetting in some cases the advance of neuropathology. There is now a little evidence from neurochemical studies with human beings, pointing directly in this direction.[17]

These three lines of evidence, inadequate though they are at present, are crucial for our understanding of dementia and for any theory of dementia care. If some degree of 'rementing' can be brought about purely through human interaction; if some sufferers do stabilize when provided with a care environment that fosters activity and cooperation; if even the ageing and damaged brain is capable of some structural regeneration, then there is ground for looking on dementia care in a very positive way. Caring is certainly much more than giving kindly oversight while witnessing the slow advance of the 'death that leaves the body behind'. Further, the idea of an inevitable progression through four or more 'stages of dementia' – the conventional wisdom that underpins a great deal of care practice and even the design of some residential and nursing homes – must be radically questioned. Of course it is possible to salvage that view by writing off all counter-examples as instances of pseudodementia or faulty diagnosis. It seems likely, though, that as expertise in dementia care advances year by year, such a position will become increasingly untenable.

Relative well-being in dementia

Evidence from the care context, then, is beginning to suggest that a dementing illness is not necessarily a process of inevitable and global deterioration. Close observation provides a far more differentiated picture. Some who have long since reached around zero score on all cognitive tests still appear to be faring well as persons. Others whose cognitive powers are only moderately impaired appear to be faring far less well. A dementing condition tends to be compounded by depression or anxiety, a sense of apathy or disencouragement. It makes good sense, then, to speak of a dementia sufferer as being in a state of relative well-being or ill-being, in a way that cuts across the dimension of cognitive impairment. On the basis of many hours of detailed observation of dementia sufferers in a variety of settings, including those which provide mainly for the very severely demented, we have drawn up a list of 12 indicators of relative well-being; each one stays close to observable behaviour. Informally we have tested the validity of the indicators by consultation with 7 experts in dementia; they have all corroborated our observations, and no further indicators that are clearly identifiable by behaviour have been proffered. The list does not, however, simply have an empirical justification, for behind it lies a conception of well-being that draws on the view of personhood we have already discussed.

The indicators are as follows. Each is illustrated by a brief vignette. Mr D or Mrs D refers to the dementia sufferer; C refers to a caregiver.

1. *The Assertion of Desire or Will*

   Mrs D has had both courses of her evening meal, and has gone to sit down in an armchair. C, not realizing she has had both courses, brings the dessert to her, and tries to feed her. Mrs D says she doesn't want the food: the carer tries to coax her. Mrs D continues to refuse. C desists. Later the truth is discovered.

2. *The Ability to Experience and Express a Range of Emotions (both 'positive' and 'negative')*

   Mrs D is at the day centre. Suddenly she looks exceedingly troubled. A caregiver sits next to her and puts an arm around her. Mrs D collapses into uncontrollable grief and sobbing. C continues to hold her, quietly and patiently. After a quarter of an hour or so Mrs D begins to recover her composure, and soon afterwards is sharing again in the life of the group.

3. *Initiation of Social Contact*

   Mr D has a small dog, a soft toy, which he evidently treasures. He goes over to a women sitting down with her zimmer frame in front of her. He perches the dog on the zimmer frame, and tries to use it to attract her attention.

4. *Affectional Warmth*

   Mrs D lives in large residential home. She often walks back and forth between wings. Whenever someone says hello to her, she stops for a moment to give them a friendly kiss on the cheek, and then continues on her way.

5. *Social Sensitivity*

C is feeling low in spirits, for reasons that have nothing to do with her work situation. Mrs D comes close to her, looks her in the face, and says 'You're not so good today, dear, are you?' C squeezes her hand, and says 'I'm feeling a bit sad, Mrs D, but I'm here.' Mrs D smiles and squeezes C's hand. Somehow Mrs D seems to understand.

6. *Self-Respect*

Mrs D has suddenly defaecated on the floor of the sitting room, in the presence of others, both men and women. She begins to wipe up the mess with her cardigan.

7. *Acceptance of Other Dementia Sufferers*

Mrs D is a vigorous wanderer; she moves fast. She catches hold of the hand of Mr D (not her spouse), who is also wandering, but much more slowly. Mr D accepts the hand and allows himself to be walked around for a while, even though the pace is so different from his own.

8. *Humour*

At the Day Care Centre a video is going to be shown about hygiene in the kitchen. There is a technical problem, and a restless atmosphere is developing. C is fumbling with the apparatus. Mr D calls out, somewhat raucously, 'Try putting a shilling in the slot'. The tension is broken by uproarious laughter.

9. *Creativity and Self-Expression*

There has been a session of singing, with accompaniment from the piano. Now the pianist is tired. Mrs D stands up and sings an old Irish song, in a trembling voice but almost perfectly in tune, and with great depth of feeling. At the end, tears are running down her cheeks.

10. *Showing Evident Pleasure*

It is an exercise event. About 10 people are sitting in a circle, each holding the edge of a parachute. The game is to change places beneath the parachute as it is lifted and slowly falling. Mrs D looks nervous; it is her turn. C helps her to start, and she makes it to her destination. People clap; she smiles and laughs, her face flushed.

11. *Helpfulness*

C, who is new to the job, enters the sitting room. She sees a group of women chatting around the fire. Mr D, who looks very stern, is wandering alone, up and down; he seems not to be showing interest in anyone. C joins the women. As there is no seats nearby, she sits on the floor. Soon afterwards, Mr D comes by with a cushion he has taken from a chair and hands it to her without saying a word.

12. *Relaxation*

Mrs D has a habit of lying on the floor, curled up and tense. Her arms and legs shake and her face is in a grimace. C gently takes her hands and guides her towards a sofa. He invites her to sit with him. In a few moments she has settled down, and cuddles close to him. Her body relaxes and her face becomes calm.

A justification for taking these indicators as marks of relative well-being can be made along two main lines. First, if we consult our own experience, and particularly those times when we sense ourselves to be faring well or ill, the indicators make sense. It is when we feel most discounted, oppressed, withdrawn or low in mood that we are the least likely to show signs such as these; it is when we are confident, buoyant and expansive that we are most likely to show them. There is, of course, some variation according to temperament and personality. For example, individuals differ considerably in the warmth that they generally convey to each other, and in their creative abilities; some find it relatively easy to assert their wishes, whereas others do not. Differences such as these can certainly be found also among those who are cognitively impaired. The indicators, then, are part of the common ground between those who are and who are not dementing. The crucial point is that the indicators are virtually independent of the complex cognitive skills that most adults continuously employ. Thus they are specific to, but not exclusive to, dementia sufferers. Because they are part of our shared experience, they have a face validity; that they are, or can be, present in severely demented persons is an empirical observation.

We may go some way further than this, however, in exploring the nature of well-being in dementia. Behind the observables, it is possible to suggest four apprehensions, or global sentient states, of which the indicators are, to varying degrees, an expression. (It should be noted here that the connections are not empirical, but based, rather, on the inner logic of mental states; ventures in this area are generally abhorred by main-stream psychology).

The first global state is a sense of personal worth, the 'deepest' level of self-esteem. The very fact of ageing almost always involves many losses, and consequent assaults upon an individual's well-being. The experience of beginning to lose cognitive skills, and all the social processes that ensue, is a formidable challenge over and above these common losses. Thus anyone who retains an apprehension of self-worth, and who is able to accept the process of cognitive impairment, can indeed be said to be in a state of relative well-being. Self-esteem is often, in psychological theory, attached to specific cognitions about the self; but it makes good sense to consider it also as a global feeling, of which a person has a diffuse awareness.

The second state that underlies the indicators is a sense of agency; the ability to control personal life in a meaningful way, to produce, to achieve, to make some mark upon others and the world. This is important for people in all stages of life; even, so developmental psychology now suggests, for very young babies. In traditional forms of dementia care an individual's agency tends to be continually diminished. The struggle to maintain it, even at the most rudimentary level, may be intense; perhaps this is how some of the so-called 'challenging behaviours' might be interpreted. So if a dementia sufferer keeps a sense of agency, and manifests this even in the smallest actions, there is good reason to postulate that he or she is in a state of relative well-being.

The third state is one of social confidence; that is, a feeling of being at ease with others, of being able to move towards them, of having something to offer to them. The everyday world, especially in societies that are highly technological and bureaucratic, requires the continual operation of highly-developed cognitive skills. Those in whom these are failing tend to be not only at a practical, but also at a social disadvantage. Again and again their attempts to make contact and to communicate are likely to be disregarded, and the 'malignant social psychology' to which reference has been made comes into play. Anyone who, nevertheless, maintains a sense that the social world is welcoming, and that he or she has a place within it, can be said to be faring well.

The fourth state is that of hope.[18] In other words, a person still retains a confidence that some security will remain even when so many things are changing, both outside and within. There is a freedom from the anxiety that pervades if many basic needs are not met. Hope is, pre-eminently, a sense that the future will be, in some way, 'good'. In many respects the dementia sufferer has little ground for hope; this is doubly the case in the light of the pessimism of prevailing ideology. To retain hope in the face of severe dementia is thus to have overcome huge obstacles. It is worth noting that hope, in the sense used here, need not be tied to specific scenarios about the future, and so require complex cognitive skill. It is nearer to the psychoanalytic concept of 'basic trust'.[19] When this is present a person can relax and the state of the 'free-child' (available to all of us but often kept right in the background) can prevail.

It is along lines such as these that the indicators of well-being receive a rational justification. There is additional support from consideration of ill-being, although this is not the main subject of this paper. Briefly, ill-being in dementia is very frequently observed, and is often taken to be the inevitable concomitant of advancing neuro-pathology. Vegetation, which according to conventional wisdom is the end-point, may be understood psychologically as a state of very severe ill-being: the individual has lost almost all that remained of self-esteem, agency, social confidence and hope, and withdrawn into terminal apathy and despair.

The 12 indicators of relative well-being, then, are both empirically demonstrable and have an underlying rationale. Some or all of them can be shown by persons who are very severely demented. Part of the relevant variability is, no doubt, neurologically based, and part is attributable to personality (in particular, to those psychological reserves that each individual brings to a dementing illness). But considering the vast differences between the behaviour of dementia sufferers in different social environments, there can be little doubt that a considerable part of the variability must be attributed to the quality of care.

The place of the other in dementia care

Persons exist in relationship; interdependence is a necessary condition of being human. Perhaps everyday life would be more fulfilling, and each individual's existence both richer and more secure, if this were widely acknowledged. A consequence would be that people would tend far more towards the psychological state characterised in this paper as fluid. As it is, many people in adulthood strive to create and maintain a sense of well-being without the deep involvement of others; in terms of our metaphor, they remain frozen. Some find fulfilment in a project: an elaborate and self-initiated plan, perhaps grasped initially at a preconscious level, and taking years to complete.

Dementia sufferers, however, are deprived of the consolation of projects, and may not even have the capacity to plan and execute the most basic tasks of daily life. The fact of dependence on others is forced upon them, whether or not it is their will. The Other is not an optional extra, but an absolute necessity. If this is true in the obvious practical matters, it is also true at the psychological level.

Everyday observation of those who are dementing, and involvement in the practicalities of care, shows how crucial it is to recognize this point. It is often the case that a dementia sufferer who is visibly withdrawing, or becoming demoralized, is transformed by a little real attention and human contact. It is as if he or she needs to be re-called to the world of persons, where a place is no longer guaranteed. At such times one or more of the indicators of well-being may be shown, only to fade quickly. Well-being, then, for dementia sufferers, often appears to be fragile and short-lived. Whereas some individuals with the full range of cognitive powers have 'inner' reserves to draw on, or at least well-developed capacities for carrying on in a 'frozen' state, those who are some way into a dementing illness do not. Often they seem to have virtually no reserves, and to be drifting towards the threshold of unbeing. Their personhood needs to be continually replenished, their selfhood continually evoked and reassured.

In some respects, then, a dementia sufferer's shattered state is like that of a very young child, who is in the primal state of fluidity. Early in life personhood is actually being created in relationship; small fragments of truly personal experience gradually coalesce, and a self, with a sense of psychological continuity, is formed. It is a process of development that absolutely needs the Other. Although the caregiver's task is demanding, in certain senses it is not difficult. It is working with a natural direction of growth, and with a given path of neurological maturation; these processes pose no dire threat. The dementia sufferer also needs the Other for personhood to be sustained. However, there are some crucial differences. Here, one might say, the natural and the social are opposing tendencies. The Other is needed, not to work with growth, but to offset degeneration and fragmentation; and the further the dementing process advances, the greater is the need for that 'person-work'. It is as if faculties which were, for a long time, the property of an individual, are now to be made over again to the interpersonal milieu from which they originated. In terms of the metaphor of states of personhood, the self that is shattered in dementia will not naturally coalesce; the Other is needed to hold the fragments together. As subjectivity breaks apart, so intersubjectivity must take over if personhood is to be maintained. At a psychological level, this may be understood as the true agenda for dementia care.

At present we know dementia very largely in a context of relative deprivation. Organizational structure, the type of training and the specification of the role of careworker all tend to require people to operate, very largely, from a 'frozen' state. None of this is specific to dementia care, although it has a particular poignancy here; it simply reflects prevailing patterns of life. From time to time in the minutiae of dementia care work episodes occur which give tiny glimpses of something far better. Already there are some hospital wards, day centres and residential homes which work with a positive and personal philosophy of care, pointing to a radically different form of social being. So a picture is beginning to emerge of what dementia care might be like in a context of psychological abundance, where interdependence is openly acknowledged, and where people exist mainly in a fluid rather than a frozen state. Perhaps, if this became the norm, dementia would not turn out to be such a tragedy, and dementia care not so great a burden. To become frail in some respect is the inescapable lot of many people in later life. To take this up into care practice is simply an acknowledgment of the truth of our vulnerability and interdependence, so often strenuously denied. Thus dementia care need not be a relatively passive attendance upon an elderly man or woman's psychological undoing. Rather, it may become an exemplary model of interpersonal life, an epitome of how to be human.

Notes

1 Kitwood, T., The technical, the personal and the framing of dementia. *Social Behaviour*, 3 (1988), 161–180.
2 See, for example, Shotter, J., *Images of Man in Psychological Research*. Methuen, London, 1975.
3 Menzies Lyth, I., *Containing Anxiety in Organizations*. Free Associations Books, London, 1989.
4 Freire, P., *Cultural Action for Freedom*. Penguin, Harmondsworth, 1972.
5 Kitwood, T., The dialetics of dementia: with particular reference to Alzheimer's disease. *Ageing and Society*, 10 (1990), 177–196.
6 Bredin, K., *A Review of Psycholosocial Interventions in Dementia*. University of Bradford, 1991. Copies available on request.
7 See, for example, Mair, M., *Between Psychology and Psychotherapy: Towards a Poetics of Experience*. Routledge, London, 1989.
8 This term, or rather 'the pathology of normalcy' was coined by Erich Fromm. See Fromm, E., *The Sane Society*. Routledge, London, 1956.
9 See, for example, Gubrium, J. *Old-timers and Alzheimer's: the Descriptive Organization of Senility*. JAI Press, London, 1986.
10 Gilleard, C. Losing One's Mind and Losing One's Place. Address to the British Society of Gerontology, 1989.
11 Kitwood, T. *Concern for Others*. Routledge, London, 1990.
12 Malerstein, A. J. and Ahern, M., *A Piagetian Model of Character Structure*. Human Sciences Press, New York, 1982.
13 Smail, D. *Illusion and Reality*. Dent, London, 1984.
14 Bell, J. and McGregor, I., Living for the moment. *Nursing Times*, 87 (1991), 18, 45–47.
15 Rovner, B., Lucas-Blanstein, J., Folstein M. F. and Smith, S. W., Stability over one year in patients admitted to a nursing home dementia unit. *International Journal of Geriatric Psychiatry*, 5 (1990), 77–82.
16 Diamond, M., The potential of the ageing brain for structural regeneration. In Arie, T. (ed.), *Recent Advances In Psychogeriatrics*, 1. Churchill, London, 1985.
17 Karlsson, I., Brane, G., Melin, E., Nyth, A-L. and Ryko, E. Effects of environmental stimulation on biochemical and psychological variables in dementia. *Acta Psychiatrica Scandinavica* (1988), 207–213.
18 We acknowledge the insight of Mr Ian Mackie, Manager of Northern View Day Hospital, Bradford, in helping to clarify this point.
19 Erik Erikson, in his theory of life-stages, sees the development of basic trust as the first task for the infant. Erikson, E., *Childhood and Society*. Penguin, Harmondsworth, 1965.

2.4

Findings relating to well-being, and findings related to ill-being (1995)

(extract from the Brighter Futures Report)

FINDINGS RELATING TO WELL-BEING

The main findings relating to the measures affecting well-being are described in this section. They are described in an approximate order of statistical significance, with the most significant first. The specific details of the statistics are outlined in Appendix 1.

Social setting

One measure of particular importance is engagement (Felce and Jenkins 1978)[1]. This represents an active and conscious link with the world around. Slumped, half-asleep in a chair is not a state of engagement; on the other hand both reading and talking with another person are. A measure of engagement was derived from the DCM data. Counted as disengaged were categories such as sleeping, sitting doing nothing, unattended distress, wandering around aimlessly and fiddling with things without paying attention. Any form of purposeful action or interaction counted as engaged.

It is important to draw a distinction between engagement and 'doing activity'. All that is required for engagement is that the person's mind is consciously active, or mindful. This can be difficult to observe at times, and it is important, for example, to distinguish between a person looking bored or disinterested on the one hand, and paying attention, looking lost in thought or day-dreaming on the other. 'Doing activity' is often taken as getting a group of people together and everybody taking part in some activity, such as a game or handicraft. This approach is only one way of creating engagement, and is often insufficiently sensitive to be very successful at meeting individual need.

There has been a great deal of work to show that providing a structure and opportunity for interaction does create engagement in people with dementia of all levels of ability (Felce and Jenkins 1979)[2]. It is therefore both possible and crucial that provision is made for a structured day, including planning for activity relating to individual need. When developing this programme, staff need to be sensitive to the normal need for people to have time out, by themselves. This need varies from person to person. However, those who prefer to be by themselves are still likely to benefit from being in a varied and stimulating environment. Some examples could include being able to watch others playing a game, having something to read, watch television, sit in the garden and so on, (depending on individual likes and dislikes). In all cases, however, it is important to avoid letting people withdraw into boredom or apathetic states. An example of this was found in some formal activity arrangements. If they went on too long, residents became bored, and switched off. This happened most often when the facilitators held the activity (and its successful completion), as more important than the relationship and social aspects.

Homes were most effective at providing a structured day when there was a member of staff with direct responsibility for the overall organization of the structure and opportunities for activity. This was especially so when that person had a strong commitment to spending time with people with dementia, and any activities were aimed at stimulating relationships. Prior organization led to a great deal more being achieved in terms of structure and interest. This planning enabled relevant people to make sure the necessary materials and space were available, and know what was expected. This does not mean that the day should be rigid; simply that people are prepared, and that momentum can be maintained.

More exciting and enjoyable days were observable where many of the people in the home were involved: staff, residents and visitors alike. However, it is important to remain clear that every person has different interests, and different social needs. To cater for this, staff need an awareness of each individual's preferences, and to give structure to the day. Activities should be chosen so that they neither go on too long, nor are too similar. Many of the people who were most engaged and confident in group settings were those who had received a good deal of one to one friendship from a group facilitator beforehand. This friendship building often had taken place over several months.

Cognitive ability

There were many examples of people faring well, despite having very damaged cognitive abilities. Well-being can be expressed in many different ways, according to level of cognitive ability; well-being is never taken away simply because of cognitive decline. However, there is a strong link between cognitive impairment and lower well-being. Since expression of well-being is possible regardless of cognitive ability, this suggests that those who are very severely impaired are less able to benefit from the style of care currently available. In order to allow residents choice and control over their own lives, current care styles often leave people to generate their own stimulation and interest. There is an assumption that residents would prefer to use the home as if it were an hotel. However those with very damaged cognitive abilities have lost much of their power for independent action, and therefore are as restricted as those who had to live in very institutional surroundings. The principal finding relating to cognitive ability is, therefore, that staff need to develop ways of enabling choice and control in people's lives, in a way which is sensitive to individual ability. One primary feature of this 'positive choice' is having something to choose from.

Dependency

For those who have forms of physical dependency which isolate (e.g. visual impairment), there is an especial need for help in maintaining contact with the social world. A person who is isolated from social contact is deprived of nourishment for their well-being.

Personality

Well-being is specifically related to two dimensions of personality, openness and conscientiousness. Perhaps surprisingly, extraversion was not a factor influencing either well-being and ill-being.

The person who is open to new experiences is better able to fare well with their changing and confusing circumstances. Those who are less open require the time and patience of others around them when dealing with change. For people who are closed to change, a structured and purposeful day is likely to be particularly important in maintaining well-being. Figure 1 below shows levels of openness and the proportion of people at each level. It is clear that only a few are 'highly open', thus showing many need encouragement and individualised structure to the day.

Conscientiousness reflects a person's 'get up and go', their commitment and sense of responsibility. All of these are important in developing an individual and meaningful life within the home community. Figure 2 illustrates how few people have high levels of conscientiousness, and those who do, are sometimes viewed by staff as interfering, and troublesome.

Relationships

Residents who were in close and regular daily contact with other residents had significantly higher levels of well-being than those who had only superficial relationships,

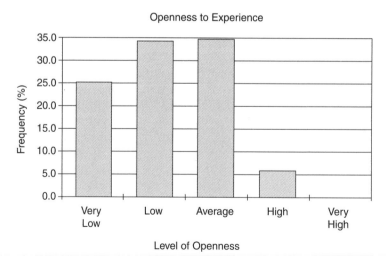

Figure 1

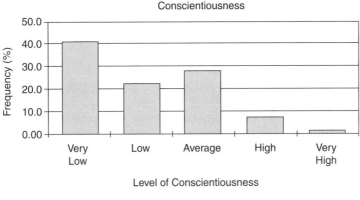

Figure 2

(see Appendix 1). Such contact was better than casual contact, regardless of whether it was close friendship or animosity. It seems, therefore that the crucial factor in maintaining well-being, is for people to have relationships which are felt to be significantly supporting. People who do not have such relationships need help in developing them, by staff and others.

Having someone close significantly increases the quality of a resident's social life, (as measured by the DCM, see Appendix 1). Good relationships between residents are extremely effective in helping people have more sociable and enjoyable days. Encouraging people to form good relationships helps to create a setting in which well-being flourishes.

Quality of social contact

This research suggests that people who have any social contact, regardless of its quality, fare better than those who are isolated and ignored. The relationship between proportion of time in a '+3' state and well-being, not surprisingly, shows that people do have higher well-being if the contact is good. People with dementia need frequent, respectful and interesting contact, though of course it depends on the individual as to exactly what works best. A dangerous state to look out for is when people are doing nothing, or being involved in a fairly minimal way, but there seems to be nothing wrong, ('+1' state). This state is 'well-being, alive but dying'. In short, where there is well-being present, it should be promoted as far as possible. Keeping the person engaged will help promote well-being a great deal. Moreover, if this can include good quality social interaction, there is a strong chance that the person will maintain or improve in their level of well-being.

Staff

Most staff described themselves as being motivated by caring, and pay was rarely cited as a cause of either satisfaction or dissatisfaction. Homes which had staff who had a personal concern for their work had residents with higher levels of well-being.

Several such staff described how they were committed to dementia care, and believed that something could be done for people with dementia. They were willing to learn new ways of caring.

Achieving a high level of commitment and willingness to learn requires a lot of effort. Most importantly the effort comes from each member of staff. This will only happen when there is motivation. Money was rarely named as a major cause of dissatisfaction; however feelings of being restricted at work and lack of support frequently were. Some staff held very high standards for their work and were anxious that they were not performing well enough. They felt they needed more support in finding out how they were doing, and opportunities for personal development.

By improving staff motivation and morale, we can improve the well-being of the residents. To achieve this increase, staff and managers need to focus their attention on the needs of the residents, and managers need to reward good person-centred care. Several approaches to this are now common: Care plans, for instance, encourage personal responsibility and help structure care and the achievement of goals. Another example is personal supervision, which although still viewed with suspicion by many, is increasingly valued by staff.

Much, much more is needed to improve the well-being and morale of staff. If residential settings are to offer a special kind of care for people with dementia, then there should be full recognition that is the staff who will make them special. Senior staff and management have a vital role in developing staff and making the role of carer fun, interesting and rewarding. Obviously, senior staff and management have similar needs for encouragement and motivation.

Physical setting

The data show that measures of physical environment had little relationship with well-being. However, there was a very mild effect relating to the physical amenities measure. The inference is that homes which had facilities such as adequate and accessible toilets, and a decent laundry were more able to enhance the well-being of residents.

No precise measure of lounge size was taken. However, it was evident that the design of the lounge had a considerable effect on the atmosphere in the home. Many lounges were large and public, which hushed conversation and inhibited friendships. In these instances there was a strong pressure to conform to group pressures. A few lounges were too cramped or were awkward, so that residents sat at strange angles, or back to back. Apathy, lack of communication and anger were more common in this type of lounge. The lounges which 'felt best' were only large enough to take everybody sitting facing each other, and have space for wheelchair access. The feeling was like having several friends round to your house and filling the lounge to capacity, but so that no one was cramped. This became impractical after about twelve people. Small group living settings were often designed to achieve this, although they could be too cramped. Occasionally, large communal settings were creatively arranged to create the small, friendly lounge feel.

FINDINGS RELATED TO ILL-BEING

This section, like the well-being section preceding, lists the conditions found to relate to the measure of ill-being. Again the findings are listed in an approximate order of statistical significance, and the actual results may be found in Appendix 1.

Social setting

One of the most important factors which led to increased ill-being was for people to be left unattended, showing signs of ill-being, for long periods of time. This lack of attention, once over thirty minutes, very significantly contributed toward a high state of ill-being. Apathy and loneliness were the most common forms of ill-being observable in those who were left unattended. These findings reinforce the need for frequent individual contact; a guideline would be at least every half hour, with a review to see if some change of activity would be beneficial. Well planned structuring of an individual's day should enable this to happen.

Some homes had a great deal of conflict and mutual disrespect among the residents. The statistics listed in Appendix 1 show that any strong relationships, good or poor will help promote well-being. So, having a row with another resident is better than nothing, but it will promote ill-being too; whereas good social contact will only promote well-being. Often the people with dementia are blamed for causing anger and fights. A common staff response in this situation is to try and get the person with dementia to keep out of the way, and not bother people. This can lead to difficulty in avoiding potential future conflict between the residents. Helping other residents to understand the person with dementia's inability to deal with certain situations could be a much more appropriate response. Promoting a good atmosphere and positive community is an essential part of minimizing ill-being.

Integration with the outside community helps keep ill-being to a minimum. Where there is integration, the home has a higher level of social interest and purpose; the residents feel less trapped, apathetic and abandoned.

There was less ill-being present when residents, as a whole, had more control and influence in the running of their home. The sense of being in control helped them deal with difficult emotional events, and feel more independent and able.

Home policies which encourage staff to leave residents to their own devices should be applied cautiously. It may be helpful to think in terms of two broad categories of people who would rather not be involved. The first are those who like to be in the background of social situations. Such people often prefer to be able to watch interesting things happening. The second group are those who feel too unsafe to join in. This is often, in part, because the atmosphere is insufficiently welcoming and supportive. Staff need to develop skills in facilitating choice. Problems arise when staff offer too much choice, or use complicated language which further confuses the person. Also, each choice needs to be backed up by sufficient support to enable the person to carry out an action. In other words, the person with dementia can only make proper choices after their disabilities have been accounted for through the skill of the staff. Therefore, each person should be considered on an individual basis, and allowance made for differing social contact and dependency needs.

Dependency

Individual dependency varies greatly, and has a direct effect on the extent to which people can generate their own quality of social life. Physical dependency can be extremely crippling, and loss of sight, hearing and language places the individual at great risk of isolation, potentially leading to extreme anger, or withdrawal and despair.

Typically those who are extremely emotionally dependent, (that is needing emotional support from others), become alienated. This is often because others around them become intolerant. Staff intervention frequently takes the form of disaster limitation, keeping the person safe from physical harm. Emotional dependency is often the most reducible of the forms of dependency, but it is also the most time consuming.

Cognitive decline varies greatly in how it affects people. In general, the greater the loss of intellectual ability, the more dependent the person is on others to generate their quality of life. Whatever the nature of the dependency, the role of the staff and those around is to compensate for that dependency so that the person is living at their highest level of independence.

Personality

Neuroticism, agreeableness and conscientiousness were three dimensions of personality which discriminated well between high and low ill-being:

Neuroticism is a tendency to view things in a negative way. People who have high neuroticism scores tend to be more anxious, but also more sensitive and emotional. When, however, there is a setting in which good relationships and support are provided, these people have a great deal to offer; they are able to transcend their state of need and support others.

Agreeableness is basically how easy to get on with, and easy going a person is. Those who are easy to get on with tend to fare better in residential settings. People seen as 'disagreeable' are in fact those who are likely to manage and implement their own ideas (Costa and McCrae 1985)[3]. In the residential setting, such people may find themselves in conflict with organizational rigidity with respect to staff and resident role. Accepting the needs for more control and a sense of responsibility may help reduce the ill-being of many 'disagreeable' people. For example, when arranging things to do, create opportunities for residents to take on some responsibility.

Conscientiousness was described above in the well-being section, and the distribution shown in figure 2. In the context of ill-being, the unconscientious person is at risk of sliding into a state of apathy, and may even want to! Such a person needs a great deal of motivating.

Relationships

The findings relating to relationships and ill-being are far from conclusive, however, by looking at the trends (see Appendix 1), some comment is possible. The statistics suggest that lower levels of ill-being are found among those with good friendships

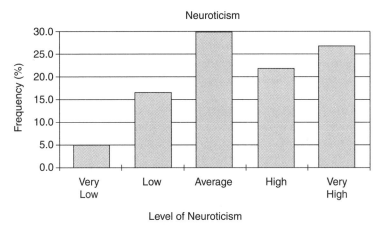

Figure 3

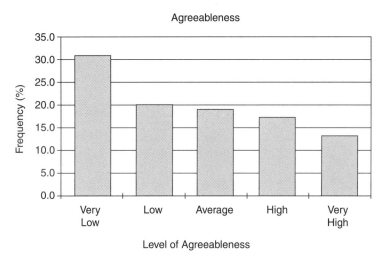

Figure 4

with other residents. Those with frequent, poor quality contact with other residents are likely to have higher levels of ill-being. This finding is somewhat circular as well-being is likely help people develop friends, and ill-being can lead to interpersonal conflict.

The type of relationship a person has with their visitors may have some effect on their overall level of ill-being. Frequent, good quality contact will help promote well-being and minimize ill-being, albeit not significantly. Frequent, poor quality contact will promote ill-being to some extent. The recommendation is, therefore, for staff to promote maximum contact between residents and visitors, while helping with relationships which are distressing, (to the resident).

Staff

Higher levels of ill-being were observable where there was an emphasis on staff routines and procedures. Furthermore staff did not enjoy their work as much where these approaches were used. Where management encouraged staff to act flexibly and creatively in meeting the needs of residents, lower levels of resident ill-being were observable, and staff had greater job satisfaction. One of the main difficulties staff encounter is in trying to meet the needs of residents, and finding themselves in conflict with the needs of routines and physical tasks. Many of these tasks were trivial and unimportant. This was mainly true for those staff who felt that spending time talking or being with residents was a very important part of their work.

Staff who lack confidence either personally or professionally often feel anxious in their work. This can lead to lack of action, sickness, avoidance of residents, and so on. Staff need to be supported in understanding that doing something, especially spending time talking to residents, is better than doing nothing, and that the main aim of their care is to develop good relationships. This approach requires commitment and a continuing willingness to improve. These attitudes are far more important than any formal training.

Physical setting

It is difficult to draw firm conclusions from the information relating to physical setting. This research, however, supports the view that physical design should be such as to enable independently living. Good lighting, easily accessible call systems, clearly marked toilets, etc. may all help to minimize ill-being.

Notes

1   D. Felce and J. Jenkins, *Measuring Client Engagement in Residential Settings for the Elderly* (Research Report No. 20, Wessex RHA, 1978).
2   D. Felce and J. Jenkins, "Engagement in Activities by Old People in Residential Care", *Health and Social Services Journal* 2 (November 1979).
3   P.T. Costa and R.R. McRae, *NEO PI-R Professional Manual* (Psychological Assessment Resources, Inc., Florida, 1985).

2.5

Toward a theory of dementia care: ethics and interaction (1998)

Of all the troubles that come to human beings, dementia is one of the most difficult to face, and one that presents some of the most intractable ethical problems. A person who has dementia is, *ipso facto*, relatively powerless, and may have to endure many kinds of mental anguish: confusion, frustration, grief, fear, anger, and despair. Moreover, the ability to understand what is happening, both within the psyche and in the outside world, may be impaired, and with that the capacity to enter fully and realistically into decisions affecting the course of life. Dementia, then, makes a person exceptionally dependent on others: not only in the physical sense, but in a psychological sense as well. It is from a recognition of this general situation that the ethics of dementia care has emerged as a large and important problem field.[1] The problems requiring ethical scrutiny range from the relatively trivial, such as how to deal with a person's preference for non-nutritious food; through intermediate levels, for example, decisions over driving or the use of potentially dangerous household appliances; and ultimately to the most serious matters of all, such as identifying the conditions under which a person with dementia should be allowed to die.

Even from the standpoint of conventional ethics, the complexities surrounding dementia are compounded by another, and largely unacknowledged fact. It is that we do not really understand the nature of the dementing conditions; even the means for bringing psychological and neurological aspects into a single coherent frame are only beginning to be developed. For many years it has been clear that the deterioration of the person in dementia is not a simple consequence of neuropathology; social and interpersonal factors enter into the process too.[2] Also, and more optimistically, we do not yet know what the course of the main dementing conditions will be when care is of excellent quality. It is now coming to light that some people who have dementia are able to pass right through the territory of rage, paranoia, and depression, and emerge into a trustful serenity that persists despite severe cognitive decline.[3] As yet we do not know how many would be able to make that journey if there were a quantum leap forward in the standards of care, and we have only the vaguest conception of the ultimate neurological constraints. Thus, the ethical problems surrounding dementia are difficult enough in themselves, but huge uncertainties are added because the true nature and course of dementia are unknown.

Much of the emphasis within the ethical discourses of Western culture has been on the question of defining a moral "ought"; and behind that, of providing some kind of rational justification for that ought. It is widely agreed by ethicists that moral judgments should be universalizable: that is, if a certain action is claimed to be right or wrong, the same claim must be made about any other relevantly similar action.[4] There are many difficulties in practice, of course, particularly over the matter of what counts as "relevantly similar," and the related question of what, among all the factors that make individuals or situations unique, might be legitimately ruled out as having no serious bearing on the issue. These matters have a particular poignancy when applied to an ethic of dementia care, where the question of the relevance of cognitive impairment becomes crucial.

Now as soon as we enter into the traditional arena of ethical inquiry, a strange transformation of consciousness occurs. It is as if the ordinary flow of life, in all its detail and infinite complexity, has been stopped. A concern or question has, so to speak, come to the surface and crystallized; it is plain to see, and can be examined in a rational (or, as Nietzsche might have said, an Apollonian) way. The matter may be difficult to resolve, and there may be a clash between the conclusions to be drawn from appeal to different discourses (for example those of Kantian and utilitarian ethics)—but at least it is possible to make a reflective exploration. Should this woman who has fairly severe dementia, and who wanders in the streets at night, be allowed to live on in her own home, as she says she wants? Should this man be subjected to a head scan that might lead to the diagnosis of a treatable condition, when he, in his confusion and fear, categorically refuses? Should this resident, who shouts out loudly and repeatedly, be given sedative medication that will reduce her capacity to live, when this will secure greater calm and well-being for 20 others? When concerns such as these have crystallized, sound conventional ethics requires a deliberation that brings forward all relevant factors, and then the results are taken back into the flow of life.

Now the reality of our day-to-day existence, whether or not in the context of dementia, is that the concerns that come to the surface and crystallize as topics for ethical consideration are relatively rare. For the greater part of the time, the ordinary process of events continues, within a taken-for-granted reality that is supported by taken-for-granted truths. Yet ethical issues are continually present below the surface; they take their form, and then dissolve or disappear subliminally, sometimes in a mere matter of seconds. In many cases when a person comes to experience chronic anxiety, or becomes depressed, the cumulative consequences of subliminal processes come to the surface; then they are usually explored, not within the discourses of ethics, but those of counselling and psychotherapy.

My argument thus far, then, can be summed up in the following way:

1. The greater part of conventional ethics, and particularly clinical ethics, has been concerned with issues that have crystallized, and that require decisions. The key question usually has the form, "What ought we to do?"

2. All decisions take place in a context, whose texture and processes usually remain outside conscious awareness.

3. The context consists mainly of near-to-spontaneous micro-actions and inter-actions, whose flow is rapid and fleeting.

4. Many ethical issues arise within that context, but they are not problematized within conventional ethical theory.

5. If we are to engage with the context as well as the issues that have crystallized, we may need some new kinds of ethical discourse; less static, more comfortable with the flow of everyday life.

So in this article I have two main aims. The first is to offer the rudiments of an "ethic of the context," in relation to the care of people who have dementia; this will serve as complementary to the mainstream of ethical debate, engaging as it does with the question "What ought we to do?" The second aim is more radical, and I shall pursue it very tentatively. It is to suggest that the problem of the context, which becomes so significant in the case of dementia, requires us to look again at the demarcations that Western intellectual culture has created in the last 400 years or so, and particularly at the sharp division between the two main value spheres of ethics and aesthetics. Perhaps new possibilities for understanding the right, the good, the true and the beautiful are emerging, from the unlikely context of psychogeriatrics, with enlightening implications for the rest of humankind.

Glimpses of everyday life

As a preliminary to analysis of the "ethic of the context," let us look at three episodes from the life of people who have dementia, each of whom had (in the short term at least) a positive outcome. Very roughly, they relate to the three main phases of dementia as conventionally defined: mild, moderate, and severe. In each case, for obvious reasons, the names have been changed.

Vignette one

George has had dementia for about 10 years, during which time he has been looked after by his loyal and loving wife, with help from their two daughters and a few friends. George, who had reached a high level in his profession, found it very difficult to cope with his cognitive impairments, at times becoming angry and abusive. He had phases of being bored and apathetic; his health was poor, and he was becoming physically frail. At a time when the situation at home was near to crisis I used to take George on outings, about three hours at a time. Our expeditions had an almost ritual quality: a drive through beautiful country, a pause by a river and a walk out onto the footbridge, a further drive to a café for lunch, and then a slow drive home.

One day, at lunch, the waitress showed us the cake trolley. Speaking rapidly, she proffered her wares: "chocolate cake, flap-jack, coffee cake, fruit loaf, lemon cake, date and walnut slice, Bakewell tart. . . ." George seemed confused; before she had finished he pointed to one item, and said, emphatically, "I'll have this." I myself was feeling somewhat dazed—perhaps in empathy with George. I pointed to an item on the trolley, and said "I'd like date and walnut slice." Now it was the waitress who looked puzzled. She said "But that's cherry and almond tart." I said "Sorry, I'm getting a bit confused. Anyway, that's what I would like."

As we settled to our cakes and coffee, George turned to me and said "That was a clanger, wasn't it?" ["Clanger" is British slang for blunder.—ED.] I agreed that it was. "Don't worry," he said reassuringly, "I'm doing it all the time." We laughed together, and there was a sense of relaxation, goodwill, and closeness between us.

Vignette two

Ethel had been in an assisted-living apartment for some time, but when her dependency became too great for her to continue there, a place was found for her in residential care. She had a very comfortable room, with toilet and bathroom facilities *en suite*. Ethel settled in well, and with her pleasant, sociable personality soon became a popular figure with her fellow residents. A problem, however, was occurring in her room: Each night Ethel urinated on the carpet. When the night staff tried to get her to go to the toilet before she went to bed she refused, sometimes angrily. Each morning the carpet was wet, and soon the room began to smell of urine. Ethel's son Peter, who visited regularly, was very upset at what he found, and complained to the manager of the home. So the efforts to rectify Ethel's toileting behavior were intensified. The staff reminded Ethel repeatedly about the *en suite* facilities, and left the light on in the toilet at night. None of these measures, however, were successful. Some of the staff began to feel deeply resentful. They criticized Ethel for being lazy, and this lowered her morale. The only feasible solution seemed to be to put Ethel into incontinence pads.

One staff member, however, made a crucial observation. This was that Ethel always urinated in the same place, near the head of the bed. He asked Peter to tell him exactly what the arrangements had been in Ethel's former apartment. Peter said that Ethel had had a commode, close by her bed. A commode was provided for Ethel in her new room, and immediately all was well; Ethel used it every night. The "toileting problems" disappeared. The goodwill of staff toward Ethel returned, and with that her social confidence was restored.

Vignette three

May and her sister Dorothy had been admitted into residential care together. May was extremely dependent and demanding, and Dorothy carried the main burden. After Dorothy died this pattern of behavior intensified; also May tended to be extremely rude to staff members, often making abusive remarks such as "You bitch." She also spent long periods shouting out "Help me, help me," in very public places such as the foyer or the lounge. At first some of the staff tried to respond kindly to May, and to discover what she was really asking for; May, however, seemed unable to explain. Others were less sensitive, and made comments such as "If you don't want anything, why do you continually ask for help?" May's behavior was generally perceived as being symptomatic of her dementia, without any attempt at a deeper understanding. Various attempts were made to "modify her behavior," particularly by ignoring her when she was shouting—but to no avail. May came to be disliked by almost everyone.

A small research team was spending time in the home, and they put forward a new hypothesis. Perhaps May's cry of "Help me, help me," really meant something like "Help me to find myself again." If so, she was pleading to be recognized and accepted as a real, unique person, and not asking for anything specific. So members of the research team started to give real attention to May; for example sitting with her, walking with her, and responding when she showed a need for physical contact. Slowly May began to show more signs of self-respect, taking greater interest in her appearance. She became more trusting, and less territorial about her chair. The repetitive shouting gradually subsided. Perhaps most significant of all, she began to call the members of the research team—and only them—by name. So May came to be acknowledged as a real human being, not a "dement," and some staff found that they genuinely liked her. The engaging and loving aspects of May's personality became apparent for all to see.

Each of these vignettes shows something of the actions and interactions that tend to maintain the personhood of people who have dementia; and conversely, of how personhood is undermined. In the case of George the speed with which the waitress proffered the cakes was unnerving. My mistake, however, helped to create a situation of equality. I was able to acknowledge my confusion, and as a result George was no longer a frail old man with dementia being helped by an omni-competent professional; he was simply one human being among others, and secure enough to own his fallibility. In the case of Ethel, she arrived in the residential home with plenty of resources for establishing herself as a social being, but these were being fast undermined as the toiletting problem induced negative reactions from the care staff. The solution turned out to be very simple, and Ethel's standing as a person was restored. In the case of May, her long-established patterns of dependency, compounded with her bereavement, provoked a situation where she was isolated and unpopular, subjected to continual misunderstanding. It was only when her repeated cries were perceived in a different way, and when a serious attempt was made to meet her intense and agonizing need, that positive changes occurred. When May appeared in a different and more attractive light, she began to receive more kindness and affirmation.

In none of these three episodes did issues arise of the kind that might be considered to fall within the range of clinical ethics as usually defined. The vignettes show something of the ordinary course of everyday life; and if other, less satisfactory, outcomes had occurred (for example George being humiliated by the waitress or myself, Ethel being put into incontinence pads, or May being reduced to silence by sedative medication), these outcomes would easily be passed off as part of the mundane reality of care practice. The "ethic of the context" does not involve problems that come to the surface as matters to be resolved by reference to moral principles; rather, it involves decisions that are reached very rapidly and intuitively, implemented without clear conceptualization in the stream of life. There are, of course, points at which ious reflection does occur, as is plain in the vignettes concerning Ethel and May. The mode of this reflection, however, is not ethical, in the traditional sense, and those who engage in it can do so very well without any training in moral philosophy. The mode is that of hermeneutics, whereby actions and utterances are assumed to be meaningful, and an attempt is made to understand them in their historical and concurrent context. George's concept of a "clanger" had resonances throughout the whole of his life, troubled as he was by his inability to do things right; Ethel's pattern of urination did indeed have a meaning, when a serious attempt was made to enter into her frame of reference; May's "Help me, help me," was a sincere and heartfelt plea, not to be taken in a wooden or literal way, but as referring to her entire existential plight. The "ethic of the context," then, is intensely particularistic: it is inseparable from the unique experience and life history of each individual. If any principle is universalizable, it would be this: "Always look for possible meaning in a person's action and utterance, even when it appears to be bizarre, incoherent, or disgusting." In this paradoxical "universalization of the particular," we are a long way from the main concerns of Western ethics.

Interaction in the care of people with dementia

It might be objected that while there can be no doubt concerning the moral significance of the context within which specific ethical issues arise, it is not susceptible to clear conceptualization beyond a general hermeneutic principle. The concern with particularistic aspects of persons and situations takes us into a realm where general theory cannot apply, and the emphasis on the fluid (or, as Nietzsche might have said, the Dionysian) aspects of human life makes rational discourse impossible. I do not believe, however, that this is the case. It is possible to produce a clear and testable account of interaction in dementia care, one in which hermeneutics is given a proper place;[5] this, however, is not our topic here. The crucial point for our discussion is that we can identify the kinds of interaction that maintain personhood, and those that tend to undermine it. The two lists that emerge are complex and many-faceted, but the number of items in each is finite, and the content is highly memorable.

In my own exploration of this topic I have pointed to 10 kinds of interaction that are clearly conducive to the maintenance of personhood and well-being.[6] Each one may or may not involve verbal communication; each is available even when cognitive impairment is severe. Together the 10 items constitute the agenda for what I have termed "positive person work" (PPW), with the implication that when skillfully employed they can do much to mitigate the disablement that so often accompanies the process of dementia. While all of the interactions entail great sensitivity, the last three move into the realm that is usually taken to be that of psychotherapy, where the ability to give free attention, and to accept the emotional processes of another person, are very highly developed. The list is as follows.

Recognition. Here a man or woman who has dementia is being acknowledged as a person, known by name, affirmed in his or her uniqueness. Recognition may be achieved in a simple act of greeting, or in careful listening over a longer period. It is never purely verbal, and it need not involve words at all. One of the profoundest acts of recognition is simply the direct contact of the eyes.

Negotiation. The characteristic feature of this type of interaction is that people who have dementia are being consulted about their preferences, desires, and needs, rather than being conformed to others' assumptions. Much negotiation takes place over simple everyday issues, such as whether a person feels ready to get up, or have a meal, or go outdoors; it takes account of the slower rate at which they handle information. Negotiation gives even highly dependent people some degree of control over the care that they receive, and puts power back into their hands.

Collaboration. Here we gain a glimpse of two or more people aligned on a shared task, with a definite aim in view; as, for example, in doing the same household chores. Less obviously, collaboration can occur in the context of personal care, such as getting dressed, having a bath, or going to the toilet. The hallmark is that care is not something that is "done to" a person who is cast into a passive role; it is a process in which their own initiative and abilities are involved.

Play. Whereas work is directed toward a goal, play, in its purest form, has no external goal. It is simply an exercise in spontaneity and self-expression, an experience that has value in itself. Because of the sheer pressures of survival, and the disciplines of work, many adults have only poorly developed abilities in this area. A good care environment is one that allows these abilities to grow.

Timalation. This term refers to forms of interaction in which the prime modality is sensuous or sensual, without the intervention of concepts and intellectual understanding; for example through aromatherapy and massage. The word itself is a neologism, derived from the Greek word *timao* (I honor, and hence I do not violate personal or moral boundaries) and stimulation (with its connotations of sensory arousal). The significance of this kind of interaction is that it can provide contact, reassurance, and pleasure, while making very few demands. It is thus particularly valuable when cognitive impairment is severe.

Celebration. The ambience here is expansive and convivial. It is not simply a matter of special occasions, but of any moment at which life is experienced as intrinsically joyful. Many people who have dementia, despite their suffering, retain the capacity to celebrate; perhaps it is even enhanced as the burdens of responsibility disappear. Celebration is the form of interaction in which the division between caregiver and cared-for comes nearest to vanishing completely; all are taken up into a similar mood. The ordinary boundaries of ego have become diffuse, and selfhood has expanded. In some mystical traditions, this is the meaning of spirituality.

Relaxation. Of all of the forms of interaction, this is the one that has the lowest level of intensity, and probably also the slowest pace. It is possible, of course, to relax in solitude, but many people with dementia, with their particularly strong social needs, are only able to relax when others are near them, or are in actual bodily contact.

Validation. This term has a long history in psychotherapeutic work; going back some time before it became widely used in the care of persons with dementia.[7] The literal meaning is to make strong or robust; to validate the experience of another is to accept the reality and power of that experience, and hence its "subjective truth." The heart of the matter is acknowledging the reality of a person's emotions and feelings, and giving a response on the feeling level. Validation involves a high degree of empathy, attempting to understand a person's entire frame of reference, even if it is chaotic or paranoid, or filled with hallucinations.

Holding. This, of course, is a metaphor, derived from the physical holding of a child who is in distress. To hold, in a psychological sense, means to provide a safe psychological space, a "container"; here hidden trauma and conflict can be brought out; areas of extreme vulnerability exposed. When the holding is secure a person can know, in experience, that devastating emotions such as abject terror or overwhelming grief will pass, and not cause the psyche to disintegrate. Even violent anger or destructive rage, directed for a while at the person who is doing the holding, will not drive that person away. As in the case of childcare, psychological holding in any context may involve physical holding too.

Facilitation. At its simplest, this means enabling a person to do what otherwise he or she would not be able to do, by providing those parts of the action—and only those—that are missing. The most facilitative interaction occurs when a person's sense of agency has been seriously depleted, or when action schemata [learned sequences of intentional body movements] have largely fallen apart. Perhaps all that is left is a hesitant move toward an action, or an elementary gesture. The task now is to enable interaction to get started, to amplify it and to help the person gradually to fill it out with meaning. When this is done well, there is a great sensitivity to the possible meanings in a person's movements, and interaction proceeds at a speed that is slow enough to allow meaning to develop.

Besides those interactions that are generated primarily by caregivers, a positive environment involves at least two kinds of interaction in which the initiative is taken by the person who has dementia; the caregiver must be open and humble enough to appreciate and to receive from one whose cognitions are impaired. The two main types of interaction are as follows:

Creation. Here a person with dementia spontaneously offers something to the social setting, from his or her stock of ability and social skill. Two common examples are beginning to sing or dance, with an invitation to others to join in.

Giving. Here the person with dementia expresses concern, affection, or gratitude, makes an offer of help, or presents a gift. Sometimes there is great sensitivity to the moods and feelings of caregivers, and a warmth and sincerity that puts the ordinary, rather frigid and intellectualized atmosphere of bourgeois culture to shame.

Furthermore, in those contexts where personhood is well sustained, there are many interactions between the people who have dementia, without caregivers' intervention: giving mutual help, forming and sustaining relationships, sharing enjoyable pastimes. In some of these interactions the verbal content may appear nonsensical; possibly it serves mainly as an ornamentation, while the really significant communication is at a non-verbal level.

On the darker side, I have identified 17 kinds of interaction that contribute to the undermining of personhood. Together they may be regarded as constituting a "malignant social psychology" (MSP). The word "malignant" has been chosen deliberately, to suggest a powerful, insidious, destructive effect—a cancer of the interpersonal environment. The word malignant does not, however imply malice. MSP proceeds more commonly from ignorance, preoccupation, or overbusyness, and it is part of a deeply embedded cultural tradition; the bad practice that springs from active ill-will is relatively rare. Since MSP has been discussed in detail elsewhere, the items are presented in extremely brief summary here.[8]

Treachery. Using some form of deception in order to distract or manipulate a person, or force them into compliance.

Disempowerment. Not allowing a person to use the abilities that they do have; failing to help them to complete actions that they have initiated.

Infantilization. Treating a person very patronizingly (or "matronizingly"), as a parent who is insensitive or insecure might treat a very young child.

Intimidation. Inducing fear in a person, through the use of threats or physical power.

Labelling. Using a pattern of behavior (for example, "smearer," "stripper") or a category such as "organic mental disorder," as the main basis for describing and interacting with a person.

Stigmatization. Treating a person as if they were a diseased object, an alien, or an outcast.

Outpacing. Providing information, presenting choices, and so on, at a rate too fast for a person to understand; putting them under pressure to do things more rapidly than they can bear.

Invalidation. Failing to acknowledge the subjective reality of a person's experience, and especially what they are feeling.

Banishment. Sending a person away, or excluding them; physically or psychologically.

Objectification. Treating a person as if they were a lump of dead matter; to be pushed, lifted, filled, pumped, or drained, without proper reference to the fact that they are sentient beings.

Ignoring. Carrying on (in conversation or action) in the presence of a person as if they were not there.

Imposition. Forcing a person to do something, overriding desire or denying the possibility of choice on their part.

Withholding. Refusing to give asked for attention, or to meet an evident need; for example, for affectionate contact.

Accusation. Blaming a person for actions or failures of action that arise from their lack of ability, or their misunderstanding of the situation.

Disruption. Roughly intruding on a person's action or inaction; crudely breaking their "frame of reference."

Mockery. Making fun of a person's "strange" actions or remarks; teasing, humiliating, making jokes at their expense.

Disparagement. Telling a person that they are incompetent, useless, worthless, and the like; giving them messages that are damaging to their self-esteem.

The vignettes given earlier in this article provide some examples of the two main types of interaction. In the first one, George was *outpaced* by the waitress, but the episode ended in *celebration* and *relaxation*. In the second, Ethel's toileting problem led to several kinds of MSP, including *labelling, accusation,* and *disparagement*. All, however, ended well, with *facilitation* and *collaboration*. In the third vignette, May was subjected to *ignoring, withholding,* and *banishment* (at the very least); the breakthrough came when she was accorded *recognition* and *validation*; at this point she was able to offer her helpers a priceless gift in calling them by name.

I would not claim that either of the two lists is exhaustive, although the latter (that of MSP) has had longer to mature. A few more items may be added to either one as experience grows. The argument here is not over detail; it is simply to demonstrate that the "ethic of the context" is not merely to be considered an *ethos* or *zeitgeist*, vague and insubstantial. Rather, it has clear content, which can be defined. Moreover, although we cannot follow the main line of ethical theory and attempt to specify right actions, it is at least possible to specify a form of good. A good care environment is one in which there is an abundance and variety of positive person work, and rich inter-actions among the people who have dementia; it is also free of malignant social psychology. A bad care environment is one where there are vast deserts of neglect, and where the malignancy that I have described has taken hold. Moreover, through a detailed observational method, such as Dementia Care Mapping, the goodness or badness of a care environment can be very roughly measured.[9] We are in an empirical domain.

The "ethic of the context," as lived, is very largely subliminal; most of the time it exists below the threshold of awareness. With careworkers who have followed the old traditions, and for whom MSP is part of the taken-for-granted world, it is often very difficult to bring about a conscious realization. Perhaps there are psychological defenses keeping difficult issues out of the experiential frame and holding "malignant" patterns of practice in place. The psyche of a really good careworker, however, seems to have a very different structure. The defenses are relatively low, and any episode can, if necessary, be brought forward for detailed and unprejudiced examination. Our aim, then, in educating careworkers is that they should engage in PPW "naturally" and in all that they do, including even the most mundane physical tasks, and, conversely, that they should be so sensitized to MSP that they have no part in it, and hold a strong commitment to its total elimination. In summary, then, the "ethic of the context" is such as to be available for reflective scrutiny, and primarily in the hermeneutic mode; but it functions at its best when interaction is relaxed, spontaneous, graceful, flexible, and assured.

The moral domain

The idea of an "ethic of the context" does, of course, apply to every kind of social setting. It simply has a particular poignancy in the case of the care of people who have dementia, because they are extremely vulnerable, and their well-being is crucially dependent on the interactions that are generated by others. So at this point we might inquire into the broader relevance of our topic. What are the general implications for the way in which we construct our ethics? The following discussion draws, in some respects, on arguments I have already brought forward.[10]

If we look at the growth of moral thinking from a historical and sociological standpoint, it soon becomes apparent that behind the abstractions of theory there usually lies a critique of existing social structures or social practices, particularly in relation to problems of power and opportunity. Morality is a meta-game (a reflective critique) upon existing mores.[11]

In Europe, during the 17th and 18th centuries, ethical theory was articulated in many new ways, and its particular concern was with what might be termed "structured domination," much of it built into social practices. There was a widespread concern to create new forms of society, free from feudalism and arbitrary privilege, justifiable on a rational basis. Each of the major discourses that emerged during this period—that of rights, that of obligations, and that of maximizing a social good—engaged in some way with this concern. Thus any human collective, whether as small as a family or as large as a nation state, might be considered as having some place on a dimension of domination (see figure 1).

Domination

High ———————————————— Low

Figure 1

Some time after these attempts to create new forms of rational ethics, another problem began to come to the surface in European culture. It first found a clear voice in Romanticism, and then to some extent in new approaches to the treatment of mental distress through hypnotism and suggestion. The issues were clarified around the turn of the 20th century, with the emergence of psychoanalysis, psycho-drama, and psychotherapy. Although there was great diversity both in theory and in practice, the central postulate was widely shared. It was that many people carry noxious memories, hidden griefs, unresolved conflicts, below-consciousness aware-ness, that create obstacles or damage to the way they live their lives. Each therapy, in its own way, was designed to promote a greater degree of psychic integration, so that a person might have an authentic emotional life, and experience more accur-ately what he or she is undergoing. The general project, then, might be summed up as that of helping a person to move forward along a dimension of expressivity (see figure 2).

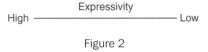

Expressivity

High ———————————————— Low

Figure 2

What happens when we bring these two areas of concern—that of the moral theorists and that of the psychotherapists—together? We can do this by treating dom-ination and expressivity as orthogonal axes, and looking at the four quadrants that are then created (see figure 3).

The first quadrant represents social settings where both domination and expres-sivity are high. This is epitomized in those situations where gross brutality prevails; where pillage, rape, torture, and even genocide form the everyday reality. The only right is that of might. It is against such a state of affairs that moralists throughout history have made their protest, hoping that an appeal to divine law or to human reason will carry conviction.

The second quadrant shows high domination combined with low expressivity. This is the state of affairs in feudal and colonial societies, for example, where people consent to some degree of oppression; where life is at least stable, and extremes of scarcity are avoided. Morality here often includes ideas of rights and duties that follow from social roles, but which avoid detailed engagement with particular issues. When domination is strong and the social order is very settled, the situation may be like a

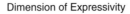

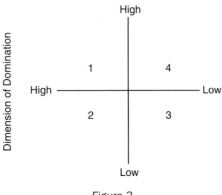

Figure 3

time-bomb, because huge resentments lie buried, and when these eventually come to the surface anarchy and terror ensue—as witness the end of colonial rule in many parts of Africa.

The third quadrant, where both domination and expressivity are low, seems to represent the state of affairs to which the greater part of Western ethical theory has pointed, and which a few liberal democracies have, to some extent, attained. As with quadrant 2, individuals are implicitly assumed to be orderly and restrained in negotiating their interests or in asserting their rights. The general project is that of creating a social order that is grounded in a universalistic ethic; but there is a relative ignorance of the expressive dimension, a failure to engage with the life of the emotions.

So we come to the fourth quadrant: where domination is low and expressivity is high. Here, it might be said, the ideals both of the moralists and of the psychotherapists converge. Generally speaking, this type of social situation has not been well theorized, even by those ethicists who have continued with the moral project of the Enlightenment in recent years: for example Rawls, in his general theory of justice.[12] Possibly the best exemplars are some of the primal societies, where strong norms existed against self-aggrandizement or the accumulation of personal possessions, and where conflict and tension were quickly resolved in the ordinary course of daily life. In Africa the Kung people of the Kalahari, or the Mbuti people of the central rain forest, seem to have had societies of this type.[13] The contemporary world has only, thus far, succeeded in creating settings with low domination and high expressivity on a very small scale, existing in the interstices of a larger social order.

This analysis, which I have offered in a general and sociological way, has great relevance to our original topic: the care of people with dementia. In the darkest days of institutional confinement, during the 16th and 17th centuries, the social setting often approximated to quadrant 1. People with mental infirmities were subjected to gross cruelty and neglect; some of the population saw their suffering as a kind of entertainment—an alternative to going to watch a hanging. The moral reforms of the 19th century might be seen as an attempt to create the kind of situation represented by quadrant 2. At least there was a social order, even if intensely paternalistic and maintained by imposed discipline. Much later, and through to the present day, the use of sedative medication provided an added stability, and a low level of expressivity could be assured. Recently, there have been many moves to make care regimes more egalitarian, approximating quadrant 3, where both domination and expressivity are low; the rhetoric of patients' rights has provided a powerful legitimation of these moves.

Situations patterned on quadrant 3 can be achieved, at least to a degree, in some rather repressed industrialized societies. They are, however, incapable of long-term realization in settings that serve to care for persons with dementia.

The necessary conditions of equality and respect require that each person be enabled to make the fullest possible use of his or her mental capacities (hence—plenty of stimulation, a variety of occupations, and no control by sedatives). When people who have dementia are given this opportunity, however, they usually recover their individuality and powers of self-assertion; their social life becomes vividly alive. The providers of care then have two main options. In fear of chaos they can re-establish a repressive regime, using chemicals to numb dissidents into silence; alternatively, they can allow the situation to develop, so that it resembles quadrant 4.

The remarkable discovery, repeated now by many practitioners, is that when the latter course is taken, chaos does not ensue. A new kind of social order comes into being and then stabilizes, almost as if it were a natural or instinctive form of human life.[14] It is full of energy; highly interactive; very sincere, accepting, and forgiving. This is not, of course, a panacea. Suffering and conflict may be more in evidence than in the over-controlled regimes. The difference is that pains and problems are dealt with openly; then they can be faced, and the necessary help provided. In this general climate of respect for persons in their uniqueness, it is only rarely that administrators have to become utilitarians, and compromise the well-being of one person for the sake of a common good. When they do so, they can more easily accept the feelings of guilt and dissonance; they recognize what they are doing.

Implications for ethics

The schema of ethical situations that I have used in this article, expressed in terms of domination and expressivity, has hints of a historical progression. There is, however, no suggestion (*pace* Hobbes and Freud) that the original state of homo sapiens was that of an anarchic horde. Quadrant 4 is the most problematic, because we know it as yet in such a fragmentary way, and the primal societies that to some extent resembled it have vanished from the earth. It is, however, the situation of low domination and high expressivity that holds out the greatest hope for humankind. Furthermore it is here that ethics, as constructed in the Western cultural tradition, comes most seriously into question.

It is clear, above all else, that as we move into the fourth quadrant, the "ethic of the context" can no longer be ignored. As soon as expressivity is clearly on the agenda, attention must be given to the flow of life, and not merely to those issues that crystallize for scrutiny in a static, reflective way. The encouraging thing for ethics is that we can understand something about the nature of everyday interaction, and become morally engaged with process.

As soon as that is done, however, a time-honored assumption begins to be challenged. This is the idea that we can demarcate two spheres of value—those of ethics and aesthetics—each with its own distinct form of rationality. We have looked at some of the kinds of interaction that serve to maintain personhood, and those that tend to undermine it, and on this basis it is possible to characterize a form of social life that is good. There can be no doubt that we are dealing here with some kind of practical morality. But each of the interactions has also an aesthetic dimension that forms a necessary part, and not a merely contingent accompaniment. Whether it is helping a person to go to the toilet (*collaboration*) sharing in the festivities of a Christmas meal (*celebration*), or providing some powerful form of comfort and reassurance (*holding*), the manner in which these things are done is of the essence. We might also note the close affinity between Stanislavsky's ideas about authentic acting and a depth-psychological approach to care: in both there is an emphasis on total sincerity, on being set free from the limitations imposed by ego, and drawing freely and fluently on one's emotional resources.[15] Care work done by deliberate reference to a code of practical morality would be as inept as the imitative, wooden manner of acting that Stanislavsky so strongly opposed.

Why, then, was the idea of two separate spheres of value so widely accepted, from the time of Kant through to the present day? One reason, almost certainly, is that philosophers have had such a resolute commitment to the Apollonian mode, and such a deadly fear of the Dionysian. Human interaction was never carefully problematized by moral theorists; for the majority it wasn't even on the agenda. Once we do so, the significance of traditional ethics, with its concern for principle and universalizability, becomes relativized, and it looks as if its discourses might need fundamental renovation. The best dementia care is, paradoxically, a paradigm for human life. The excellent caregiver is, so to speak, a moral artist, and sets an example to all of us as we search for the right and the good.

Acknowledgment

Vignette two was supplied by Roy Edward, and vignette three by Brenda Walker. I would like to thank them both for contributing to this article this way.

Notes

1 S.G. Post, *The Moral Challenges of Alzheimer's Disease* (Baltimore, Md.: Johns Hopkins, 1996).
2 T. Barnes, J. Sack, and J. Shore, "Guidelines to Treatment Approaches," *Gerontologist* 13 (1973): 513–27; T. Kitwood, "The Dialectics of Dementia: With Particular Reference to Alzheimer's Disease," *Ageing and Society* 10 (1990): 177–96.
3 T. Kitwood, "Positive Long-Term Changes in Dementia: Some Preliminary Observations," *Journal of Mental Health* 4 (1995): 133–44.
4 J.L. Mackie, *Ethics* (Harmondsworth, England: Penguin, 1977).
5 T. Kitwood, "Towards a Theory of Dementia Care: The Interpersonal Process," *Ageing and Society* 13 (1993): 51–67.
6 T. Kitwood, *Dementia Reconsidered: The Person Comes First* (Buckingham, England: Open University Press, 1997).

7   N. Feil, *The Validation Breakthrough* (Baltimore, Md.: Health Professionals Press, 1993).

8   T. Kitwood, ed., *Evaluating Dementia Care: The DCM Method*, 7th ed. (West Yorkshire, England: Bradford Dementia Group, 1997).

9   Ibid.

10   T. Kitwood, *Concern for Others* (London: Routledge, 1990).

11   D. Wright, *The Psychology of Moral Behavior* (Harmondsworth, England: Penguin, 1971).

12   J. Rawls, *A Theory of Justice* (Oxford, England: Oxford University Press, 1972).

13   C. Turnbull, *The Forest People* (London: Paladin, 1961).

14   J. Bell and I. McGregor, "Living for the Moment," *Nursing Times* 87, no. 18 (1991): 46–47; J. Tooth, "A View from Australia," *Journal of Dementia Care* 5, no. 2 (1997): 12–13.

15   T. Kitwood, "Lowering our Defenses by Playing the Part," *Journal of Dementia Care* 2, no. 5 (1994): 12–14; D. Margashack, ed., *Stanislausky on the Art of the Stage* (London: Faber, 1961).

Part 3

PERSONHOOD

Personhood

Co-authored with Alison Phinney, Barbara Purves, Deborah O'Connor and Habib Chaudhury of the Center for Research on Personhood in Dementia, Vancouver, and Ruth Bartlett, Bradford Dementia Group.

Readings

Kitwood, T. (1970) The Christian understanding of man, in *What is Human?* London: Inter-Varsity Press.

Kitwood, T. (1993) Towards a theory of dementia care: the interpersonal process, *Ageing and Society*, 13(1): 51–67.

Kitwood, T. (1994) The concept of personhood and its relevance for a new culture of dementia care. In Jones, G. and Miesen, B. (eds) *Caregiving in Dementia*. London: Routledge.

Kitwood, T. (1997) Personhood, dementia and dementia care. In Hunter, S. (ed.) *Research Highlights in Social Work*. London: Jessica Kingsley.

Kitwood, T. (1997) On being a person, in *Dementia Reconsidered: The person comes first*. Buckingham: Open University Press.

Critical commentary

Central to Kitwood's work on dementia is the concept of 'personhood', as the maintenance and promotion of personhood form the primary aim of 'person-centred care' (see Kitwood 1997a). For Kitwood, the conceptualization of personhood was more than an academic, philosophical debate as the stance taken on this issue had serious implications for practice. Indeed, in developing his theory of personhood, Kitwood explicitly stated that any such theory should 'shed light on the psychological predicament of people who have dementia and suggest what they might need . . . [and] . . . it should be able to tell us something about the nature and meaning of good dementia care' (Kitwood 1997b: 14/237). For Kitwood, then, the work of developing a theory and model of personhood and person-centred care were inextricably woven together, each informing the other (praxis).

In this chapter we shall explore Kitwood's (albeit, we shall argue, incomplete) theory of personhood. In so doing we will explore some of the possibilities that this re-theorization of personhood opened up, the religious roots of the theory and highlight some of the criticisms that have been made of Kitwood's view of personhood. In conclusion, we shall suggest and briefly explore some of the work that we think needs to be done in order to more fully understand 'personhood', especially in regard to people living with dementia. We will, no doubt, raise more questions than we could possibly answer within the confines of a single chapter – indeed, this is our intention – and readers expecting a fully articulated theory of personhood will inevitably be disappointed, as Kitwood was still developing and articulating his theory of personhood prior to his untimely death. We hope, however, that readers willing to be stimulated, challenged or even provoked into taking up some of the issues raised will find the chapter a useful starting point for their own ongoing reflection.

A note on personhood

The concept of personhood has been, and still is, highly debated in philosophical circles (see for example Fleischer 1999; Kittay 2005). The interest in personhood lies partly in a desire for self-definition – a partial answer to the question of 'Who am I?' – and partly in the guidance that any answer might give for moral action – an answer to the question, 'How am I to treat others and be treated by others?'

The question, 'What is a person?', is an exercise is setting boundaries. By definition there will be those who fall within and those that fall outside those boundaries – that is, there are persons and non-persons. The implication that follows from this definitional exercise is that it is permissible to treat non-persons differently (that is, usually, less well) than we do persons. The framing and answering of these questions take different forms in different discourses – for example, personhood as legally defined might be very different from personhood as ethically or psychologically defined – and also within discourses – for example, compare the differing views of personhood held by ethicists Dan Brock (1993) and Stephen Post (1995). We shall return to competing views of personhood later. For now it is enough to recognize that Kitwood was aware of differences in discourses and the 'personhood' they produced (see later) and attempted to combine insights from different discourses into a more complete theory of personhood.

Kitwood's theory of personhood

Although personhood forms the basis for person-centred care, it was not until the mid-1990s that Kitwood actually started to draw together and articulate a relatively cohesive theory of personhood to underpin developments in person-centred care. In so doing, Kitwood conflated the notions of metaphysical personhood (personhood as a purely descriptive category) and moral personhood, that is, the moral standing of those who are defined, metaphysically as persons. (For a discussion of metaphysical and moral personhood, see Beauchamp 1999.) In other words, Kitwood's definition of personhood stemmed not from an abstract philosophical analysis as to the nature of personhood (regardless of whether personhood brought with it moral standing or not) but from his prior view that people living with dementia were, per se, of moral standing and that any definition of personhood had to include people with dementia.

For Kitwood, personhood lies at the meeting point between three discourses: transcendence, ethics and social psychology (Kitwood 1997a). From the discourse of transcendence he takes the idea of being-in-itself, a sense that life is sacred; from ethics, the Kantian principle that persons should always be treated as ends in themselves and never as means to some other ends; and from social psychology, an understanding that individuals exist within a network of relationships.

While the first two of these are basically taken for granted in Kitwood's theory, he does explore what would be required of a suitable theory of personhood at the social psychological level, laying out seven criteria (Kitwood 1997b). For Kitwood, any theory of personhood must:

1   be reflexive: 'the categories that are used to describe or explain one group of people (in this case, those who have dementia) must be applicable in principle to the "professionals" who use them' (p.13/236)
2   view the person as a social being
3   be developmental, showing how people can change, for good or ill, throughout the lifespan
4   bring out some of the most relevant psychological differences between people
5   be compatible with what neuroscience tells us about how the brain develops and functions both in health and disease
6   shed light on the psychological predicament of people with dementia and suggest what they might need
7   be able to tell us something about the nature and meaning of good dementia care.

The model of the person that Kitwood then goes on to sketch out focuses on the social psychological discourse, attempting to bring together symbolic interactionism and depth psychology (Kitwood 1997a, 1997b). In attempting this, Kitwood argues that there are two aspects to the person: the 'adapted self' and the 'experiential self', the former referring to the socialized aspect of being and the performance of given roles, the latter to relations based on equality, mutual attention and mutual respect. The details of these two aspects can be found in the 'Readings' section (Kitwood 1997).

A further step in the development of a theory of personhood was then to link the experiential self with Buber's notion of 'I–Thou' relationships: to be a person is to be addressed as Thou (Kitwood 1994) and that 'I–Thou', relationships are predicated on self-disclosure and spontaneity with meetings between Thous based on openness, tenderness, presence (being in the present) and awareness. Such relationships are in contrast to 'I–It' relationships that imply coolness, detachment and instrumentality. In making this association, Kitwood implies a recursive link to the Kantian notion of persons as ends in themselves and fulfils his own requirement that a theory of personhood view the person as a social being.

Kitwood thus arrives at his, now famous, definition of personhood: 'It [personhood] is a standing or status that is bestowed upon one human being, by others, in the context of relationship and social being. It implies recognition, respect and trust' (Kitwood 1997a: 8/246).

While Kitwood acknowledges that the above theory is but a sketch and that much more could be said, it does constitute the most comprehensive outline that he developed before his death. It is thus this theory that we have to work with, criticize and move forward. Before embarking on a critique of Kitwood's theory of personhood, it is helpful to explore the possibilities opened up by this view of the person.

Possibilities

In the debates about personhood, there are, roughly speaking, two camps: those who believe that individuals are persons because of some capacity or capacities they possess and those who contend that being human is the same as, or at least equivalent to, being a person. This debate is sometimes described as one between personalism and physicalism or vitalism (see Fleischer 1999). For those in the personalist camp there is a distinction to be made between the human being (a descriptive term signifying belonging to a particular species) and personhood (an evaluative term signifying and granting membership to a moral community). In these terms, it is possible to be human but not granted moral status. Similarly, some would argue that it is possible to be non-human but granted moral status.

For those in the physicalist or vitalist camp, a focus on capacities requisite for being granted the status of personhood is too narrow in that it, by definition, excludes those who cannot 'measure up' and also takes too narrow a view of what it means to be human. For example, Stephen Post criticizes traditional bioethics on the grounds that in focusing on cognitive capacity it both excludes people with dementia and fails to recognize the importance of the affective aspects of being human (see Post 1995).

When Kitwood was developing his theory of personhood the debate was dominated by those in the personalist camp.[1] At that time, influential ethicists and authors such as Dan Brock were arguing strongly for a capacity and interest-based view of personhood that explicitly denied the personhood of people with dementia:

> I believe that the severely demented, while of course remaining members of the human species, approach more closely the condition of animals than normal humans in their psychological capacities. In some respects the severely demented are even worse off than animals such as dogs and horses, who have a capacity for integrated and goal-directed behaviour that the severely demented substantially lack. The dementia that destroys memory in the severely demented destroys their psychological capacities to forge links across time that establish a sense of personal identity across time. Hence, they lack personhood. (Brock 1993: 372–3)[2]

Kitwood's work on personhood and person-centred care clearly and accessibly challenged the biomedical, capacity-based view of the loss of personhood with the onset and advance of dementia (see Kitwood 1990a; Kitwood 1993a, 1993d; Kitwood and Benson 1995; Kitwood and Bredin 1992a). This view of the self remaining throughout the progression of dementia is becoming far more established:

> There is growing empirical research which affirms that people with dementia retain a sense of self despite cognitive impairment. Mills and Coleman (1994), using coun-

selling skills and reminiscence work, present case study evidence that personal awareness of an individual self remains. 'Dementia may fragment the personality of the sufferer, but the personal awareness of individual uniqueness of being remains until death' (Mills and Coleman 1994: 213). Sabat and Harré (1992) present an account of the construction and deconstruction of self through the late stages of Alzheimer's disease. Based on interviews with and observations of three people with dementia, they argue that one's private sense of self persists into the late stages of the illness, and that the loss of self commonly attributed to the disease process is the loss of the public or social self, which they attribute to how others respond to and treat the person with dementia. Their research provides some empirical basis for the less empirically-based assertions of Kitwood. (Downs 1997: 599)

A second possibility opened up by Kitwood's reformulation of personhood was that of engaging with people with dementia in order to understand that lived experience. Following research into the abilities of people living with dementia to express their views and preferences with regard to research and service design and evaluation it is now generally unacceptable to exclude them (see Downs 1997). Indeed, people with dementia are to be assumed to have capacity unless judged otherwise on a decision-by-decision basis, according to the Mental Capacity Act 2005 and all practicable efforts are to be made to elicit the views and preferences of the person living with dementia (Mental Capacity Act 2005). The literature on dementia is increasingly populated with works on eliciting the experience of people living with dementia and engaging them in matters that concern their care and well-being (see, for example, Downs 1997; Goldsmith 1996; Wilkinson 2002).

A third potentiality in Kitwood's theory of personhood is that it forms a productive framework for exploring the social interaction of persons with dementia and their carers (Hamilton 2005). His inclusion of criteria from social psychology, in particular his insistence on reflexivity, the relational basis of personhood and the psychological predicament of people with dementia, is consistent with the theoretical stance of interactional sociolinguistics, that is, that meanings are created through social interaction. It is not surprising, then, to find Kitwood's theory of personhood cited in various studies of conversations with people with dementia (for example, Müller and Guendouzi 2005; Sabat 2001; Small et al. 1998). The possibilities of conversation as care within Kitwood's theory of personhood have also been explored by Ryan and colleagues through an examination of person-centred interactions in recorded conversations between people with dementia and their carers:

As person-centred conversations lead to reciprocity, contributions on the part of the person with dementia are also shown. The real value of positive care interactions is that they reinforce the position that individuals with dementia, even those who are in the more advanced stages, retain communicative competence and are active contributors to interpersonal relationships. (Ryan et al. 2005: 18)

A final possibility within Kitwood's work on personhood lies in his usage of Buber's 'I–Thou' relationship and is touched on in one of his last works; that is, there is a symbiotic relationship between caregivers and people living with dementia, the personhood of each being potentially enhanced through their mutual interactions. Although Kitwood does not draw on this aspect of the 'I–Thou' relationship, 'Buber insists that the relationship involves the preservation of the other as an end and the confirmation of the self, that is, "I become who I am" through my relationship with the other' (Malloy and Hadjistavropoulos 2004: 153).

In *Professional and Moral Development for Care Work: Observations on the process*, Kitwood talks about the moral agent being 'one who can engage consistently in right action, even in the face of countervailing pressures; moral character is learned primarily through practice, by facing up to real opportunities, difficulties and dilemmas' (p. 401/ 321). Engagement with people living with dementia is thus a moral project, not just in the sense of caring for the Other whose personhood is made vulnerable, but in its contribution to the development of the carer. Engagement in practice and reflection is a formative process: by recognizing, maintaining and enhancing the personhood of the individual living with dementia, the caregiver is developing moral sensitivity and character. As Malloy and Hadjistavropoulos (2004) state:

> Both the patient and the caregiver have the opportunity to grow authentically through the caring process. In cases of extreme dementia, it may only be the caregiver who is capable to grow – to take this opportunity away from the caregiver by putting emphasis upon institutionalization and frozen roles and procedures is to lessen the authentic possibilities of the health care profession. Moreover, the caregiver finds meaning in his or her authentic relationship with the patient and this 'role' (e.g. nurse, physician) also becomes a means through which the caregiver's own personhood is developed and authenticated. (pp. 153–154)

The religious roots and failings of Kitwood's theory of personhood

The theory presented earlier, drawn from the two main Kitwood texts, is very much a humanist approach to the question of personhood. On first reading of these texts, Kitwood seems to have moved away from his previous theological, Christian understandings of what it means to be human (see Kitwood 1970). Even when he draws on the language of theology to support his view of personhood, as he does with his reliance on Buber and the 'I–Thou' mode of relating, the concepts are shorn of their theological context and import. By the same token, Kitwood cannot quite abandon the notion of transcendence, grace and the divine, all of which make fleeting appearances in *Dementia Reconsidered*. In this section we will explore some of the roots of Kitwood's theory of personhood, as found primarily in his first, most overtly theological, book, *What is Human?* (Kitwood 1970).

In *What is Human?*, his only overtly Christian publication, Kitwood sought to compare and appraise three competing views of what it means to be human: humanism, existentialism and Christianity. While trying 'to give a fair account of humanism and existentialism, seeking not only to present the facts but to enter into their spirit', it is clear that Kitwood was writing as a Christian minister, a bias he readily acknowledged, as reading openly declared, biased accounts was, in his view, 'certainly more instructive than reading those who, claiming to have no bias, conceal their prejudice beneath a professed objectivity' (Kitwood 1970: 9).

The view of man [sic] put forward in this text is a fairly orthodox, fundamentalist one: man is made in the image of God and 'any attempt to build a life for man which ignores God cannot in the long run succeed or satisfy' (p. 93/189). This means that man bears some of the characteristics of God (such as a capacity for love and a will of his own). Being made in God's image also means that life has both meaning and purpose:

> What then is the meaning and the purpose in the Christian view? The meaning is love. Every human being is uniquely loved by God. All are of equal value in his sight. Man made in God's image is endowed with a sufficient God-likeness to be able to enter into communion with him. He can find God's love constantly encountering him through people and situations and beauty, and is able to make a response of love. (p. 98/191)

And:

> The purpose is service. The Christian seeks to serve God with all his faculties, in all his motives, words and actions. The mundane and trivial are included as well as the noble and spiritual . . . Serving God is never, in the Christian view, to be set in opposition to the service of mankind. The one includes the other. (p. 98/191)

Furthermore, still in accordance with Christian orthodoxy, man is viewed as 'fallen' or alienated from God, through his own fault and bearing the responsibility for that. Christianity, however, offers a way of overcoming this alienation through grace, the bestowal of new life by God. It is through grace that man can once again become fully human.

As with both humanism and existentialism, Christianity views suffering (anxiety, despair, hopelessness, fear, isolation) as part of the human condition. It is, indeed, an evil to be overcome but it is not simply a pragmatic problem as it is for the human-ist; nor is it part of the meaninglessness of life as it is for the existentialist. For the Christian, suffering is a mystery which, if faced with humility and fortitude, can be 'one of the most creative experiences' (p. 119/202) and can arouse and exercise the greatest of human qualities: 'Certainly, if human existence were made up of day after day of comfort and pleasure . . . there would be no scope for our highest and our best. Thus sometimes it is only through the facing of disaster and anguish that we come to know our true humanity' (p. 119/203).

The suffering and alienation that are part of the human condition are, paradoxically, those things that make us human and bring us together. In this fallen state we are called to 'unlimited liability for one another' (citing Douglas Steere: 117/201) and this liability is fulfilled in the 'I–Thou' relationship: 'It is in the encounter with the other that we discover what life really is, we discover ourselves, and we meet the one who is address-ing us in every human encounter, God himself' (p. 65).

Although in his later publications Kitwood shed the language of Christianity, the themes he deals with, especially in relation to dementia, echo those he raised in *What is Human?*: the equality/equal worth of all human beings (Kitwood 1998b) the uniqueness of individuals (Kitwood 1994, 1997a, 1997c, 1997d), the necessity of relationship – in particular the 'I–Thou' relationship (Kitwood 1997a, 1997b), the subjectivity and suffering of individuals (Kitwood 1988c; Kitwood 1994; Kitwood and Bredin 1992a), the link between personhood and caring (Kitwood 1994; Kitwood and Bredin 1992a), the importance of love (Kitwood 1997a).

The move to a more humanistic framework is perhaps explainable by the fact that Kitwood resigned his orders in the late 1970s and became more immersed in the social sciences. Perhaps, also, by reframing his work he thought his message would reach and be taken up by a wider audience. This speculation is perhaps less important, and certainly less interesting, than an examination of the impact this move has on Kitwood's theory of personhood. It is our contention that by removing some of the key elements of the theory from their original context (a context in which they retained their full meaning and import) the theory of personhood presented by Kitwood loses some of its coherence.

For example, although Kitwood refers to transcendence in *Dementia Reconsidered*, this is linked only to a sense of the importance of being-in-itself and is not rooted in any philosophical or religious tradition. As such, it remains unfounded and un-theorized as a fundamental aspect of personhood. Furthermore, without these roots, transcendence is merely an alternative for physicalism, adding nothing to our understanding of personhood. It is interesting to note that although Kitwood relies on the notion of transcendence to give weight to his theory of personhood, he does not argue that spirituality is integral to personhood.[3]

Similarly, by removing the notion of the 'I–Thou' relationship from its original theological context, the rationale for that relationship (the meeting of man and God through relationships with others) is also removed. The 'I–Thou' relationship, whatever its merits in humanistic terms, is thus a pale reflection of what it originally meant and cannot bear the theoretical weight accorded to it by Kitwood in his later writings. For Buber, the 'I–Thou' relationship was related to the purpose, or telos, of man, that is, the relationship with God. Shorn of this purpose the concept has no vital force driving man towards self-fulfilment.

Without these two (which we see as critical) planks to his argument, Kitwood's theory of personhood begins to lose its apparent coherence. Personhood, as a status bestowed by others, thus becomes a precarious status – if it can be bestowed, it can, without firm foundations, be equally easily withheld. We are not suggesting that Kitwood would have ever countenanced such a withdrawal of personhood, merely that the theory he presents no longer has the firm foundations of the original concepts. Commitment to the theory is thus predicated on a more relativist ethics (and is thus more vulnerable) than if it were rooted in the traditions from which it emerged.

We are not, however, saying that because of these failings, we should abandon Kitwood's theory of personhood. Indeed, as we have seen already, it has done much to open up constructive and creative areas for research and practice and has, indubitably, contributed to the well-being of people living with dementia. Instead, we suggest, that work needs to be done on developing the philosophical foundations of the theory. Such developments would, we believe, strengthen the theory and argument for person-centred care. Furthermore, areas such as spirituality that are increasingly recognized in consideration of what it means to live with dementia and what constitutes good dementia care, thus become integrated into the general theory of personhood, giving weight both to the theory and the practice. In so doing, the fit between the theory and Kitwood's seven criteria is strengthened.

Moving forward

Kitwood's theory has been the subject of some criticism. While some of this is no doubt valid, some, we believe, is based on a less than full understanding of his work. In this section we shall examine some of these criticisms with a view to introducing pathways that might go some way to addressing those limitations and developing a more comprehensive, cohesive theory of personhood.

A number of criticisms of Kitwood's theory of personhood can be made:

* Although the proposed theory of personhood is relational, Kitwood only captures a unidirectional realization of that theory. Consequently, the theory and its realization in person-centred care are individualistic and focused on the person living with dementia to the exclusion of those caring for the person living with dementia. Thus the theory is uneven in the sense that people living with dementia have personhood bestowed on them but are not seen as bestowing personhood on others. They are thus made more dependent on and more vulnerable to the vicissitudes of others (Nolan et al. 2002; O'Connor et al. forthcoming).
* The sustaining of personhood creates a further burden for family carers and runs the risk of generating further guilt while, at the same time preventing family members the opportunity to grieve for the lost relationships that will never be recovered (Davis 2004).
* Personhood is an essentially non-political concept and thus limited in scope and impact (Bartlett and O'Connor 2007).
* Kitwood failed to provide the necessary empirical support for his theory (Adams 1996; Adams and Bartlett 2003).

In addition, it is possible to identify areas that impact on personhood that Kitwood never addressed, such as the relationship between embodiment and personhood and the role of place in constituting personhood.

In raising these criticisms, we acknowledge that it is easy to criticize authors for what they have not done. That has not been our intention here. Rather, in the spirit of Tom Kitwood, we have raised the questions in the hope of finding ways of moving things forward. Things change and Kitwood recognized this. He would not have wanted his theories and arguments to be embraced uncritically but to be engaged with, developed and put into practice for the benefit of people living with dementia and their carers. In this section, we hope to be true to that spirit, indicating what we think are the limitations of Kitwood's theory as an introduction to moving forward with the theory of personhood. Our contribution to this, here, will focus on four aspects of personhood that we think need to be included and developed: personhood as process; the embodied person; personhood and citizenship; and personhood and place.

Personhood as process

While Kitwood's theory of personhood is clearly relational, the concepts both of the reciprocity of relations between people with dementia and their carers and of developmental aspects of personhood have been relatively underdeveloped. Nowhere is this so apparent as in considerations of the implications of Kitwood's views of personhood for family carers, in part because it is this context which offers rich possibilities for appreciating both these aspects of personhood. In the context of family care, the merging of social psychology's concepts of personhood (focusing on what it means to be a particular person) with those of transcendence and ethics (focusing on the moral standing of persons in general) is problematic to the extent that it obscures fundamental differences between these two views, that is, the ever changing status of particular persons versus the enduring moral status of persons in general. The tension between these two differing perspectives of personhood captures the very dilemma facing family carers as they seek ways, first, of reconciling the person they have always known with the evolution of that person into someone with dementia and, second, of resolving their moral obligations to that evolving person. Davis (2004) challenged Kitwood's claim that personhood can ultimately be sustained, arguing that, for family carers who were in relationship with the person prior to the onset of dementia, such a claim risks creating a further burden of guilt if they fail to support the personhood of their kin, while at the same time denying them the opportunity to grieve the loss of a particular relationship that is no longer recoverable. He suggested that 'the seductive nature of Kitwood's arguments should be resisted so that debate can continue as to the status of people with dementia and how they are positioned with respect to their loved ones' (p. 377). While agreeing with the need for such an agenda of research, we would argue that it constitutes a further elaboration of Kitwood's theory of personhood, rather than a refutation of it.

One approach to examining personhood in the context of family care is to conceptualize it, not as a fixed status, but rather as a process grounded in social interaction. Attention to family talk can reveal how evolving roles and relationships are negotiated among family members as they try to come to terms with their kin's dementia. A key point here is that, in discursive approaches to understanding social interaction, roles are not fixed, determinate categories. Rather, they are constructed through talk that positions participants in particular ways, thus allowing for 'a diversity of selves' (Davies and Harré 1990: 47). As Davies and Harré pointed out, positioning oneself and others in interaction is not necessarily intentional, nor is it necessarily consistent; it is a dynamic process that positions not only the other but also, relative to that positioning, oneself. By their utterances, 'persons locate themselves and others within an essentially moral space by using several categories and story-lines' (Harré and van Langenhove 1991: 396), that is, a person who positions another in a particular way has (or thinks she has) the moral right to do so. This moral right is usually linked to people's social or institutional roles; for family members, these roles are complicated by the onset and progression of dementia. For example, in positioning oneself as a family caregiver, one necessarily positions the other as 'person with dementia' (O'Connor forthcoming), yet, because positionings are contextually bound, one may also continue to position that person as, for instance, wife, father, husband. Further, one's positioning of another may be resisted or contested by that person (or others), necessitating accounts and justifications that themselves contribute to the construction of person-hood. Analysis of everyday talk offers insights into how family members caring for kin with dementia challenge, mitigate and negotiate different positionings, constructing their own and each other's evolving personhood in a dynamic process (Purves 2006). Given the complexity of Kitwood's theory of personhood, such insights are critical if we are to articulate fully that theory and its implications for care, not just for persons with dementia but also for their families.

The embodied person

At the same time that Tom Kitwood was starting to draw together his theory of person-hood, the sociology and phenomenology of the body were beginning to attract increas-ing attention in academic circles (e.g. Featherstone et al. 1991; Leder 1990). As these lines of thought have continued to develop, they have contributed to an elaborated understanding of the self in dementia, as not only socially constructed, but also embodied.

But what exactly does this mean? Certainly, Kitwood himself used the language of embodiment in *Dementia Reconsidered*, although it was largely in reference to neuro-logical features of the physical body. He argued that psychological events (e.g. human interactions) could, in theory at least, also be described in terms of certain kinds of brain activity and that developing a theoretical model of personhood was ultimately a matter of 'finding a way of bringing the discourses of the human and natural sciences together' (p. 16/253), linking mind and body, as it were. By articulating the problem in this way, Kitwood confined the body to the realm of the natural sciences, viewing it implicitly as a biological entity, an object body with no inherent significance in and of itself, other than perhaps as a vehicle of expression.

While relatively few writers have followed up on this aspect of Kitwood's work, the significance of embodiment is a clear thread in more recent thinking about personhood in dementia. Here we are drawing on work by scholars in Canada and the UK, including Davis (2004), Hughes (2001), Kontos (2004, 2005) and Phinney (Phinney and Brown 2004; Phinney and Chesla 2003), all of whom seem to view what Kitwood had to offer as necessary but insufficient for a theory of personhood. They are claiming, in one way or another, that what has been missing is an account of how personhood is constituted in and through the lived experiential body. Drawing variously on philosophical and social theorists including Bourdieu, Merleau-Ponty and Taylor, this body of work is focusing attention, not on the biological or corporeal body, but on the 'pre-reflective' or 'taken-for-granted' body as it is engaged in the usual habits and practices of daily life. Moreover, it is situating the body in a social and cultural world that not only provides the sources of these bodily practices but also serves as the background against which they make sense and are meaningful. In short, this work has expanded on Kitwood's model by taking first steps toward articulating a view of personhood that foregrounds an embodied self existing in dialogue with others in a socio-cultural context.

At this point in time, what exists in the literature is largely theoretical. Limited empirical evidence exists to support further development of these ideas, although there is work being done currently that may help move this thinking forward. Kontos and

Hughes both speak to the implicit understanding of 'personhood as embodied' that they have seen among carers, claiming that the embodied perspective has intuitive appeal and that it is therefore important to clarify what exactly the theoretical claims might be, and to figure out what the implications are for care. Kontos (2004, 2005) takes this a step further, arguing that the theory itself needs to be better understood by practitioners so they might provide more appropriate care that takes into account how personhood is embodied. She is currently conducting research to develop and test ways to expand models of person-centred care that take the embodied self into account. Phinney and colleagues are also conducting research to better understand the embodied experiences of people with dementia. Her past work articulating how symptoms are experienced through the lived body and her current research examining involvement in meaningful activity and social interaction have the potential to further contribute to a theoretical model of personhood that takes into account the inescapable fact of our essential embodiment.

Personhood and citizenship

Another area where Kitwood's conceptualization of personhood has been critiqued lies in its inability to fully realize its potential as an agent for political change. There are several aspects related to how personhood has been understood and applied that limit its application in the political arena.

First, despite the recognition that personhood exists and is developed within social relationships, both Kitwood and others applying his theory of personhood have tended to focus narrowly on the individual within his/her immediate environment. Although not inherently antithetical to Kitwood's conceptualization, with few exceptions, limited attention has been given to considering how personal experiences with dementia are shaped within a broader socio-political context. For example, after 10 years of research involving people with dementia a great deal is known about micro level issues such as quality of care (Brooker 2003; Netten 1992; Tune and Bowie 2000); communication techniques (Killick and Allan 2001) and individual coping strategies (Bruce 2004; Bruce et al. 2002). Much less is known, however, about macro-level issues such as the impact of social structures related to disability, age, gender, ethnicity and social class on people's experiences (Cantley and Bowes 2004; Hulko 2002; O'Connor and Phinney 2006). Failing to attend to these contexts can give the impression that the dementia experience occurs in a vacuum, ignoring the importance of socio-cultural values, norms, beliefs and assumptions for influencing how this experience is interpreted and responded to, by both afflicted persons and their social partners.

The net result is that the personhood lens remains fixated on what happens within narrowly defined relationships rather than leading to broader investigations of why persons with dementia are treated as they are within our society. This gap raises concerns that a focus on relational personhood may simply shift blame for the treatment of persons with dementia from the disease process to those within that person's immediate environment, thereby failing to adequately capture how wider social problems and structures help construct the lived experience of dementia.

Moreover, because personhood is essentially an apolitical concept it does not provide the language for discussing people's situation in terms of power relations.

For example, although Kitwood uses the language of equality, his theory of personhood does not provide a language for exploring the possibility that 'caring' might sometimes have more to do with power and control than with values of trust and giving. Similarly, this lens really is not able to describe relationships in the context of wider social structures. Consequently, socio-political matters such as experiences of disempowerment and discrimination tend to be personalized as individual issues rather than seen as exemplifying public problems.

Finally, although Kitwood's theory of personhood is grounded in the idea that a person with dementia is someone who counts, this lens does not necessarily promote the vision of someone with agency and multiple social identities. Rather, drawing on the definition of personhood most commonly cited, personhood is conceptualized as something that is 'conferred on' a person with dementia, conveying a unidirectional understanding which arguably continues to position a person with dementia as passively dependent upon others for affirmation. As Downs (1997: 598) noted, maintaining the personhood of people with dementia is essentially 'the responsibility of those who are cognitively intact'.

In his conceptualization of personhood, then, Kitwood revolutionized thinking about the dementia experience to recognize that persons with dementia do indeed have something to say. However, the need to move further, to integrate an understanding that facilitates a political analysis and societal-based change, is increasingly being recognized. In some ways, this is undoubtedly an expectable progression – Kitwood's focus on personhood opened the space to hear the voices of persons with dementia, now, increasingly, there is a demand that these voices indeed be heard. Furthermore, with the advent of new health technologies and approaches, such as anti-dementia drugs, which may help slow the progression of the disease and/or help persons with dementia feel better about themselves for longer periods of time (Ibbotson and Goa 2002; Rockwood et al. 2003), expectation that persons with dementia will – and should – be able to contribute as active agents for longer periods of time is anticipated.

The notion of citizenship offers a lens for extending notions of personhood into a political arena. Kitwood's writings on personhood give lip service to notions of equality but a focus on citizenship introduces 'rights'-based talk that moves beyond the immediate care environment. Citizenship recognizes that all who possess the status of citizen are equal with respect to the rights and duties that the status bestows and is fundamentally concerned with the (mis)use of power. It has been proposed as being more apposite than personhood for understanding and combating discrimination (Shotter 1993). Given the extent to which people with dementia are discriminated against as individuals and as a client group the time for applying a socio-cultural – and political – framework to dementia practice and research has definitely come (Downs 2000).

Developments in the field suggest that struggles for citizenship are indeed happening. For example, organizations such as the Dementia Advocacy Support Network International (DASNI) (see http://www.dasninternational.org) – run by, rather than for, people with dementia – are emerging with a focus on challenging discrimination and improving services for people with dementia. Such work parallels the self-organizational activities of older people, people with physical disabilities and people with mental health conditions and arguably, mark the 'growing collective self confidence of (people with dementia) to put the issue of institutional discrimination on to the public agenda'

(Barton 1993: 245). These activities constitute a struggle for citizenship because by choosing to talk publicly about their experiences of living with dementia, individuals are in effect repositioning themselves (Sabat 2003) as active citizens rather than as tragic victims of a disease. The fact that people with dementia themselves are beginning to call for social change is significant, not least because it suggests people with dementia are making political the personal experiences of stigma and discrimination associated with dementia.

Incorporating a theory of citizenship into dementia practice and research is indeed challenging. Certainly, while the understanding that persons with dementia should be accorded full citizenship may be accepted, it must also be acknowledged that deteriorating cognitive abilities may limit a person's abilities to exercise associated rights and practices (Karlawish et al. 2004). It is here that the intersection between personhood and citizenship may occur. The challenge will be to move beyond personhood while simultaneously retaining a focus on it.

Home, self and dementia: exploring the nature of intersection

Just as personhood can be embodied, or established in relationships with others, so, too, it can be regarded as being founded, undermined or supported by our relationship with place, particularly our sense of 'home'. The home environment provides the central context of our life experience contributing to various dimensions of meaning of home including refuge, sense of belonging, social status and self-identity. Over time, we develop affective relationships with our homes, as well as other personally meaningful places. Also, the never-seen house, – created in our longing, the faraway land that we call our home and may never actually live in or the garden that awaits as the abode in the hereafter, are all in our personal or collective imagination and potentially as real as the places that we physically experienced in the past. They become part of our mental landscape, serve as anchors in memories of our lived experiences and become part of our self-identity – who we see ourselves as persons. Memories of homes have the significant function of mnemonic pathways of not only recollecting and remembering the homes themselves, but also, and more importantly, the larger life experience grounded in events, people, emotions, perceptions, values and meaning. The process of recollecting homes from the past is a way of preserving our self-identity.

The relationship between self, identity and personhood is complex and contentious. While not synonymous with each other, these concepts do, it seems to us, at least overlap in significant ways and each is tied in with the notions of process, embodiment and citizenship that we have already discussed. There is evidence to suggest that a sense of home is strongly associated with selfhood (Frank 2005) and, indeed, many of Brummett's characteristics of home – connectedness/belonging, privacy/territoriality, control/autonomy, choice/opportunity (cited in Frank 2005: 172) – are obviously convergent with Kitwood's positive person work based on relationships, respect, collaboration and empowerment (see Brooker and Surr 2005). However, we know very little about the nature and evolution of memories of home in self that is also experiencing the condition of dementia. While some work has been done in conceptualizing the relationship between self and place (Chaudhury 1999, 2003) this area still requires much further work.

Based on empirical work on memories of home in residents with dementia in care facilities, we believe that 'home' has an extremely rich potential in understanding the condition of self in dementia, as well as offering opportunities in connecting to the self that is veiled behind the realities of dementia. A sense of home remains in the minds of those living with dementia (Frank 2005) and eliciting that sense of home – for example, through art (Chaudhury 2003) or reminiscence (Chaudhury 2002) – can serve as a re-affirmation of self. As such the physical and emotional environment experienced as 'home' can act therapeutically in the maintenance of personhood.

Concluding remarks

Tom Kitwood's work on personhood helped to change dementia care. By placing the person at the centre of his work, he challenged the prevailing view of those living with dementia as 'non-persons'. The theory of personhood he developed served its purpose well, but things have moved on and there are developments in the theory of personhood that can be usefully and creatively combined with Kitwood's theory: personhood as process, as embodied, as citizenship and in its relationship to place. These aspects of personhood are more than theoretical speculations – each has its implications for dementia care and research.

Notes

1   Ten years on, some authors are of the opinion that the debate is still dominated by the personalist camp. See, for example, Kittay (2005).
2   In the year of publication (1993), Dan Brock was, among his many other appointments, Professor of Philosophy and Biomedical Ethics and Director of the Center for Biomedical Ethics at Brown University, a member of the Ethics Working Group of the White House Task Force on National Health Care Reform, a member of the Rhode Island Hospital and Miriam Hospital Ethics Committees and a member of the Executive Board of the American Association of Bioethics.
3   It is interesting to note that, although the two main texts in which Kitwood developed his theory of personhood appeared in the same year, the notion of transcendence only appears in *Dementia Reconsidered*. While this might reflect Kitwood's ability (and perhaps desire) to write persuasively for different audiences, it may also reflect an ambivalence towards spirituality as an aspect of personhood. For example, on page 55 of *Dementia Reconsidered*, he says that a theory of personhood 'must be valid in terms of a psychology that focuses on experience, action and spirituality', yet on page 69 he leaves open the idea that there is a spirituality, stating that if there is a spirituality, 'it will most likely be of the kind that Buber describes, where the divine is encountered in the depth of I–Thou relating'.

3.1

The Christian understanding of man (1970)

'A man is only a man when he is like God and lives in fellowship with him.'

Stephen Neill.

'To come into the field of force of God's infinite caring is to feel . . . unlimited liability for one another.'

Douglas Steere.

Existentialism and rational humanism, while radically opposed in many respects, do at least have one thing in common: their total rejection of religion in its usual theistic sense. The non-existence of God is the practical starting-point of humanism; it is also the basic experience from which existentialism has grown.

Although Christianity accepts a number of insights from both, it has a totally different starting-point. A first-century writer defending Christianity in comparison with the secular philosophies of his day advised his readers: 'Shake off the hidebound notions which can only lead to error, and put yourself in the position of a brand-new man on the point of hearing a brand-new language.'[1] Christianity has always involved an unfamiliar way of thinking which comes strangely to those who throughout their intellectual training have lived with the assumption that there is no God. It does so still today. We must understand at the outset why the Christian approach is so different.

Humanism and existentialism are man-made systems of thought; they claim nothing more. But Christianity purports to be God's self-declaration. If God is infinite, man by himself can never find him. God must reveal himself. This claim for Christianity may seem laughable in view of the endless wranglings between Christians of different denominations. It may reasonably be claimed, however, that there is an essential Christian religion that has existed right from the days when the New Testament was written. It has been present in the Christian church ever since, despite a great variety of outward expressions and the fact that at some periods parts of the church have deviated far from the basic faith. The authentic Christianity is that of the Bible, in which there is a record of God gradually revealing himself to the Jews until they had a sufficient understanding, and then his ultimate self-declaration in Jesus Christ. That, at any rate, is the Christian claim.

It is natural, therefore, that there should be an element of dogmatism in statements of Christian belief, which is not present, or should not be, in non-religious philosophy. But if God has indeed revealed himself, a note of authority is altogether reasonable. The possibility that this is so must at least be allowed as a prerequisite for an honest examination of Christianity. Then, as with the other two views of man which we have considered, the Christian one must be looked at whole before it is judged.

Christianity thus involves a reversal of the secular starting-point, and a denial of many secular assertions. The critics of religion tend to say that belief in God is a prop for the immature or insecure, an illusion grown from wish-fulfilment. That sort of remark has been made as easily by Bertrand Russell as by Friedrich Nietzsche. But the Christian holds that God, far from being an illusion, is the reality from whom all truth originates. Therefore in Christian understanding any attempt to build a life for man which ignores God cannot in the long run succeed or satisfy. What the atheist considers to be an unnecessary, indeed an imaginary, prop, the Christian sees as an integral part of the structure. A thoroughgoing atheist looks down on the man who prays as immature, abnormal, maimed. But the Christian holds that it is the man who refuses to believe who is immature.

One further caution must be given. The Christian religion is not, fundamentally, a structure of theoretical ideas. Its assertions are generally founded upon experience; of a succession of men who believed God had spoken to them; and from those who were with Jesus when he lived and died. Whether the Christian interpretation is correct is for the reader to judge. But it must be remembered that religious language can never be separated from experience. It speaks of things which, though they lie beyond the possibility of accurate definition, are apprehended by the whole person. Some religious statements therefore may appear to be indirect or metaphorical. In theology, it has been truly said, we can only babble and mutter. Yet there are those who claim to know Theos, the subject of all theology, with a conviction that goes beyond the reach of words. It is the understanding of man which comes from that conviction with which we have to deal.

Existence with meaning

Man is God's creation. The Christian understanding of man must begin here. According to Christianity, man is not just a collection of chemicals that came into being by an intricate process and then evolved mind and consciousness. Man owes his whole being, his physical vitality and his spiritual aspirations, to God from whom all life derives. His existence is no chance or accident.

The early chapters of Genesis describe creation in evocative pictorial language, more akin to poetry than science. The whole natural order, the primaeval energy, the earth, the sea, the plants, the animals, and finally man himself, are declared to be the work of God, and good. God is described as forming man from dust and breathing into him, giving him life. That is to say, it is God who has designed man to be what he is: thinker, artist, scientist, builder; above all, worshipper. Man's enormous creative capacity comes from the Creator. The most creative act of all is a response to him. That, as Christians understand it, is why men of every race and culture seem to feel for God, even when the expression of their search is crude and superstitious.

The Christian doctrine of creation is not concerned with the biological details of man's origin. That is the proper field of study for the zoologist and anthropologist. But Christianity does assert that by whatever means man has come into being, it is the work of God. The theory of evolution is at present generally considered to be the best description of the development of living things that science can give, though like all scientific theories, it is open to criticism and will need modification as new evidence comes to light. But at best it is only a description of the process. The belief of Christians is that, whatever the process, the author is God. It would be a misunderstanding, incidentally, to think that creation by a process is less divine than a series of mighty acts that do it all at once.

Science describes processes and relates apparently unrelated facts, but its accounts are always incomplete, for they can never in the ultimate sense be explanations. Genesis, however, purports to be an explanation of man's existence, not in terms of science but of meaning, by referring it to God's creative act.

Man was formed by God. Genesis also teaches that he was made in the image of God; he bears a reproduction of some of God's characteristics. This means, first, that man has a capacity for love and self-giving. The theologians have long pondered over the question, Why did God bring his creation into being at all, if he is self-sufficient and in need of no other? The beginning of an answer can be given by analogy with love between a man and a woman. Though there is the deepest satisfaction in their love, they wish it to overflow into having children who will be both the fruit and the object of their love. So also, perhaps, it is with God. The creation was the overflowing of his love.

A human analogy has been used here, but really the analogy is the other way round. It is man whose creative love reflects that of God. Though pale and weak by comparison, and never entirely freed from self-interest, human love can have some of the quality of true self-giving. There was no common word in the ancient world for this kind of love. That presumably is why the early Christians had to take the word *agapē* and give it a new meaning of their own.

Man's capacity for love and self-giving must be used, in response to other human beings and above all in response to God. Existentialism denies that this is possible. But according to Christianity not only is it possible; it is the great task of life.

'In God's image' means, second, that man has a will of his own. Returning to the analogy of human love, we may say that no parents would want a child who was a machine with unalterable fixed reactions, even if those reactions were of total obedience. One thing is certain: the reactions could never be those of love. No-one can be conditioned to love, for love is the free response of an independent will and can only be voluntary. So if we are indeed the creation of God, it is reasonable that we should have our own autonomy. He has given us the power either to respond to him or to turn away. Man, says Genesis, was placed in a garden where he was free. Round the forbidden tree there was no electric fence. Though man could give all love and obedience freely, he was also free to eat the fruit and reject the authority of God. In the Christian view, the abuse of this freedom is the fundamental error of mankind.

Third, it means that man has a position of authority, under God and over the rest of the creation. All authority derives from God, but some is delegated to man to whom so many talents are entrusted. He is given the commission to become master of the world. He is expected to find out the potentialities of earth, air and sea, to use nature and its resources. He is required to give names to all living creatures. In this we can see the scientific quest foreshadowed, whose aim is to understand and classify the natural world. Here is the divine charter for the immense variety of human activity: agriculture, technology, industry, craft and art. These, according to Christianity, are God's gifts for the enrichment of man's life.

But authority can be misused. If science and technology have not turned out to be an unmitigated blessing it is not because the pursuit of them is unworthy, but because they have often been used godlessly, without care or compassion. Polluted atmospheres, man-made deserts, nuclear stock-piles and many other blights on our environment are the direct result of human selfishness and greed. When man exerts his authority without reference to God he does so at his peril. For though in authority he is still a creature and, as Christians see it, to usurp the place of God is the crowning folly.

If the Christian understanding of man as God's creation, in God's image, is true, it means that man's life has both meaning and purpose. Nietzsche the atheist held that all meaning, all significance, comes from God. Christians believe that too, but they also believe in God. Man finds his meaning in God. This would certainly explain why it is that, when he tries to live his life apart from God, he discovers it to be meaningless, as Nietzsche so tragically realized. The poignancy of so much existentialist writing is that it describes exactly what would be expected if men who are made in the image of God deny him and try to live on their own.

What, then, is the meaning and the purpose in the Christian view? The meaning is love. Every human being is uniquely loved by God. All are of equal value in his sight. Man made in God's image is endowed with a sufficient God-likeness to be able to enter into communion with him. He can find God's love constantly encountering him through people and situations and beauty, and is able to make a response of love. Many humanists too would assert that the meaning of life is love, but there is this difference. For them, the love is their own initiative. For the Christian, the love is a response to a greater which is there already.

The purpose is service. The Christian seeks to serve God with all his faculties, in all his motives, words, and actions. The mundane and trivial are included as well as the noble and spiritual. When all of life is seen as God's service, pleasures gain in richness and sorrow is borne with more stability. Life, instead of being a fragmented collection of joys and pains, fits together and begins to make sense.

Serving God is never, in the Christian view, to be set in opposition to the service of mankind. The one includes the other. A man 'cannot love God, whom he has not seen, if he does not love his brother, whom he has seen'.[2] Humanism has a high ideal of loving one's brother, and here it holds much common ground with Christianity. But Christians believe that the most effective and selfless service is given to mankind when it is seen as part of the service of God.

Christianity thus makes assertions which are totally opposed to the philosophy of meaninglessness. Moreover the claim that 'God is, therefore life is meaningful' is no less consistent than the statement of the existentialist: 'God is dead, therefore life is meaningless.' It is also made on the basis of experience. If the existentialist could find himself believing, he would have a full cure for his predicament. Certainly there are many who have been kept from despair because even in desolation they were still able to believe in a God who loved them.

But there is another reason why Christians assert that human life has meaning. They believe that God himself entered human existence; not as a legend, handed down from generation to generation; not as a myth, as with the Greek stories of theophany; but as a fact of history, soberly recorded, whose date we can estimate to within three or four years, and in a town which we can visit today. Man is in God's image, but Christ is the Image of God.

In the man Jesus, Christians believe, God entered human existence, living it on the same terms as ourselves. In so doing he not only expressed in human terms what God is like (that is why he is called the Word, or expression of God), but also showed how a truly human life should be lived. Pilate, when Jesus was up for trial, exhibited him to the crowd and in derision cried out: 'Look! Here is the man.' Christians endorse that, but in a very different sense. Here they see true manhood; here in the strict sense is the normal man, the man to be followed. Though some of the details have been eroded away, it is still possible to know a great deal about his life from the records which were written down either by men who knew him or had intimate contact with those who did. The stories that have come down to us are quite sufficient to offer a very comprehensive pattern for human living.

From conventional standpoints it was a very ordinary life, just that of a small-town carpenter turned preacher in one of the least important outposts of the Roman Empire. The conflicts which it raised were provincial and trivial. But when that life is examined more closely, it may be seen to have a stature which no other man has equalled, through its power, gentleness, boldness, tenderness, poise and self-giving. It is clear that Jesus lived out what he preached, a fact which his accusers could never deny. Although the Gospels show a life that has been called perfect, however, they do not portray a demigod. They portray a man.

If it really was the life of God on earth, as his followers came to believe when they pondered on its quality, it alters irrevocably our understanding of our own. This life shows the nature of God, not in abstract words or ethical precepts, but in concrete terms of human character, speech and action. A man is showing what God is like. A man is bearing unmarred the image of God. As we look at him perhaps we shall understand not only what is divine, but also what is human.

The humanism of Christianity

Man was formed by God, and the purpose of his life is to serve his Creator. But how is he to do that? In the creation story we have already considered, a very interesting phrase is used which, though pre-scientific, is very much in accord with a modern understanding of personality. God makes man from dust, gives him life, and man becomes, as the older translations put it, 'a living soul'. This bears the meaning of a unity in which the various functions of man are intimately fused. 'Soul' is not here used in the Greek sense of a spirit distinct from a body; it means, rather, a single functioning unit in which what we term physical, mental and spiritual interpenetrate one another completely. This concept underlies the humanism of Christianity.

A pious Jew would have thought it inconceivable that farming or singing should be activities qualitatively different from prayer. All are expressions of the living soul. It would be meaningless to offer some of these activities to God and not them all. There is no true distinction between secular and sacred. Either the whole of life is offered to God, in which case the whole is sacred, or the whole is held back, in which case even 'religious' activities are not sacred at all.

The Bible therefore is the most earthy of all the great religious books. Even its spirituality is firmly grounded, with insistence on worship from the heart mentioned in the same breath as condemnation of sharp practice. The good life is certainly not seen as that of a contemplative mystic withdrawing himself from an evil world. Man, rather, seems to feel very much at home in the world, enjoying his part in the created order. He finds great satisfaction in the skill of the craftsman and the work of the artist. He loves music, both for pleasure and refreshment, and for praising God. He delights in the harvest and the seasons, in the power of nature and the curious ways of the wild animals. Probably the reverence and wonder that many European poets have felt about nature is a direct inheritance from the Jewish-Christian tradition, while appreciation of it is often lacking in cultures which have no clear belief in a Creator. The strength of the greatest nature poetry is that, beyond the splendour of the visible, it feels towards God revealing himself in beauty and wisdom.

The whole-hearted embracing of life as God's gift is clearly seen too in the biblical picture of marriage and family life. It is true that some of the early Christians, in their zeal for purity in an environment that knew very little sexual restraint, almost went so far as to deny that sexuality was God's gift at all. But in the Bible attraction, courtship, marriage and the delights of love physically expressed are all extolled. Like any gift they may be misused, but in themselves they are thoroughly good and to be thankfully received.

But in the biblical view man can never truly enjoy the world unless he enjoys it as a worshipper. He must gratefully acknowledge that all the richness of life is God's gift. He must see beyond the creation to the Creator. Prayer and worship must have their rightful place among all man's activities, for it may be that they are the most distinctively human thing about us.

Christians, therefore, like the humanists, can fairly claim that 'our concern is with this life'. But the Christian concern is different. Christians see themselves as guests in the universe, there to use responsibly and to enjoy what has been given. Humanists, rather, see themselves as hosts, to do with their existence what they will. And while humanists see life as bounded by the physical environment, Christians are always feeling beyond it. They are at home in the world, thoroughly at home. But no-one who has experienced God can feel that the world is his ultimate resting-place.

The religion which Jesus lived and taught endorses the life-affirmation of the Old Testament. He himself was a Jew and had breathed this tradition from childhood. His love of life can clearly be seen in the Gospels. His stories and illustrations frequently show his pleasure in the natural world. He was extremely sociable, to such an extent that his critics called him a glutton and a drinker. He certainly expressed his emotions: anger when he threw out the crooked businessmen in the Temple forecourt; grief when confronted with the death of a friend; fear as he anticipated the horror of crucifixion; compassion when he met with all forms of human need. It is possible still to detect his irony and humour despite the fact that his words have gone through two successive translations. The force of his personality, like that of Nietzsche's superman, was released creatively into life.

There is a common misunderstanding of Christianity at this point. Swinburne once wrote:

'Thou hast conquered, O pale Galilean;
the world has grown gray from thy breath.'

Somehow, contrary to all the evidence of the Gospels, Jesus is made out to be a dreary figure, one who made life insipid and robbed human pleasures of their vitality. But the following of Jesus may be claimed to be an enhancement of life because, while acknowledging a secular humanism to the full, it never rests there. It adds a spiritual dimension, and offers as reality that for which the human spirit longs. This may be why some of the greatest works of art, music and architecture have turned out to be those with a Christian theme or motive, and even in the twentieth century a number of artists, though themselves not believers, have turned to Christian subjects. It is also true that very little art of merit has come from within the framework of an explicit secularism, perhaps because there the spirit of man is limited and tied.

But the teaching of Jesus is not a simple life-affirmation. It certainly has its stern and challenging aspect. He was calling people to something beyond this world, to the 'kingdom', to obedience and faith in God. And he taught unequivocally that it was worth sacrificing anything – riches, pleasures, prospects and even human love – to enter that kingdom. He did not offer his followers an easy time, for he spoke of self-sacrifice and of 'taking up a cross', which in his day was the common gallows and therefore a mark of shame. In other words, his followers were to be prepared to be openly known as such, even when it brought mockery and opposition. The 'cross' meant unashamed committal, and sometimes following a road alone and misunderstood. Christianity requires a man to stand by his convictions, which is not always easy. It might even be necessary to die for one's faith as Jesus himself did. Therefore if Christianity is 'life-affirming' in one sense, it is 'life-denying' in another, for it teaches that God must come first at all costs.

At this point the teaching of Jesus almost seems self-contradictory. The paradox is summed up in one of his most famous saying, the only one to be recorded in all four Gospels: 'Whoever tries to save his own life will lose it; whoever loses his life will save it.'[3] He is teaching that the way to a truly rich experience of life is through self-forgetfulness, and being absorbed into a purpose bigger than ourselves. Self-interest often defeats its own end. The rich man is often miserable, the pampered bored and frustrated. Conversely, those who whole-heartedly give themselves up in concern for others are among the most joyful. Christianity teaches that the one in whom we are to lose our self-interest for ever is God. Then we find our life again, the same yet subtly transformed.

Humanists put humanity first. In the Christian view that ideal is disastrously incomplete, for it can easily become a sophisticated selfishness. Christians seek to put

God first. This in no way lessens the call to be of service to humanity, but it puts that call into a different perspective, showing it to be part of something greater.

We have seen how Christianity has an ideal of personal self-expression, but directed God-wards. It must also be with discipline. Uncontrolled self-expression can be moral anarchy, as modern society knows all too well. There must be a direction, a channel, a structure. Christians believe the structure to be the law of God, a set of timeless principles given to man to live by, and within which to find his freedom. Seen in this way the Ten Commandments, far from being restrictions, are the very safeguards of liberty. Christianity here differs sharply from humanism, whose provisional moral codes often appear permissive and vague.

'Honour your father and mother' protects the integrity of the family and communication between the generations. 'You shall not commit adultery' defines the right and wrong use of sex so that this immense drive may be expressed without reservation in a context of love and security. 'You shall not steal' enables community living. 'You shall not bear false witness' makes possible free and trusting human relationships. 'You shall not covet' paves the way for true contentment. 'You shall not' is not, as is sometimes imagined, the statement of an attitude to life; rather, it is a definition of the boundaries, so that within them there may be a fulfilment free from shame.

This can be seen in the first four Commandments also, which deal with man in relation to God. They ensure that man shall be a worshipper of the right God, in the right way. For whether a believer in God or not, man finds himself a worshipper. If he does not worship God, he will find some form of idolatry, to success or wealth or comfort, or even to himself. The first two Commandments therefore determine the object of worship, God alone. The third, not to take God's name in vain, deals with the nature of that worship, which must be sincere. The fourth, the sabbath law, ensures that there shall be time for it.

Jesus had a great deal to say about the law. His judgment was thoroughly to endorse its relevance, extending its scope beyond conduct to the realms of thought, motive and desire. The moralists of his day had defined and refined the details until the law had become a dead set of rules, obedience to which could lead only to self-righteousness. Jesus did exactly the opposite. He showed that the law was fundamentally concerned with man's attitude before his actions, so that outward conformity meant nothing without obedience from the heart.

Teaching about God's law or absolute moral standards often sounds strange to our modern age of expediency. It is often assumed that fulfilment can be found only in rejecting moral codes, though the evidence is often to the contrary. Certainly the experiments in moral lawlessness of the twentieth century have not been conspicuously successful even in bringing happiness. The Ten Commandments and the teaching of Jesus come from a culture very different from our own, which means that care and ingenuity may be needed in applying them to, say, trade union ethics or student revolt. But this is perfectly possible, though the Christian church has been slow to apply God's law to a changing world.

The humanism of Christianity, therefore, like that of the secularist, is an ideal of personal fulfilment and self-expression, of service to humanity. But Christians believe that these are only possible when man himself bows down to God and makes him the supreme end of his life.

A moral failure

Modern existentialism, as we have seen, holds that man is in an acute state of isolation from his fellows. We are compelled to live close to others, but their presence is a source of irritation and anxiety, an intrusion and a threat. Sartre, in one of his plays, sums up the human predicament in the famous line, 'Hell is other people.'

This is clearly true to part of human experience, as anyone who has faced working with an incompatible colleague, suffered persecution on grounds of race or creed or, worse, lived through the failure of human love, can testify. The Christian faith here agrees with existentialism that this is a common state of affairs, but asserts that it need not always be so. Christianity sees man's alienation from his fellows as due to a deeper alienation. He is separated from God. Because God is the source of all being and self-giving, it is natural that those who are alienated from him should find it hard to make relationships with each other. In the Christian view, no radical solution to the conflict between man and man is to be found unless this deeper problem is solved. The existentialist simply has to accept the fact of alienation and live with it. The humanist often blandly ignores it. But Christianity claims both to give a correct diagnosis of the sickness of man's spirit and even to offer a cure by which men will be brought out of alienation from God and again into true relationship.

The Christian faith does not flatter at this point, for it asserts that mankind has deliberately turned away from God. Given an autonomy and some power of self-determination, he has wilfully abused it. Genesis speaks of man eating from the tree and being cast out of the garden; that is to say, he has taken upon himself the right to choose what is good and evil – by making himself into a god he has rejected the true God; he has broken the relationship and thwarted the purpose which God intended for him. Even the law of God, given as a guide for fruitful living, serves to catalogue the failure that has ensued.

Jesus once said this about the human heart: 'It is what comes out of a person that makes him unclean. For from the inside, from a man's heart, come the evil ideas which lead him to do immoral things, to rob, kill, commit adultery, covet, and do all sorts of evil things; deceit, indecency, jealousy, slander, pride, and folly – all these evil things come from inside a man and make him unclean.'[4] He is saying that the cause of our moral failure lies in the spring of our willing and desiring. We have turned from the right we do know; we have hidden from the little of God that we did understand. We have kept ourselves in a selfish comfort and security, refusing to have any master but ourselves, with the result that our actions are poisoned at their very source.

The humanist will not admit this because in general he holds too hopeful a view of human nature, or regards a moral lapse as merely the unfortunate result of heredity and conditioning. Christianity, however, like existentialism, holds a clear doctrine of human responsibility. When the fullest allowance has been made for circumstances, men are still guilty of a deliberate turning from God and breach of his law. Christian values, though, are not the conventional ones. It may well be that in God's sight a religious man who is thoroughly self-righteous has rejected God much more completely than another whose conduct simply goes against the social taboos. The former stubbornly refuses to humble himself before God, while the other makes no pretence of goodness. Only God knows what allowances need to be made for individual cases.

But judged according to the true scale of values, all mankind has failed and is guilty before him.

'There is not one who understands,
Or who seeks for God.
All men have turned away from God,
They have all gone wrong.
No one does what is good, not even one.'[5]

So wrote the apostle Paul. These words do appear at first sight to disparage so much that seems self-evidently good in human effort. But Paul is speaking of a divine judgment on the human heart which, until any individual is willing to admit is true about himself and even his own attempts at goodness, he will not find the way to restoration. Though no-one has the right to make that sort of judgment upon another, it is necessary for each, personally, to acknowledge his responsibility for selfishness and godlessness, his accountability to the Creator who is also his Judge.

Nietzsche and others claimed that this doctrine made men morally sick. Christianity, rather, suggests that it is only when men are realistic about their condition that they will wish to consult the doctor. But they should not then let their mind dwell on the illness. Having begun to apply the remedy, they will concentrate on health and vitality.

Deliberately so far I have not used the word 'sin' at all. Traditional theology and traditional religious language would put it thus: all human beings are born with the taint of original sin and go on sinning throughout their lives. This brings its inevitable consequence of spiritual death, which is separation from God. Original sin (though this is not meant to be an exhaustive definition) can be seen as the tragic fact that we are born into a world of alienated people. From birth and possibly before, the alienation of man from man is with us. First experienced in the fallibility of parental love, then in childhood quarrels, then in the gulf which separates the growing person from his parents, then perhaps in difficulties in marriage and, finally, in the loneliness of old age, this sense of alienation is with us, and as the existentialist writers so clearly understand, it goes as deep as anything we know of ourselves.

I have suggested that Christianity offers a way out of this predicament. The Christian church, when it is true to its own ideal, claims to be a group of human beings once alienated but now related to one another because they have come into a relationship with God. It is a plain fact, open to verification, that within a Christian group people of very different ages, colours, races, status, income and intelligence are able to co-exist in deep mutual understanding and harmony. Paul put it that in Christ 'there are no Gentiles and Jews, circumcised and uncircumcised, barbarians, savages, slaves, or free men, but Christ is all, Christ is in all'.[6] That list contains some of the most mutually prejudiced groups that this world contained. It is a bold claim, but despite the manifest failure of parts of the institutional and visible church, anyone who has been within a genuine Christian fellowship knows that it is true.

How, then, is it possible for man to come again into relationship with God? By himself, man cannot do it. But God from his side has done it already. The clue to understanding this is to be found in what Christians believe to be the starkest expression of alienation ever to be uttered, Jesus' cry while he was dying on the cross: 'My God, my God, why did you abandon me?'[7] Here is a question springing from a terrible anguish, equal in quality to the darkest experiences of existentialism. It is almost a cry of 'God is dead'.

The words of theology are always approximations, and this is particularly true when we try to speak adequately about the spiritual dynamics of the cross. Christians believe that in the death of Jesus, God was bearing himself the alienation that has come into our world. He took upon himself the consequences of what we have done. Like anyone who has been wronged and seeks a reconciliation, he bears the pain and loss himself. God took the alienation fully upon himself, going to its very depths and exhausting it. In so doing he abolished it and made a way of peace for any who would accept what he has done.

All this has great relevance to the problem of guilt, with which perhaps Kafka was dealing in *The Trial*. Christianity says unequivocally that all are guilty before God. But we must make a clear distinction between guilt-feelings and actual guilt. There are certain actions, the transgression of a social code more than of divine law, which can be highly charged with guilt-feelings, while some evident inhumanity may have no association of guilt at all. For example, someone might feel very guilty about not going to church twice on Sunday and perfectly at ease about his neglect of his children. The first step in the Christian healing of guilt is to attribute it rightly, to distinguish between scruple and disobedience. Then Christianity offers a full forgiveness for the actual guilt because in Jesus God has taken the consequences of it upon himself.

Those who receive pardon for their true failures, and really accept that they are forgiven, can then find release from their irrational feelings of guilt. The objective removal of guilt, Christians believe, is instantaneous; but the deliverance from guilty feelings – the cleansing of the conscience – may take time. You are accepted by God, says Tillich; now 'accept that you are accepted'. That is why the Christian religion speaks of salvation by grace, which means that God in his kindness gives to man what is beyond his power to work for or achieve; forgiveness, reconciliation, the restoration of the relationship which has been lost.

But every individual who wants it must receive it personally. God does not deal with humanity in the mass, but with individuals. Therefore I must accept my own responsibility for my own failure; whatever help and guidance I have received from other human beings, I must come alone to God and cast myself upon his mercy. Although this will be the most solitary thing I ever do, it brings me into company, possibly the first real company I have known.

The overcoming man

The idea of grace, of a loving initiative from beyond man, has no counterpart in humanism or existentialism. We have seen how Christians believe that the reconciliation between God and man is an act of grace from God's side. But more than that; in grace God not only does for man what he does not deserve, but makes him what he could not otherwise be. Against philosophies of man making himself, Christianity speaks of God working within, making new persons, giving life in a new mode.

No amount of religion or self-improvement, no accumulation of good deeds can achieve this. It is something which comes from God, to which man can only respond. The Christian ideal of the overcoming man, to borrow Nietzsche's phrase for the man who has gained mastery over life and self, is of one made new by grace.

There is a strange interview recorded in the Fourth Gospel, in which an eminent teacher of religion, a good and fair-minded man named Nicodemus, comes to Jesus one night to question him. While Nicodemus is still on his preliminaries Jesus seems to cut him short, comes straight to the point, and tells him that he must be 'born again'. Even to a highly-trained Jewish theologian those words have an unfamiliar ring. Nicodemus is puzzled. 'How can a grown man be born again? . . . He certainly cannot enter his mother's womb and be born a second time!'[8]

Jesus is using a metaphor. He is describing a change, or renewal, so total that it can best be pictured in this way. Among all the biblical illustrations of this change, the second birth is the most graphic. There can be no question that here is the heart of the New Testament message: the claim that God in his grace bestows a new order of life to those who will humbly accept his gift. Sometimes false emphasis in the teaching of the church or popular misunderstandings have obscured the teaching of the New Testament and reduced the Christian religion to a moral struggle or a following of the example of Jesus with the help of prayer. But anything less than the offer of restoration and re-creation is sub-Christianity. Christianity purports to be good news before it is an ethical code.

The new birth occurs at the point where a human being, knowing his failure and inadequacy, comes to God for forgiveness and life, and offers himself to God's re-creative power.

For some the new birth is traumatic, accompanied by great inner conflicts and agonies. Paul's was like this. Conversion for him meant a total re-orientation of his values. He had, in effect, to come to the point of admitting that his effort was utterly misdirected, and his way of life unhappiness and folly. For a man openly committed to the persecution of Christianity this was no easy thing to do. The result of his inner struggle was so devastating that it involved a temporary collapse of his very forceful ego, after which he went away alone for a period to think out the implications of what had happened to him, and was another ten years before he set out on his intensely active work as a missionary. The new birth cannot but be traumatic for those whose attitude has hardened in ways that are un-Christian. To deny what one has accepted for half a lifetime, and to affirm what one has laughed at or denied, is painful and costly. The subsequent adjustments may take years.

For others the new birth is so quiet and unobtrusive that it is hardly noticed at the time, although the results that gradually follow are momentous. This is often the case for those who come from Christian homes and feel that faith has been theirs since childhood, or for some who become Christians in adolescence, before their personalities have set in some definite mould. There are many Christians who can put no date or time to the new birth, but are in no doubt that it has happened.

When a person has been born again the signs become clearly discernible: a hunger for spiritual nourishment; an understanding of Christian language as if it had become real and three-dimensional; an assurance of being reconciled with God; an inner sense that Christ is a living person. Just as many an existentialist has said from his experience 'God is dead – for me', so the born again may say: 'God is very much alive and real – for me'.

The new life grows through months and years. There will be many falls and discouragements, as much as any child finds when it tries to crawl, walk, run, swim. There will almost certainly be one-sided growth at some stage – an immature enthusiasm or a claim to too much knowledge – just as with any growing person. Sometimes there will be revolt, like that of an adolescent who has to do so to test his convictions and establish his own identity. Almost certainly doubt and questioning will come, for that is the means of deeper understanding. The growth to maturity is gradual. But in spiritual life there is no growing old. When the body becomes fragile and exhausted, and even the mind loses its clarity, spiritual vitality and growth may continue.

At this point the Christian religion is empirically verifiable. Anyone who has been able to observe a church or movement which keeps to the Christianity of the Bible can see for himself the changes made in individual lives, and the difference between the unbeliever and the Christian in extreme old age, when most of the comforts and hopes of life have gone.

The new birth does not mean that a person's fundamental endowment of temperament or individual psychology is altered. Those things are the raw material of our existence. Christians may suffer as much as any others from the illnesses of body or mind, or from the stresses that can come to a sensitive personality. Christianity is no insurance policy against the vicissitudes of life. But the new birth does mean that the character is gradually changed, for character is what the raw material becomes as it is influenced. The dishonest becomes truthful; the idle, hardworking; the fearful, bold; the sullen, sweet-tempered; the shiftless, reliable; the selfish, concerned for others. This is a slow process, and it is never complete in this life. God does not go about his new creation in a hurry, any more than he did the first. But he does recreate from within, until the qualities of the life of Christ, love, joy, peace, patience, kindness, goodness, faithfulness, humility, self-control, are produced as spontaneously as fruit by a tree. Paul lists these virtues as being produced by the Spirit,[9] meaning by the natural outworking of a life in which the Spirit of God dwells; that is, a life made new.

I have suggested that the new birth does not alter temperament. A better use, however, can be made of it. If Christ gives self-control, we are less at the mercy of our natural waywardness. If Christ brings joy and peace, we are less vulnerable to our natural moods and discontents. Perhaps, too, the restoration of a relationship with God means a greater measure of self-acceptance and self-forgiveness, which are most necessary for inner peace.

The New Testament frequently uses the phrase 'eternal life' as another way of speaking of that dimension of life which a person enters when he is born again. Translations are incorrect when they render the phrase as 'everlasting life', implying simply a long duration in time. Rather, it means life that belongs to a dimension beyond this world. Perhaps men came to believe in its everlastingness because of what they had experienced of its quality – rather like the feeling of lovers that their love is of such a nature that it can have no end. Certainly there was a time when the Jews had only a very dim concept of life after death, but a burning sense of the reality of God in the present.

So eternal life in the New Testament sense begins here and now. But it is of such an order that it goes on beyond death. The life after death as Christians believe in it is not a shadowy reflection of this present life, a kind of dismal Hades. If anything, it is the exact opposite. This life is the shadow, the threshold, the incomplete, while the life to come is the full-blooded, the solid, the real.

C. S. Lewis fancifully pursued this idea in *The Great Divorce*. A bus-load of the occupants of hell are taken on a visit to heaven, and may stay there if they wish. The visitors find that by heaven's standards they are insubstantial – they barely exist at all. Heaven is immensely solid: the raindrops weigh tons; the blades of grass are strong as steel. The more in accord with the spirit of heaven the visitors are, the more substantial they too become, but those who cannot face its ways fade away to nothing.

This is why Christians affirm in the Creed, 'I believe in the resurrection of the body', not 'I believe in the immortality of the soul'. The body of course does not mean the atoms and molecules of which we are at present composed. They are only borrowed from a general pool and we return them within a very few years anyway. It means the real us, the whole us. Beyond this affirmation, Christians may not claim a fuller knowledge. The heightened language of the end of the book of Revelation is not giving a description of the geography and furnishings of heaven. It is teaching that heaven is the ultimate best, the supreme bliss, the satisfying of all desire and yearning, the meeting with God face to face and the worship of him eternally.

All this is implied in the doctrine of the new birth. Although it is a profoundly other-worldly doctrine, it is not, as some detractors of Christianity say, a sort of insurance policy; a basic premium paid now in the form of unwelcome duty and discipline to attain a considerable endowment hereafter. The evidence is very strong that far from incapacitating people for the present, a Christian faith brings new motivation and hope, a zest for living, and stability and resilience for those who suffer.

Moreover, no-one can be genuinely a Christian without feeling what Douglas Steere has called 'unlimited liability for one another'. A glance at world history in the last few hundred years will show that many of the major breakthroughs of science, and almost all the serious attempts to spread medicine and education to those without them, have been made by Christians. Indeed, it may be argued against the humanist view of history as the gradual conquest of superstition by reason that the development of science and the widespread practical application of human compassion could occur only within a culture that believed in a loving and rational God. Christianity when practised in the manner of its founder is neither escapist nor futuristic. The founder himself spent the greater part of his public work in deeds of kindness, and the greater part of his teaching was about a style of life in which love was the driving force. He did, however, constantly give warning that those who view this present life in material and intellectual terms only are blind and foolish.

The overcoming man, as the Christian sees him, is the man who has been reconciled with God, has received new life, and is being inwardly transformed. Not in his own strength, but by the grace of God, he is able gradually to master himself, is given power to live and love and finally to face death with confidence.

Immersed in suffering

The humanists' approach to suffering is simple. They feel bound to remove it where possible, with all the energy they can muster and with all the means at their disposal. As we have already seen, men and women of essentially humanist conviction are to be found at work in all humanitarian causes: the relief of famine, medical practice and research, and education – frequently with an altruism that appears to transcend the pedestrian tenets of their creed. The fact of suffering presents no intellectual problem; there is only the pragmatic one of what to do about it.

The existentialist position is very different. Suffering, despair, anguish are simply part of the meaninglessness within which man has to live, and if possible live courageously. Again there is no intellectual problem, merely the practical one of living as a sufferer and mastering despair. If existentialists are less involved than humanists in the relief of suffering, this is the direct consequence of the extreme individualism of their approach to life.

But the Christian cannot look at suffering in quite so simple a way. Suffering is a mystery, if by that we mean a problem in which we are personally involved, and through which, though we do not understand it fully, we can gain a deeper insight into our existence. Suffering, like love and joy, is too profound for mere rationalistic discussion. We can never stand back from it as if it were a problem in mathematics.

Intellectually, of course, there is the question of how to reconcile belief in a good, almighty God with so much in the world that seems to be destructive, wasteful and meaningless. It is only for those who believe in a good God that such a question arises at all. This is not a new problem, however, discovered, as is sometimes implied, by the agnostics of the last 100 years. All the time man was coming to believe in a good God, he was suffering too. Chronologically, it is probably true to say that the experience of suffering preceded the formulation of any doctrine about God, and that belief in a good God has come about in the face of pain.

At the level of experience, therefore, it seems that men can both suffer and believe in God. But although Christianity can go some way to meeting the intellectual question, it cannot offer a complete solution. We will first see what it does have to say about the problem of suffering and then later become more practical.

Consider a few examples of suffering: thousands killed or made homeless by an earthquake; starvation and death to innocent people as a result of war; the loneliness and anxiety of old age; the anguish of depression and other mental illness; the birth of deformed or idiot babies due to unforeseen complications from a drug; the breaking up of a marriage; the encroachment of a slow and fatal illness. In some of these, possibly the majority, human selfishness, weakness or negligence are involved. A great deal of suffering has been brought by man himself, and therefore man is to blame for it. But there is also much for which there is no human cause at all.

Suffering can be one of the most creative of all experiences, if faced with humility and fortitude. Indeed, would it be possible for the greatest human qualities to be aroused and exercised without it? The greatest heroism may be found in a patient enduring a long and painful illness; the greatest devotion and care may be shown in the family with a deformed or retarded child; the greatest patience by those who deal with an imbecile; the greatest long-suffering by the persecuted. Adversity does not always arouse these qualities but often it does, and in the most unlikely people. Certainly, if human existence were made up of day after day of comfort and pleasure, if our life really was what the humanists sometimes appear to want to make it, there would be no scope for our highest and our best. Thus sometimes it is only through the facing of disaster and anguish that we come to know our true humanity.

To say this sort of thing is dangerously near callousness, for it appears almost to welcome suffering, and it is much more easily said by someone in good health and spirits than by one who suffers. But Christians are never asked to welcome suffering. They are always committed to the utmost activity in the relief of it, as Jesus himself was. They will never treat calamity with resignation as something God has sent. But where suffering is inescapable or irremediable they seem to have resources to face it and even to use it creatively, accepting it as something God has permitted. Jesus shrank from the prospect of the cross but, convinced that there was no other way, went through with it in peace.

These two points, that suffering is often caused by human failure and the fact that suffering can evoke man's best, alleviate the intellectual problem but do not solve it. There remains much that appears to be simply destructive. Why does a good God allow that? It is here that we come face to face with the mystery.

In the Bible this question is very powerfully and dramatically treated in the book of Job. Job is a good man, yet he has to suffer. We meet him first in the height of his prosperity and happiness when, suddenly, his comfortable existence is shattered. His flocks are stolen; his possessions are destroyed; his nearest and dearest are killed in a tornado; then Job himself is afflicted with a disfiguring and painful disease. Thus, poignantly, the question is posed. Why does God allow even the innocent to suffer? Is he in control and is he just?

Job's friends come and offer advice – it can hardly be called sympathy – based on the assumption that his suffering is the result of his wrongdoing and that he should mend his ways. But Job, though he knows his imperfections, also knows that he is not disproportionately worse than his friends. Feeling that the justice of the universe has been violated, that life is meaningless, he enters the darkest experiences of doubt, anguish and near-total disillusionment, a despair that is almost suicidal.

But gradually he comes to see further. His soul reaches out towards belief in immortality; perhaps the final justice is beyond this life. He comes to believe in a deeper way that God is still mighty and just, and it ill behoves man to argue with him. Then at last Job finds satisfaction. God speaks to him from a whirlwind, reminding him that he is a mere man who has no right to question the ways of the Almighty. He points Job to the many questions that man cannot answer, the wonder of creation in the earth, the sea, the snow, the storm, the stars. He reminds him of the power and freedom of the wild animals, and such apparent absurdities of nature as the ostrich, the hippopotamus and the crocodile. In a roundabout way God is telling him that the true scheme of things is much grander than is encompassed by Job's little philosophy. So Job is humbled and he acknowledges: 'I know you can do all things, and no purpose of yours can be thwarted. . . . I had heard of you from others, but now I see you myself. . . . Therefore I repent from the bottom of my heart.'[1]

Thus Job sees himself as he truly is, and understands something of God as he is. After this moment of truth his prosperity is restored. The point of the story surely is this: not that Job regained his riches and security, but that in the encounter with God he found the answer for which he was looking. His intellectual problem about the cause of his suffering was never rewarded with a solution. There was no solution, but there was an answer; God himself, whom Job had to learn to trust in the darkness. This met his need at a much deeper level than that of mind. It met his emotions and will and loyalty, the point where suffering had occurred.

It would be possible to deride all this by saying that it simply sidesteps a major obstacle to belief in God by placing the answer beyond the mind. But that is too superficial. It is a plain fact of experience that, though suffering is intellectually inexplicable, it is often the dimension in which faith becomes really faith and men come to maturity. And those who trust God are frequently able to face great suffering without bitterness, with patience and even humour. Christians, too, have always been known to die courageously, as bear witness a succession of heroic men and women from the martyrs thrown to the lions in the first century to the many who have lost their lives for their faith in Africa in the last 100 years. Confronted with suffering, it is really the humanist view that seems inadequate because it scarcely reckons with the mystery of it; confronted with a sufferer, it may well be the humanist who has nothing to say.

The Christian faith adds an important insight to the message of the book of Job, which leaves us with a mystery and an almighty God. The Christian religion asserts that God himself is involved in the suffering of his creation. In the person of Jesus, God entered human life on the same terms as ourselves, including the experience of suffering. It is well known that how much a person suffers depends on his sensitivity. May we not suppose then that, as the supreme man, he knew the fullest pain? Insult and rejection would give him greater sorrow; being flogged and nailed to a cross would hurt him more. In his darkest hour, he cries out as if God has abandoned him; he, too, feels the desolation and meaninglessness of the abyss. Only, he feels it with an intensity granted to no other man.

If it is true that in Jesus God was suffering, there is comfort and reassurance. Whatever we may go through, however dark and inexplicable, God knows and understands, through experience; in a sense he goes through it with us too.

'I am poorly paid, I am unemployed, I live in a slum, I have tuberculosis. . . .
I am cold, God says, I am hungry, I am naked,
I am imprisoned, laughed at, humiliated . . .
I moan, riddled with shrapnel; I collapse under the volley of machine-gun fire,
I sweat men's blood on all battlefields,
I cry out in the night and die in the solitude of battle.'[2]

Christians, then, first see suffering as an evil to be overcome. They are followers of one who took great trouble with the sick, the insane, the hungry, the anxious, the rejected. Christians have been and always will be committed to the same work. Their effectiveness at it is beyond question, as many a hospital, hostel or refuge for social outcasts will bear witness. There is, in fact, a Christian way of caring which, because it is sensitive to the mystery of suffering, may bring a greater comfort than the easy answers of secularism could ever do.

But, for the Christian, suffering can never simply be an evil to overcome, nor can it simply be a way in which life's meaninglessness confronts us. Like the existentialists, Christians see suffering as something inescapably bound up with our existence. It is, paradoxically, one of the things that makes us human. Anyone who has been through acute suffering knows how it strips away all superficial covering and exposes the core beneath. But, if the core is exposed, it need not be exposed for destruction; rather it may be exposed to the love of God.

John, in his Gospel, has a curious habit of referring to the suffering of Jesus as his 'glory'. To John the most glorious moment does not seem to be the resurrection morning, but the lifting up of Jesus on the cross. And so Christians cannot only see suffering as a problem to be dealt with; certainly they do not seek to revel in it masochistically. But when unavoidable suffering does come they seek to use it creatively. In John's sense, they use it gloriously.

The Christian way of knowing

In the first part of this book we saw how the humanist position is based fundamentally on reason, to such an extent that humanists themselves now admit that they make an act of faith in it. Then we saw how the existentialists, in believing that this life has no meaning or rationality, repudiate the idea of objective knowledge and deny reason any ultimate validity. Each is setting out a way of 'knowing'; the first by reason and the second by intuition or arbitrary choice. What is the Christian way of knowing? On what sort of ground does a Christian hold beliefs such as those we have just considered?

The Christian way of knowing is through the combined exercise of reason and faith. Both are necessary for a mature Christian outlook, one that is genuinely faith and not a form of rationalism overlaid with piety, but yet which at the same time is not mere subjectivism, at the mercy of changing moods and fancies. First, then, we must look at the rational case for Christianity and see how far this takes us. Although this in itself is a subject for one book or several, an outline will be given here to show at least the sources from which the evidence comes.

A few hundred years ago, and in some quarters even until recently, much was made of the 'proofs for the existence of God'. It was claimed that by a process similar to Euclidean geometry the existence of God could be deduced from the natural world. Influenced as we are today by linguistic analysis, we would certainly no longer speak of 'proofs' in the sense of logical steps leading to the conclusion that God is. Proofs of this sort need axioms, and no statement could be more axiomatic, more supra-logical, than 'God is'. This could never be deduced.

The 'proofs' for God's existence really stand as a witness that in all lands and cultures there are men who find themselves believers in God and, finding themselves so, have used their rational faculty to try to prove what they already believe. The 'proofs' or arguments for God are in methodology more like those of natural science: inductive, seeking to provide explanations that fit the facts. And as such they still have some validity.

The ontological 'proof' sought to argue from the presence of the idea of God in the mind to the existence of God himself. Although such a step is logically impossible, the fact remains that almost all peoples do have a concept of the Deity. At least one explanation is that God has implanted the idea of himself into men's minds that they might search for him. This is no bolder an explanation than that of the psychologist who suggests that it is all wish-fulfilment.

The 'proof' from design was an attempt to argue from the order and pattern in the universe to the existence of a designer. It is logically not possible to prove it, but this is at least one explanation of the beautiful complexity of the world as revealed by science. Even the adaptation of living forms to their environment, which is sometimes presented as a process of blind chance, can be seen as part of God's technique.

Another 'proof' of God was based on the moral sense, the feeling of duty, of obligation, of 'ought', that all or most men possess, which goes far beyond the dictates of prudence or reason. One explanation of the presence of the moral faculty is that it was implanted by a moral God. The psychologists are fond of discovering the origins of morality in the relationship of the infant with its parents. This is perfectly acceptable to the Christian who simply holds that, in so far as theory is correct, it has described the way God works.

This brief account of the arguments for God is totally undeveloped but perhaps shows the sort of way in which they are relevant. The induction that 'God is' is for each argument at least a possibility. Of course there is nothing specifically Christian in these arguments, which could apply to any theistic religion.

But Christianity makes a distinct historical claim, by which it stands or falls. It is that God entered human life within recorded history, and that there is a reliable record in the New Testament both of what happened and of its impact on the men who thus met with God on earth. The New Testament has been subjected to the most searching and sceptical scrutiny during the last 100 years, to which it has stood up very well. The abundance of manuscripts and the early date of some mean that there can be little doubt about what the authors actually wrote. Those parts of the New Testament which can be verified by archaeological remains and the secular writings of contemporary historians, strongly support the substantial historicity of its background. I say 'background' deliberately, because there is very little about the central events of the Christian gospel to be found in early documents outside the New Testament.[3] (And why should there be, considering that Christianity for its first fifty years was generally thought of as a mere sect within the despised Jewish faith?) But we do know a good deal about the leading characters and places of the time: Pilate, Caiaphas, Herod the Great, Gallio, Jerusalem, Antioch, Corinth. The New Testament is verifiably accurate over these, Luke especially having been shown to be a thoroughly reliable historian. If so, it is reasonable to claim a similar degree of accuracy for the biblical account of the birth, life, death and resurrection of Jesus. Certainly it is prejudice, not reason, that dismisses this as impossible.

Suppose, then, that the Gospels and Acts are at least a fair record of events as judged by the standard of the historical writing of the day. Then we must provide an explanation of the person of Jesus as portrayed there. We must account for the absolutely central claim about his resurrection, which it seems was never effectively controverted at the time, and then the rapid spread of this faith all over the then civilized world. One very reasonable explanation of all this is simply that Jesus was God and Christianity is true.

There is another source of evidence for the truth of Christianity which we may term pragmatic, the evidence of faith at work. I have several times made statements about the effects of Christianity, suggesting that they are empirically verifiable: the unity and brotherhood that Christians can experience; the transformation of character which occurs through conversion; the radiance of the elderly who have Christian faith in contrast to those who do not; the capacity of Christians for compassion and self-sacrifice; the courage with which they generally face suffering and death. If these claims are correct, here again is a strong argument for belief. If Christianity works, it may well be true.

None of these evidences, inductive, historical, pragmatic, is in itself sufficient to compel assent. None of them is complete by itself. But they do all converge; it is this, rather than any single argument in isolation, that forms the intellectual case for the truth of Christianity.

Thus reason may take a man part way to Christian conviction, but by itself it can never make him a Christian. At some point faith and commitment must take over. Existential Christians have sometimes likened faith to a leap in the dark, an idea which can be dangerously misunderstood. It does not mean simply leaping out in a desperate hope that there might be something there. It is not a plunge across an utterly dark abyss. Of course a leap must be made, but it is made from reasonable ground. Faith is, rather, the considered commitment of a thoughtful person using all his faculties. Though it goes beyond reason, it does not violate it. And when Augustine wrote, 'I believe in order that I may understand', he implied that anyone who has made the step of faith has entered a wider field for the use of his reason.

Now it was at this point that Kierkegaard parted company with the general Christian tradition which followed Augustine in laying emphasis on both reason and faith. Because Kierkegaard found that the Christianity of his time had become largely a matter of 'man's wisdom', in his extreme reaction he emphasized faith so much that reason was neglected or even positively denied. He went so far as to say that Christianity is absurd, but yet must be believed. Kierkegaard's religion requires a continual crucifixion of the intellect. This means that the believer, never being convinced in his mind, cannot give the full assent of his personality to God. He cannot believe with integrity. This is a serious departure from the Christianity of Christ who, though proclaiming what purported to be a revelation of God's truth, constantly appealed to the mind and critical faculty.

On the other hand, some theologians have gone so far in their emphasis on reason that real faith has become unnecessary. There have been various attempts in Christian history to create complete theological systems, the two most famous being the *Summa* of Thomas Aquinas, which is still the corner-stone of Roman Catholic theology, and the *Institutes of the Christian Religion* by John Calvin. Both these thinkers were far too wise and subtle to forget about faith. But at times the result of their systematization has been to diminish the necessity for it. If every problem that concerns you deeply has a neat answer, completely tied up, which can be found on a certain page of a theological encyclopaedia, where is the need for faith? Christianity so treated always runs the danger of becoming just another glib rationalistic system, only with God as the key idea; as inadequate for the deep needs of humanity as rational humanism itself.

A Christian reared in this sort of religion once asked me: 'I used to know the answer to the problem of evil, but now I have forgotten it. Could you please remind me?' It was against the devastating shallowness of this sort of attitude that Kierkegaard revolted. There can be neither lasting security nor satisfaction within an enclosed system of thought. God's truth is far larger than any man-made theological framework. A number of times in history it appears that God has set aside the accepted theology and made some new truth known outside it. He refuses, it seems, to be contained within our systems.

Earlier we thought of faith as a leap. Now we must change the metaphor to something more personal. Faith is trusting. Faith in a human being implies a trust, a willingness to leave one's interest in his hands, a committal. Christian faith is a personal committal to Christ. Like human trust it is something which goes far beyond reason and, like human trust, it is the entry into a realm of rich experience and personal knowledge that transcends the logical. In Christian understanding, committal to Christ is the entry into eternal life; it is the beginning of that personal knowledge whereby Jesus becomes a friend, not an idea, and the sense of forgiveness not a theory but a fact.

So Christianity differs from both humanism and existentialism in its way of knowing. It does not, like extreme existentialism, deny the validity of reason; nor, like humanism, does it give it first place. It claims not to violate reason, but to go beyond it. The Christian's deepest knowledge is reached through an act of faith that is completely personal. In this sense Christian truth is existential.

Notes

1   *The Letter to Diognetus.*
2   1 John 4: 20. Unless otherwise indicated, biblical quotations in this chapter are from *Good News for Modern Man* (The New Testament in Today's English Version, Fontana Books).
3   Luke 17: 33.
4   Mark 7: 20–23.
5   Romans 3: 11, 12 quoting Psalm 14.
6   Colossians 3: 11.
7   Matthew 27: 46.
8   John 3: 4.
9   Galatians 5: 22, 23.

1   Job 42: 2–6 (a loose paraphrase).
2   M. Quoist, *Prayers of Life* (Gill).
3   See Michael Green, *Runaway World* (Inter-Varsity Press) for a survey of such evidence as there is.

3.2

Towards a theory of dementia care: the interpersonal process (1993)

ABSTRACT

A description of the microstructure of interpersonal processes is developed, based on the analysis of interaction as a succession of reflexive triadic units. This account can be modified in some aspects so as to provide a detailed theory of the process of dementia care. The theory is particularly relevant to moderate and severe dementia, and to formal care settings. A key concept is that of facilitation. The idea of a 'culture of dementia' is explored. Cautiously optimistic conclusions are reached about the possibilities for enabling dementia sufferers to remain in a state of relative well-being.

Introduction

Throughout the history of the dementias of old age the actual process of caregiving has remained opaque, mysterious, uninformed by theoretical insight. Some attempts have been made to outline a general psychology of caring. Recent work has, for example, examined such aspects as the components of caregiving, the caring relationship and the feelings that accompany the giving and receiving of care.[1] In relation to dementia many family members have offered accounts of their experience, and there have been some valuable studies of the nature and consequences of caregiving.[2] Much more is required, however, if this vital and creative work is to come out of the shadows. We need a social psychology which reveals dementia care as a true process of meeting between persons; which shows what that meeting consists of, how it comes about, and what might prevent it from occurring.

It might be argued that theory in this field is not really necessary: that good caring springs spontaneously from our human nature, and that what is really important can be learned simply and directly, through example. This view, however, will not suffice, for several reasons. First, caregiving of the kind we are considering requires a level of insight that goes far beyond commonsense, and it may even be beyond that for which our species is instinctually prepared. Second, the ageing of populations and the concomitant vast increase in the prevalence of dementia are so recent that there has been no cultural preparation; the good caregiver is, in some respects, a person who is ahead of the times – perhaps one who beckons us on to a gentler and more compassionate age. Third, while there can be no substitute for learning through experience, mere copying is not enough; there needs to be a *prise de conscience*, a 'grasp in conscious-ness', if work is to be done with a confident intelligence. Caregiving – whether in family or institutional contexts – needs to find a voice.

Neither psychiatry nor clinical psychology have provided the foundations for a theory of dementia care. Generally they have preferred to remain on more solid ground, assigning individuals to diagnostic categories, codifying their various impair-ments, and searching for correspondence with defects in the structure or functioning of the brain. Behind this, there is the relentless search for causes, construed almost entirely at a neurological level. Nursing, for its part, has made great advances in recent years, moving away from its former subservience to medical science and developing a body of theory that is genuinely its own. As yet, however, the issue of caring for a person with dementia has scarcely been addressed. In none of these areas is it possible to find the kind of social psychology that meets our requirements. While the issues relate to all contexts, in this paper we shall mainly be concerned with those of formal care.

It is outside the fields dominated by medical discourse that the beginnings of a practical social psychology of dementia care may be discerned. Perhaps the earliest hints are in the work of Feil, and the practices that she came to call Validation Therapy.[3] There are problems in her theoretical frame, as we shall see; but Feil was the first person to insist, loudly and clearly, that the subjectivity of the 'confused old-old' (to use the term she first favoured) must be taken seriously. Feil developed her ideas partly in reaction to Reality Orientation as she encountered it, with its simplistic emphasis on mundane facts. As a contemporary practice, however, Reality Orientation has moved on a long way from this; and when it includes such matters as the 'reality' of relationships, feelings, and immediate sensory experience, it gives hints of a much more sympathetic social psychology.[4]

Reminiscence work also has proved valuable with those who have a dementing illness, particularly in group contexts.[5] Here, however, the benefit may not mainly be from the kind of 'internal' work we associate with Reminiscence Therapy; it may well be that memories mainly provide a resource that dementia sufferers can draw upon in order to communicate effectively in the present.[6] A recent arrival on the scene is Resolution Therapy, with its typically Rogerian emphasis on accepting the validity of dementia sufferers' experience, its insistence on looking for the meaning that may be present in their utterances, and hence its concern to identify real, present need.[7]

Approaches such as these give many valuable pointers towards understanding good dementia care; when practised with skill and kindness they do undoubtedly provide some basis for a real meeting between the dementia sufferer and the Other. At the level of theory, however, they have been bounded in a common limitation, one which they share with most of psychiatry and clinical psychology. It is as if a radical divide has been made between 'us' (the cognitively intact, and fundamentally sound members of society) and 'them' (the damaged and deficient). 'The problem' of dementia is attributed to 'them', while 'we' are let off the hook. The dementia sufferer is thus a kind of alien, and caregiving tends to be viewed as action by superiors – a modern version of old-time charity. Matters look very different when 'the problem' of dementia is seen as something that belongs to us all, whether or not we have cognitive impairments. The damage and deficits that 'we' bring come clearly into view, and behind that the ageism, fear, greed and hypocrisy endemic in society.[8] Positively, this view opens up a much more hopeful, much less deterministic, prospect for dementia care.[9]

A less clinical account of dementia has also been adumbrated by Gilleard, emphasizing the point that mind itself is social rather than individual.[10] More recently Sabat and Harré have questioned the idea of 'loss of self' in dementia.[11] They argue that if a dementia sufferer is to sustain his or her part in the social world, other people, with their corresponding expectations and performances, are required. Often those others do not provide what is needed. When they do, however, some personae can be sustained by the dementia sufferer and self, in this sense, is not lost. This analysis is valuable and certainly moves towards a social psychology of caregiving. It may, however, be in danger of trivializing the ravages inflicted at the neurological level in severe dementia. Correspondingly, it may have seriously underestimated the part played by the caregiver; if this were simply a matter of providing the corresponding personae to sustain social acts, dementia care would be a relatively simple matter. If our theory of dementia care is to be adequate to the task, we need to inquire more deeply into the nature of the shattering of subjectivity that a dementing illness may entail.

Understanding processes: a note on method

The problem of how to develop a theory of a process is one that has engaged the natural sciences for centuries. In general, the tactic which has proved to be outstandingly successful is as follows.[12] A thorough exploration is made of the problem field, including those aspects which might at first seem to be trivial, ephemeral or circumstantial. Next, through an act of the intellect, a 'thought experiment', a coherent account is created, one which has its own 'inner' logic or consistency. Then this account is tested as carefully as possible at those points where it makes contact with observables. In physics the account almost always draws on mathematics, using such devices as the differential equation; in chemistry and biochemistry use is often made of some kind of model also; the process is thus made capable of visualization.

Something analogous, it may be argued, is required when attempting to create a theory of processes that occur in the social world. It will not suffice to use a crude empiricism, which simply takes measurements at different time points, without attempting to discern an 'inner' rationale. Moreover, since we as persons actually occupy a world of meanings, and since we successfully engage in interpersonal processes every day, we are already immersed in that which we seek to investigate; we do indeed have 'privileged access'. So in order to create theories and explanations related to our social being we do not need to find the resources in natural science, with its ultimate agnosticism about what its subject-matter really consists of. The raw materials for generating appropriate theories are already to hand, even if they have to be refined considerably for a specialist task such as the one we have in mind.[13] Empiricism comes afterwards, as a way of checking the validity of theories created 'from within'.

There is a large body of theory and investigation in social psychology, related particularly to interpersonal communication, whose underpinning consists of electromechanical analogies.[14] Its basis might be termed 'the morse code model of communication'. The central thesis is usually set out in a manner such as that shown below,

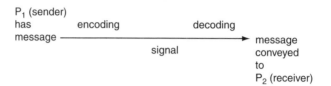

A model such as this does, undoubtedly, have value, especially perhaps when dealing with non-verbal communication within a tightly-bounded cultural context. More generally, however, it is deeply unsatisfactory. It seems to presuppose, for example, that in any communicative act there is a pre-existing message, independent of the code; that a code exists, independent of the communicative context; and that the code is understood similarly at some level (even if preconscious), by both 'sender' and 'receiver'. Among its further drawbacks are that it does not give sufficient space either for creativity or reciprocity, or for understanding misunderstanding.

This kind of theory has been applied to the development of a model of communication with dementia sufferers.[15] The use of electromechanical analogies may assist in sharpening our understanding of the ways in which information-processing is restricted as a result of neurological impairment. Such an approach, however, fails to grasp that commonality of personhood that underlies all true meeting, and it fails to do justice to the subtlety and fragility of the communicative act.

In developing a process theory of dementia care it may be much more fruitful to draw on a body of knowledge created entirely by consideration of the social world: that of symbolic interactionism. Here the basic unit of interpersonal communication is generally taken to be a reflexive triad, of the form shown below.

(i) P_1 makes an action
(ii) P_2 interprets P_1's action and responds
(iii) P_1 interprets P_2's response and reflects upon it

The fabric of everyday social life may be considered to consist of triadic units of this kind, in which meanings are continually being created and negotiated. The idea of the triad needs to be greatly elaborated, as we shall see, for its full explanatory power to be deployed. But we have here the basis for giving an account of social acts so simple and non-problematic as an exchange of greetings, or so complex and convoluted as the attempt of two people of different culture and language to make contact with one another. From it we can also develop a rich understanding of the interpersonal process in dementia – both when it succeeds and when it fails.

The reflexive triad – in more detail

If the basic unit of communication that we have been considering is analysed in more detail, it has a form such as that shown below.

P_1 – (a) an individual with a given temperament, constitution, etc
  (b) carrying his or her unique legacy from past experience
  (c) in a particular sentient state (referring here to mood, emotion, feeling, etc)
  (d) defines the situation in a certain way and
  (e) having various assumptions (about others' expectations, states, etc)
  (f) and with certain desires, intentions, expectations, etc.
                                   – makes an action
P_2 – (a, b, c, d, e)
  interprets P_1's action and (f)
                         – responds
P_1 – interprets P_2's response and
                         – reflects
  checking in various ways whether the act he or she is trying to bring off with P_2 is likely to be successful.

At this point the next initiative may be taken by P_1 or P_2 – or, of course by some other person. In the light of what has happened, any of factors c–f, with any participant, may change.

This framework is, of course, highly analytic; its purpose is to illuminate what is going on as social acts are carried through. During the process a great deal is being registered at a preconscious level: it is not present in conscious awareness, although it can be made to be so.[16] Behind this lies the domain which depth psychology terms the unconscious. It has a particular relevance to (b), the legacy from past experience; for this may be regarded as a unique cluster of personal resources and psychic defences, formed in situations where the individual has had a sense of power and competence, or of impotence and threat. (All this, together with (a), is often gathered together under the term personality.) The emphasis, then, is on the human being as one who anticipates and constructs, while also acknowledging (as in mainstream psychoanalytic theory) that the past is still present, shaping a person's thought and action.[17]

Besides showing how it is possible for social acts to be successful, this framework also offers many insights into why communication between persons may break down. Definitions of the situation may be at variance, expectations may not be complementary, emotions or moods may be misconstrued, a sense of threat may be created with the corresponding activation of defences, and so on. This whole approach clearly has far greater explanatory power than one which is based on the 'morse code model', with its simplistic assumptions about encoding and decoding.

Before we apply these ideas to dementia care, one communicative context deserves special consideration. It is that of 'good' psychotherapy (whether or not it is done under that name). Here one person (say P_2) is able to give sustained 'free attention' to the other (P_1). He or she is able to develop an empathic understanding of P_1's frame of reference (essentially a combination of factors a–e), and is aware of some of P_1's conflicting desires, defensive manoeuvres, areas of high vulnerability, dislocations and developmental blocks. In order to be able to do this for others, P_2 needs to be aware of these things in his or her own being, and to have done some work upon them; if so, then awareness of P_1 is less likely to be blanked out defensively, and the disturbances created by P_1's communicative attempts are more likely to be used constructively. The more open P_2 is to his or her own experiencing, the greater is the possibility of therapeutic interchange. Conversely, the more 'blocked' P_2 is, the less P_1 will be helped to develop new personal resources.

That, so to speak, is the microstructure of therapeutic communication. The larger and continuing context is a relationship in which a high level of trust has been established. P_2 is providing a safe space for P_1's hidden pain, fear, shame, conflict, to emerge, there to be faced in a climate of honesty and kindness. While this is occurring P_2 may be described as 'holding' P_1. Holding is, of course, a metaphor. Its original reference is to the holding of an infant, where the physical and symbolic actions of providing a place of safety come together.[18]

Application to dementia care

The general framework we have been considering needs to be developed further when it is applied to those situations where one person has a dementing illness. Some of the presuppositions of everyday communicative contexts may no longer be applicable. New skills will have to be added to those which ordinarily suffice. Although their cognitions are in disrepair, dementia sufferers have a rich and powerful emotional life. Often, too, they are very sociably inclined.[19] In many cases the psychological defences which gave stability and protection against that which might overwhelm the psyche are breaking or have broken down; thus they are liable to be 'invaded' by grief, rage, fear, a sense of terrible menace or desolation. Dementia care, then, provides a unique communicative context, which merits consideration in its own right. What follows applies to some extent to all care contexts, but particularly to formal care.

Suppose that P_1 is the dementia sufferer, and P_2 the caregiver. P_1 makes a gesture: an utterance of some kind, or a bodily movement. It is the beginning of the construction of an action; it may be an attempt to make contact with another, or the expression of a desire. To an even greater extent than a person whose cognitions are intact, P_1 cannot make the action alone. If the dementia is severe P_1's capacity for defining the situation, for holding intentions and expectations in place, is failing and fading. Perhaps he or she gets as far as a proto-definition; but the action is blurred, confused, virtually from its beginning. One thing, however, is not in doubt: P_1 did initiate something – there was a reaching out into the social world.

So P_2's part involves at least the following:

1. To recognize P_1's initial gesture and to honour it with a response.

2. To have some empathic understanding of P_1's inwardly 'shattered' state; to have a sense of what P_1 might be experiencing.

3. To fill out a definition of the situation in collaboration with P_1; not 'correcting' it to fit institutional convenience.

4. To appreciate and respond to the desire or need that P_1 may be expressing: to help to convert it into an intention.

5. To use interaction to sustain P_1's action; to keep it from falling into the void because of P_1's memory deficit.

6. To respond sensitively to signs that P_1's proto-definition of the situation may be changing, and to move with that change.

7. To 'hold' P_1 through whatever emotional experience the interaction may entail, so that it becomes a completed act in the social world.

There are many ways in which P_2 might prevent the communicative act from being successfully completed. The following are particularly common.

1. Failing to recognize the gesture: writing it off as 'agitation', perseveration, 'naughtiness', etc.

2. Failing to operate at the level of feeling and diffuse awareness.

3. Imposing his or her framework (or that of the institution) upon P_1.

4. Being over-committed to a single and definite course once the interaction is in progress.

5. Rushing the interaction, rather than letting it go at its natural pace.

6. Blocking P_1's communicative efforts, or distancing P_1, at some point where they arouse anxiety, or a sense of personal threat, or a feeling of inadequacy (in P_2).

There are great limitations, then, in models of communication in dementia care which assume pre-set social acts with a more-or-less standard form, or social personae which are stable throughout. The more severe the dementia, the less these ideas apply, and the greater the degree to which communication with a dementia sufferer becomes an open-ended and unpredictable adventure.

If a successful communicative act is to occur, then, P_2 must play a rather different part from that required in everyday communication. He or she will need some of the qualities and skills of a therapist or counsellor, and some that are special to dementia care. The more severe P_1's dementia, the greater will be the need for P_2 to have these additional communicative competences. To use a simple analogy, P_2 is rather like a very resourceful tennis coach, keeping a rally going with a novice (or – an even closer parallel – a deeply discouraged older person); whatever shot is attempted, provided it goes over the net, the coach will create something from it, and make a return that can enable the rally to continue. The coach needs attitudes and skills very different from those required to win a game with a player of the same standard; but this kind of play can be creative, demanding and intensely satisfying.

The analogy may be illustrated by three vignettes, each of which describes events in the context of formal care. In each vignette, also, we can gain a sense of the triadic sequence taking its course.

The first concerns a woman (Mrs A) who had been a widow for some years; she was still living at home, and attended a day centre. There she often presented, without obvious emotion, a simple narrative line, of the form 'My husband died six weeks ago and I'm still right upset about it'. On one occasion a caregiver listened to her attentively, and responded with such words as 'You're missing him, aren't you?', 'Yes', she said 'I am'. Then she repeated her narrative, this time with a little more detail, soon returning to the original line. Again the caregiver gave her an empathic response, to which she gave a fuller version of her story, with more sign of emotional engagement. The cycle was repeated several times, each iteration bringing greater elaboration and animation, until it approximated to a clear and rational account of her husband's death and its aftermath. A little later she collapsed in deep sobbing; another caregiver held her in her arms and comforted her until the wave of grief had dissipated.

The second vignette concerns a woman (Mrs B) who was receiving respite care in a residential home. Apparently she had woken up in a 'bad mood', and was thoroughly uncooperative. She had been left in her room for a while; eventually she was brought down in her dressing gown, after all the other residents had had their breakfast. She sat alone in the dining room, shouting, and pounding on the table with her fists. When given a bowl of porridge she refused to eat it; later she started to throw spoonfuls of it around. In due course the bowl was taken away. She swore at the care assistant, and attempted to hit her. A few minutes later another caregiver came and sat beside Mrs B at the table. She swore at him too, and began to hit him. He said to her 'You're angry, aren't you? You're wanting to hit someone. Alright, hit me then', and he offered her his hands; (an extremely risky offer; not one which could be recommended for general use). She did indeed hit him, and continued to swear, rudely and angrily, for a while. Eventually she began to quieten down. He offered her a cup of coffee, to which she replied 'Yes please'. When he returned with the coffee and three biscuits she seemed again to be enraged. She started to break up a biscuit and throw it on the floor. He took another biscuit, and did the same. From this point forward her rage abated, and she became increasingly calm and sociable. With the exception of one small episode where she was clearly provoked by a careworker who disliked her, she remained so for the rest of the day.

The third vignette concerns a woman (Mrs C) who had been in residential care for some time. She spoke only occasionally, and her state seemed to alternate between tension and withdrawal. Since she caused hardly any disturbances she received very little attention. Often when seated her arms produced wiping or drumming movements, which appeared to be only partially under voluntary control. Her face was generally sorrowful and haggard. In conventional terms, her dementia was far advanced. One day she was sitting alone at a table, drumming with her hands. A caregiver sat with her for a while. Then he took a teaspoon; very gently, he began to drum on the table also, responding to her rhythm. Her face began to brighten, and her drumming became louder. Gradually the sounds developed into a kind of duet, one in which both persons were highly engaged. For a while no words were spoken, but the level of contact, both through the 'music' and through the language of facial expression, was high. At a break in the duet she turned to him, coyly and shyly, calling him 'Daddy', and began to talk to him as if she were his little girl.

Episodes such as these are commonplace in settings where dementia care is centred on the person. Undoubtedly they involve 'holding', or the provision of a safe space where an individual is not going to be overwhelmed by painful emotion.

Also they involve 'validation', in the sense of acknowledging the reality of the dementia sufferer's experience, and within his or her frame of reference. It seems highly unlikely, however, that what is occurring approximates to the process suggested by the theory of Validation Therapy: the working on, or even working through, of issues left unresolved from earlier stages of life. It makes much more sense of the facts to suppose that in each such episode a dementia sufferer uses whatever action resources he or she still has available, from a diminishing repertoire, so as to do whatever is still possible in order to remain, even if minimally, a person.

Mrs A had a story line; perhaps she needed to repeat it often, or it might be lost for ever. The single line could be amplified when another person was truly present for her. Mrs B had some of the learned habits of an angry child, which she could employ with considerable effect, especially considering her physical strength. Mrs C had some simple bodily movements, perhaps the vestigial remains of many actions habituated in the running of her home. Each of these three women, with their differing degree of impairment, needed the presence and help of another human being in order to continue to be a person. Each needed 'holding', in order for their emotional lives to be tolerable. Each needed 'validation', in order for their private experience to become real. But also each needed what might be termed 'facilitation': that form of enabling provided by another person, in order for acts to be accomplished, and for a place to be reserved for them in the social world.

Facilitation: the missing concept in dementia care

Much of what we have been considering here has parallels in the psychology of infancy and early childhood.[20] Here also cognitions are not stable, emotional life is rich and powerful, and defences are not elaborated. Much of what has been learned about the conditions under which personhood emerges can be applied to the dementing process, where personhood is potentially in demise.

The infant makes a gesture. It may be an incompletely coordinated body movement, a cry, a gasp, or the beginning of a little game. The sensitive caregiver sees the gesture and responds to it, destroying nothing of its originality and direction, but helping to fill it out with meaning and make it into an action. A central hypothesis is that such joint ventures, successfully completed, convey to the infant that he or she is an agent; one whose movements, coming increasingly within conscious control, have meaning, and one whose intentions count for something in the world. The infant must be 'held' also, in order to feel safe when overwhelmed by powerful emotion. When these conditions are present the infant acquires the sense of a rich 'inner' world; the stability of that world is guaranteed by memory, and its validity is open to continual reality-testing. Thus the infant comes gradually to intuit that he or she belongs to the company of persons.

What happens, in contrast, if gestures continually meet with no response, perhaps being ignored, or over-ridden, or simply not being noticed? For a while the infant will continue, making colossal efforts to be heard and recognized. Compliance is a last resort, when there seems to be no other way to be recognized by the Other. The cost, however, so depth psychology suggests, is enormous. The growing person is handicapped by a tendency to over-conformity, unable to hold up as an agent in the face of neglect, pressure or opposition. One of the key elements of true personhood is impaired, because the necessary facilitation was missing.

Ideas such as these make sense, and are loosely corroborated by developmental data, although they are not testable in every detail. They suggest powerful analogies for our understanding of dementia care, as is clear from the three vignettes we have examined. Just as the infant needs facilitation, while the nervous system is in a crucial process of maturation, so also does the dementia sufferer, while the nervous system is in a crucial decline. The most poignant parallel is to those occasions where the gesture meets with no response. Those who are dementing are relatively powerless, and cannot give a detailed description of the terms on which they would like to live from day to day. If, then, their gestures repeatedly fall to nothing, their predicament is a terrible one. They have only dwindling 'inner' resources on which to draw, and their confidence to make an appeal to others is draining away.

This is one way of interpreting the later stages of a dementing illness, when an individual appears to be vegetating. It may be construed as a state of compliance enforced by psychological neglect, when all hope of reaching out to others has been abandoned. Before this occurs there may be a period of protest. Those who are at this point use such means as are at their disposal. Sometimes these are not so unlike those which are available to a young child; particularly shouting and crying, repetitive movement, sleeplessness and the use of the excretory function.

There is, however, a very serious difference for older persons whose mental powers are failing. Those who are forced into compliance early in life may have the possibility of creating a rich 'inner' world; for some this may be the seed-bed of artistic and creative work, and of certain kinds of religious experience. The dementia sufferer, it seems, cannot have such compensations, because his or her subjective world is in chaos and ruin. As neurological impairment advances, the only richness will be that which is discovered in the company of the Other; the only creativity will be that which emerges through facilitation by the Other; and if there is a spirituality, it will be of the kind described in Martin Buber's theology, where the eternal Thou addresses us in the human experience of true meeting.[21]

A culture of dementia

Thus far the discussion has focussed on interactions between dementia sufferers and caregivers. There is another aspect to dementia care, one which has been almost totally neglected in the literature. This is the interaction between dementia sufferers themselves. It is evident that in some care environments there is virtually no contact between one dementia sufferer and another; or that contact, when it does occur, tends to be destructive. In other environments, however, where the persons concerned are cognitively impaired to roughly the same degree, there is a great deal of contact and communication that is clearly enhancing; in fact, what might be termed a 'culture of dementia' has developed.

One dementia sufferer takes another to the toilet, and patiently waits outside for her to finish . . . a man and a woman form an unspoken bond, which has some of the appearances of a long-standing marriage . . . a man tolerantly allows the looting of his little supply of sweets . . . two women sit side by side, doing 'pseudoknitting' . . . one person senses that another is still hungry, and brings him an extra plate of food . . . conflict occurs, and there is a real reconciliation . . . three people go out together, perfectly at ease, relaxing in the sun. Here we have glimpses of a situation where the caregivers have done their work so well that for a while they have receded right into the background. To return to the tennis analogy. It is as if the deeply discouraged would-be players have gained sufficient confidence to play together, accepting that they all make many errors. Their attempts at rallying, however, have a special kind of rhythm and fluency, and can continue for hours and hours.

The nature of communication within a culture of dementia is a topic that deserves to be studied closely. At a purely verbal level many of the interactions seem to make very little sense by the standards of everyday conversation, or even by those of Resolution Therapy. Yet it would be a great mistake to suppose that these are 'collective monologues' (to use Piaget's somewhat disparaging phrase in referring to the conversations of four-year-olds). The point is, rather, that human contact is supremely important, and almost any means can be adapted in order to obtain it. Dementia sufferers sometimes seem to have a heightened awareness of body language, and often their main meanings may be conveyed non-verbally. In the case of those who are very severely impaired in cognition, it seems probable that the words and sentences are at times more of an accompaniment or adornment than the vehicle for carrying the significant message.

It would be very worthwhile to enquire systematically into the question of why a culture of dementia develops in one context and not in another. The answer seems to be a simple one, but it is not based on systematic comparative evidence. When a person-centred approach to care has been used consistently over an extended period, the dementia sufferers have developed a general sense of well-being and personal security. Individuals have received a more or less enduring facilitation, and their personal resources are no longer dwindling; the spectre of vegetation has vanished. Instead they are, to varying degrees, self-respecting, socially confident, hopeful agents. They feel able to reach out to each other, to take some risks, to find ways of establishing contact even when the verbal channel has only limited use.

A culture of dementia, then, is a vast distance from that dullness and deadness which generally characterizes poor care settings, where troublesome behaviour is often controlled by drugs. Also it does not require an environment where every need is supplied upon demand. This is not how adult life is, and it is not a model for the life of those who are cognitively impaired in old age. Where there is a culture of dementia, founded upon general well-being, the participants are more able to deal with conflict, challenge, change, frustration, disappointment; not unlimited, and in a milieu that is fundamentally safe, sound, and simple enough for its pattern to be grasped.[22] There is an endemic danger, then, of underestimating what dementia sufferers can do when continual facilitation is provided. The illusion of incapacity comes because life has so often been set up for them on impossible terms.

A person-centred approach to care

In this paper we have been looking at the microstructure of dementia care, focussing attention on the communicative act and its vicissitudes. It is clear that caregiving, far from being something merely done 'to' or 'for' a needy person, is a truly cooperative and reciprocal engagement. The theory, when explicated in full detail, becomes rather complex; its roots lie in centuries-old discussions about the nature of science, and the problem of how we are to understand the social world. It is possible, however, to express many of the key ideas in a simple and accessible way, especially through the use of appropriate analogies and illustrations.[23]

The theory presented here has incorporated some of the key social-psychological ideas that already inform good care practice. For example, there is the concept of 'validation', in its original sense of making real, making strong, of acknowledging the subjective truth of another person's experience.[24] I have suggested, however, in contrast to Validation Therapy, that it is extremely unlikely that a person will genuinely 'work through' or resolve developmental issues from the past during a dementing illness. The central idea of Resolution Therapy is present also: that is, taking a dementia sufferer's message seriously, and trying to find the need that is being expressed.

It may be the case, however, that some communicative gestures do little more than express a broad need for aliveness and human contact; meaning may actually be created as the gesture becomes an action. In contrast to some of the more established ideas, I have attempted to take into account the transient, moving, ever-changing nature of the 'situation', and the corresponding open-ness and flexibility that are required of the caregiver. Above all I have given attention to what it means to take seriously the personhood of those who have a dementing illness; thus creating an interpersonal – and indeed moral – psychology, far removed from the behaviouristic crudities that have so often been used in this field.

The theory sheds new light on why dementia care, whether in family or in institutional settings, has often failed. So many gestures have passed un-noticed, or been ignored or discounted; so many communicative acts have been aborted; so many gross impositions have been made upon the dementia sufferer from others' frames of reference. The hope for dementia care, within new patterns that are currently being created, is that a far higher level of communicative competence may be possible than has generally been believed. The key concepts here are 'holding' and 'facilitation'. Although all this may appear to make extra demands upon the caregiver, the general experience seems to be that the kind of approach I have described here makes care work less exhausting; it can even, at times, be stimulating and refreshing.

In an earlier paper in this journal (see ref 9) Kathleen Bredin and I looked at the matter of relative well-being in dementia. We identified 12 indicators of well-being, which can be operationally defined. Behind these, we postulated four 'global states', grounded in the life of emotion and feeling rather than that of elaborate cognition. The states are self-esteem, agency, social confidence and hope. The links with the theory presented in this paper can now be made. *A communicative act was carried through successfully*. The dementia sufferer felt recognized as a person: *self-esteem was enhanced*. A gesture was transmuted into action: *agency was confirmed*. The dementia sufferer moved towards the Other and was welcomed: *social confidence increased*. Confusion and disorder within the psyche were met with order and stability in the social world: *hope was sustained*. It is the repetition of this experience, we may hypothesize, that can establish well-being even in the face of severe cognitive impairment.

None of this amounts to 'therapy', although some of the concepts and skills derive from psychotherapeutic work. There has been an inflation of terminology. Whether there can be a further set of interpersonal processes that genuinely meet the criteria for calling them therapy for dementia sufferers is an issue worth examining in its own right. The problematic which this paper has addressed, however, is a simple and straightforward one: the actual process that is involved in providing person-centred care. If the theory presented here is sound in its essentials, we have greater ground for optimism than tradition has allowed, and carers of all kinds can take heart.

Acknowledgement

I wish to thank Kathleen Bredin for the many contributions she has made to the development of the ideas in this paper, and for her collaboration in collecting the data that form its empirical base.

Notes

1 Hall, J. N., Towards a psychology of caring. *British Journal of Clinical Psychology*, 29 (1990), 129–143.
2 Willoughby, J. and Keating, W., Being in control: the process of caring for a relative with Alzheimer's Disease. *Qualitative Health Research*, 1 (1991), 27–50.
3 Feil, N., *Validation: the Feil Method*, Edward Feil Productions, Cleveland, Ohio, 1982 (now available from Winslow Press, Bicester).
4 Holden, U. and Woods, R., *Reality Orientation: Psychological Approaches to the Confused Elderly*. Churchill Livingstone, New York, 1988.
5 Coleman, P., Issues in the therapeutic use of reminiscence with elderly people. In Hanley, I. and Gilhooly, M. (eds), *Psychological Therapies for the Elderly*. Croom Helm, London, 1986.
6 Sutton, L. J., Discursive critique and discourses in our study of memory and dementia. Department of Clinical Psychology, Moorgreen Hospital, Southampton, 1992.
7 Stokes, G. and Goudie, F., Counselling confused elderly. In Stokes, G. and Goudie, F. (eds), *Working with Dementia*. Winslow Press, Bicester, 1990.
8 Kitwood, T., The dialectics of dementia: with particular reference to Alzheimer's Disease. *Ageing and Society*, 10 (1990), 177–196.
9 Kitwood, T. and Bredin, K., Towards a theory of dementia care: personhood and well-being. *Ageing and Society*, 12 (1992), 269–287.
10 Gilleard, C., Losing one's mind and losing one's place: a psychosocial model of dementia. Address to the British Society of Gerontology, 10th Annual Conference, 1989.
11 Sabat, S. R. and Harré, R., The construction and deconstruction of self in Alzheimer's Disease, *Ageing and Society*, 12 (1992), 443–461.
12 Harré, R., *The Principles of Scientific Thinking*. Macmillan, London, 1970.
13 Harré, R. and Secord, P. F., *The Explanation of Social Behaviour*. Blackwell, Oxford, 1974.

14 Shannon, C. and Weaver, W., *The Mathematical Theory of Communication*. University of Illinois Press, Illinois, 1949.

15 Jones, G. M. M., A communication model for dementia. In Jones, G. M. M. and Miesen, B. M. L. (eds), *Caregiving in Dementia*. Routledge, London, 1992.

16 Epstein, S., Some implications of cognitive-experiential self theory for research in social psychology and personality. *Journal for the Theory of Social Behaviour*, 15 (1985), 283–309.

17 Kitwood, T., *Concern for Others*, Chapter 3. Routledge, London, 1990.

18 Clancier, A. and Kalmanovitch, J., *Winnicott and Paradox*. Tavistock, London, 1987.

19 Dobbs, A. R. and Rule, B. G., Behaviour of dementia patients: implications for environmental design and patient management. Paper presented to Geriatric Psychiatry Workshop, Edmonton, Canada, 1990.

20 Kagan, J., *The Nature of the Child*. Basic Books, New York, 1984.

21 Buber, M., *I and Thou*. Clark, Edinburgh, 1958.

22 Bell, J. and McGregor, I., Living for the moment. *Nursing Times*, 87 (1991), 18, 45–47.

23 Kitwood, T. and Bredin, K., *Person to Person: A Guide to the Care of Those with Failing Mental Powers*. Gale Centre Publications, Loughton, 1992.

24 Laing, R. D., *The Politics of Experience*, Chapter 2. Penguin, Harmondsworth, 1967.

3.3

The concept of personhood and its relevance for a new culture of dementia care (1994)

Before the term 'care' was annexed to the twin vocabularies of nursing and social work it belonged, essentially, to the field of ethics. In this context, to care for others means to value who they are; to honour what they do; to respect their unique qualities and needs; to help protect them from harm and danger; and – above all – to take thoughtful and committed action that will help to nourish their personal being. In such ideas there is a strong recognition of the interdependence of human life, the fact that no one can flourish in isolation; the well-being of each one is linked to the well-being of all. Moreover, the noun 'carer' did not exist. That was a later accretion, a kind of debasement.

There are no techniques for caring, in the original sense, for the highest that any person can give to another is on the ground of wholeness and spontaneity. Diagnosis, assessment, care planning, therapies, care interventions, and so on are, at best, mere aids or supports; at worst, they are 'fixes', mainly serving the function of evasion and buck-passing.

Behind the masks of confidence and competence, behind the proud ideology of individualism and self-determination, perhaps every human being yearns to be truly cared for and to care. The wisest parenting, the richest friendships, marriages, part-nerships, seem to come close to this high ideal. Perhaps, as a highly social species, we are actually endowed with instinct-like tendencies to develop strong and affectionate social bonds. The work of Bowlby (1979) and others, drawing on insights from etho-logy and psychoanalysis, certainly suggests that this is the case. Even self-reliance, so highly valued in western societies, is based on relationships that are experienced as secure. If these assertions are true, it must also be said that whatever nature has given us is always completed, filled out with meaning, in a culture. Thus caring is facilitated in some cultural settings, and is marred and distorted in others. Paradoxically, then, we are faced with the task of creating environments in which caring feels natural, and so, eventually, bringing about a new culture of care.

Those who have dementia, we can say without a shadow of doubt, need to be cared for in the true and original sense. In fact, however, this need is very rarely met, either when they are being looked after by members of their family or in formal settings. The traditions that we have inherited from the past contain many false beliefs and inept practices: there is much to lay aside, and much learning to be done, in creating a new culture of care. Also we should take into account the possibility that we do not have instinct-like drives to help us when it comes to looking after those who are old and frail, whereas we do for looking after children. If motive is to be found, it may have to come primarily from a culture that embodies a very strong ethical ideal.

The concept of caring can be linked to another, that of personhood. Here too the fundamental matrix is ethical: it implies a standing or status that is accorded by others. Thus one can be a human being, and yet not be acknowledged as a person. We have all had experiences of this, to a greater or lesser degree: we have known occasions where we felt discounted, devalued, violated, used, abused. Fortunately, most of us have also had experiences of the opposite kind, where we felt that our personhood was acknowledged. Even if these have not been as frequent as we would have liked, we have a record of them in our emotional memory; we can draw on them in our attempt to recognize the personhood of others, and in our hope of developing into people who really know how to care.

Two ways of being and relating

Perhaps the most profound account of personhood in this century is that given by Martin Buber (1923), in the small book originally translated into English as *I and Thou* (Buber, 1937). Here he makes a contrast between two ways of being in the world, two ways of forming a relationship. The first he terms I–It, and the second I–Thou. Relating to another in the I–It mode implies coolness, information-getting, objectivity, instrumentality. Here we engage without there being any commitment; we can maintain a distance, make ourselves safe. Relating in the I–Thou mode, however, requires involvement: a risking of ourselves, a moving out and a moving towards. 'The primary word I–Thou can only be spoken with the whole being. The primary word I–It can never be spoken with the whole being' (1937: 3).

It should be noted here that Buber is not telling us of the existence of two classes of object in the world: 'Thous' and 'Its'. He is describing two contrasting ways of relating. Thus, as we have already noted, it is possible for one human being to relate to another in the I–It mode, and, alas, this is all too common. Buber also suggests that it is possible to relate to a non-human being in an I–Thou mode: an old woman whose dog is her sole companion, perhaps, or a Japanese man who faithfully attends to his bonzai tree day by day.

Many languages make a clear distinction between 'Thou' and 'You'. 'Thou', when sincerely used, is a form of intimate address, as if whatever is said or disclosed is for one person only. 'You' is more general, and far less personal. In the English language 'Thou' has virtually disappeared, its last vestiges being still found in a few dialects and in the language of certain religious groupings. The Quakers were very reluctant to relinquish their use of 'Thou', and for good reason. It is a curious irony that the best-known translation of Buber's work into English bears the title *I and You* (Buber, 1970). Without 'Thou' the essence of his meaning is much harder to apprehend.

The connection between Buber's ideas and the concept of personhood is self-evident. We misunderstand him if we think he is telling us that every individual needs a 'Thou' in order for his or her life to have meaning. He is saying, rather, that to be a person is to be addressed as Thou. In other words, the I–Thou mode of relating actually constitutes personhood. We can approach this idea from another angle by considering Buber's famous dictum 'All real living is meeting' (1937: 11). What is the nature of this meeting? It is not that of one intellectual exchanging opinions with another; it is not that of a rescuer, doing something for a needy victim; it is not even that of two practitioners, co-operating on some task. The meeting of which Buber speaks is that of making contact with the pure being of another, with no distant purpose, explicit or ulterior. The words we might associate with such meeting are awareness, openness, presence (presentness) and grace. Grace is a gift not sought or bought, a benediction that simply happens because one is in the right place at the right time.

This brings us to the way Buber speaks of freedom. 'So long as the heaven of Thou is spread out over me, the winds of causality cower at my heels, and the whirlpool of fate stays its course' (1937: 9). Here he points poetically to one of the most rich and mysterious of all human experiences. When we are addressed as Thou – when all instrumentality and manipulation are removed – we experience a profound expansiveness and liberation. Here – perhaps here alone – we can grow beyond attitudes, habits, scripts, poisonous expectations – all that others have imposed upon us in their zeal for utility. In contrast to this, to live exclusively in the I–It mode, whether as giver or receiver, is to be perpetually at the point of death.

It should be noted that Buber is not offering a psychology, in the ordinary sense. There is no way of demonstrating empirically, through experiment or observation, the truth or falsehood of his basic assertions; attempts to do so would involve a trivialisation so gross that it would be a travesty. Buber's work might be taken, rather, as a prelude to a psychology, or perhaps as an underpinning; it should be viewed as metaphysical. The point is this: before any empirical science or any form of systematic inquiry can get under way, some assumptions have to be made. If they are made openly and with awareness, they may or may not turn out to be valuable, but at least they are open to criticism. If the task of examining assumptions is avoided (as has so often happened in psychology), there is the risk of building an edifice on weak or inept foundations. Sartre (1939), in his account of the emotions, suggested that much of psychology is doomed to failure because it seeks to achieve a definitive understanding of human nature as 'the crowing concept of a completed science'. The truth is that the given world will not order the facts for us. We cannot avoid making choices about how to view human nature, how to bring structure into the domain. If we avoid these issues, we may simply end up by making bad choices. Psychology must begin, then, with a clear commitment to a view about what it is to be human.

So, Buber is offering us some basic assumptions about our humanity. We cannot prove or disprove them; we can only give our assent or dissent, according to whether they seem coherent and whether they accord with our experience. Here, at any rate, is a clear conceptualization of personhood, a possible basis for a psychology of caring. And there is a very sobering fact to take into account, in relation to those who have dementia. It is that the most thorough assessment can be carried out, the most efficient 'care planning' undertaken, the most comprehensive service provided – totally in the I–It mode, without any of the meeting of which Buber speaks ever having taken place.

The I–It mode

If Buber's ideas, formulated some seventy years ago, still strike us as revelatory, it is surely because the I–It mode of relating is so common that it is often taken as 'normal', and the I–Thou mode has been exiled to the margins. Psychiatry as it has developed during the twentieth century, principally under the influence of medical science, scarcely knows the meaning of Thou. The person who is suffering from mental distress comes under the objectifying gaze of a powerful professional, there to become an instance of a disease category. It is not uncommon for someone placed in this situation to feel the last remains of hope and self-esteem ebbing away to nothing. A person may indeed go through a full course of psychiatric intervention without ever feeling heard, acknowledged, understood, comforted; he or she is simply given a diagnostic label and passed on for a 'treatment' that is of a predominantly technical kind. There are, of course, many individual examples that go against the norm. It is encouraging to know that there is an informal affiliation of doctors who are committed to the 'medicine of the person', as originally set out by the Swiss psychiatrist Paul Tournier (1957).

Psychology, too, as it has self-consciously developed into a 'science', has virtually no place for the I–Thou mode of relating. For some psychologists in training, who had hoped to develop a profound understanding of persons, this can be a cause of great disappointment. In the main frameworks of observational and experimental work the human being is a 'subject' (read – 'subjected to a set of rules in whose making he or she had no part'). It is relatively rare that we find mainstream psychology really making an attempt to understand persons on their own ground, and it is virtually unknown for it to have any serious concern with meeting, in Buber's sense. The great exception, of course, is psychotherapy, at least in some of its more homely forms (for example Hobson, 1985; Lomas, 1992). In therapeutic work, despite many failures and abuses, there is a serious commitment to meeting. It is disturbing to note, however, that orthodox psychology tends to exclude and dismiss psychotherapy as hopelessly unscientific and 'subjective' (for example Eysenck, 1985). In other words, orthodox psychology does not have a sufficient commitment to the I–It mode.

The patterns of so-called caregiving that we have inherited from the past are contaminated in a very similar way. It is a strange and tragic paradox that so much 'care' has been practised without real meeting; and even today, in a relatively enlightened age, it features only to a minute extent on any official agenda. Those with dementia have been among the worst affected. It is as if the presence of what used to be called 'organic mental disorder' places some kind of veto upon normal human encounter, and justifies an I–It mode of relating. The malignant social psychology that I have detailed elsewhere (treachery, disempowerment, infantilization, condemnation, intimidation, stigmatization, outpacing, invalidation, banishment, objectification) epitomizes this disastrous devaluing of persons (Kitwood, 1993).

If we search historically, the reasons for this and parallel corruptions of the idea of care are easy to discern. For the institutional practices that were accepted in asylums, hospitals, nursing homes and the like are the product of a long evolutionary development. According to Foucault (1967), in his history of madness in Europe, we need to go back to the seventeenth century, the period when society in its modern form was coming into being. In order for the new, more centrally governed, more 'rational' state to function effectively, all that smacked of disorder must be suppressed. So in that remarkable phase which Foucault termed 'the great confinement' huge institutions were built; large numbers of the mad, the dissident, the flagrantly immoral, criminals, beggars and witches were locked away. The regime of the new institution resembled in many respects that of an old-time zoo. The inmates were forced to work or left to their own devices in violence and squalor – on view to a prurient public on high days and holidays. Later, mainly during the nineteenth century, initiatives were made to reform the institutions and convert them into places of moral correction. Where this occurred the regime was softened and humanized, even if its style was patronizing to the point of stultification.

Then, from around the turn of the twentieth century, a new way of framing disorder gained ground. What had previously been moral inadequacy became a medical condition, and a strenuous attempt was made to reclassify aberrant thought and behaviour into a category frame of diseases. Accompanying this, of course, was a search for corresponding lesions in the nervous tissue. The success of this project in some instances such as tertiary syphilis promoted the view that the organic disease process would be found in every case. Within psychiatry it was Janet, and later Freud, who questioned the universality of organic aetiology, causing a frisson of doubt about the validity of this project at its outset (Gay, 1988). The reverberations of this scepticism have never died away.

This is the complex and self-contradictory tradition of 'care' that western society has inherited. In each of the three main phases of the history of mental institutions (bestialization, moralization, medicalization) the norms of practice had virtually no place for the personhood of the inmate, no recognition of the necessity of real meeting if a human life is to flourish. Of course there were some who went against these norms, attempting to develop forms of practice liberated from the dead hand of the I–It mode (for example Laing, 1961). But they were no great threat to the system; under the prevailing regimes of truth it was easy to consign them to the ranks of eccentrics or subversives.

The crisis of postmodernity

This is not an easy time to create a new culture of dementia care. There are many signs that western civilization has now entered one of its major phases of dissolution and re-formation. In some ways this may be comparable to the change that ushered in modernity, when many of the social forms we know so well were coming into being: nation states, centralized government, global trade, machinofacture, capital accumulation on a large scale, subordinate women, powerful associations of doctors, lawyers and financiers. The formation of the asylums was part of this first transition; the end of the asylums is part of the second.

Now the recognition is growing that the grand project of modernity has been, in some respects, a failure. Technology, developed mainly under the joint imperatives of profit and war, has solved the basic problem of scarcity, while bringing a host of new environmental and social problems. The economic–political process for delivering sufficiency, security and peace to the world population has not yet been discovered.

Very few of the institutional forms in which such high hopes were placed – for example medicine, education and welfare – have worked successfully. In many countries, the state, which had taken on such huge burdens, has been divesting itself of its responsibilities as fast as it can. The pursuit of social order has produced an underlying chaos. The pursuit of reason has produced a profound irrationality (Smail, 1993).

This is the context for the restructuring of social care, which has taken different forms from one society to another. Although it would be a great mistake to ignore the genuinely humanistic concerns that have contributed to some of the changes, there can be little doubt that the one main motive has been financial. In relation to those whose mental powers are frail and failing, the worst possibility that lies ahead is that new institutional forms will emerge, no more respectful of personhood than those they were designed to replace. An older person living at home, receiving so-called packages of 'care', may turn out to be just as imprisoned and depersonalized as the former inmate of an asylum – and possibly a great deal more isolated and alone. A new-style residential or nursing home, despite all its appearance of comfort and efficiency, may reproduce many of the worst features of the older institutions; and – in some cases at least – with the additional dehumanizing tendencies that accompany the relentless pursuit of profit.

Nothing, however, is fixed or fated. If the crisis of postmodernity presents dire possibilities, it also holds out new opportunities (Murphy, 1991). There is, undoubtedly, a new humanism around, even if it thrives at present mainly on the margins. The last twenty years or so have seen a vast growth in counselling and psychotherapy, a new and widespread concern with the interpersonal domain. The cynic may say that this has happened because of the need to contain the stresses of impossible social conditions. If people were to be made redundant, or extremely insecure, or exploited by the imposition of impossible burdens at work, or excluded from a valued future, their anxieties would need to be eased if the whole system was not to be called in question. The radical consequences of this new exploration of experience, however, will not be easily dismissed. For there has emerged a new recognition of personhood, a new knowledge about what makes for its weal or woe. The disappearance of morons, imbeciles, idiots, mongols and cretins is far more than an exercise in cosmetics: it bespeaks a genuine social change. The improvements that have occurred during the last ten years or so in the care of those who have dementia are part of a similar growth in compassion and responsibility. The uncertainty and lack of direction that provoke so much bewilderment also provide a space for the emergence of a new culture of care. The dismantling of some of the old structures, although deeply unsettling, has created the opportunity for a radical and more benign redistribution of power.

Dementia and personhood

It is not possible to create a culture through utopian speculation, by some ungrounded act of the imagination. We can, however, already have some inkling of what a new culture of dementia care will involve, because enough has already been learned in action (Bell and McGregor, 1994). The chaos of the last few years has provided the condition for questioning long-held certainties, for challenging deeply embedded practices. Certain guiding themes related to personhood have now clearly emerged, each in its own way challenging a cherished tenet of modernity. I shall discuss three of them briefly here.

The uniqueness of each person

It is paradoxical that an epoch which has exalted individualism virtually to the supreme value should have had so gross a disregard for individuality. Behind the ideology it was, of course, merely an economic individualism that was espoused. The truth is that we have each of us, our own history, personality, likes, dislikes, abilities, interests, beliefs, values, commitments, and our unique identity is made up through some combination of these. In asserting this we are no longer on the ground of metaphysics, but of perfectly orthodox social psychology, where propositions are testable, at least to some degree (Harré, 1976). It is amazing how far the individuality of those who have dementia has generally been expunged, even where rigorous methods of record-keeping, assessment and care-planning have been in place. In the older traditions of 'care' it was as if the single category 'primary degenerative dementia' rendered obsolete all other forms of differentiation; there is a mind-set here that is very difficult to overcome. Now, however, we are gradually beginning to make the joyful discovery that the more we truly recognize aspects of individuality such as those that I have mentioned, the less important the dementia seems to be.

The strong recognition of individuality is, then, the ground of true meeting, of addressing the other as Thou. It is not a matter of having a large collection of facts; but rather, of having a diffuse awareness, of being open to the uniqueness of the other's way of being.

Subjectivity

This is the second theme, clearly related to the ideas we have just explored. This is to say that each person has his or her own special way of experiencing events, relationships, change, places, atmospheres, familiarity, newness, surprise – and so on. There are particular kinds of things that tend to cause anxiety or fear, particular sources of pleasure, joy and satisfaction. All this, and much more, is summed up in the concept of subjectivity. Each of us acquires our subjectivity as a result of the accumulation of layer on layer of experience. For some persons, subjectivity is rich in feeling and emotion, whereas for others this domain is very largely occluded. No one can know the subjectivity of another, although at times it may be possible to develop rudiments of an empathic understanding. The failure to recognize differences in subjectivity is a major cause of the breakdown of relationships. The modernizing project placed its emphasis, of course, on objectivity, with the consequence that those who saw this as disastrous folly tended to be forced into extreme positions of protest.

An emphasis on subjectivity has a particular piognancy for the care of those who have dementia, because they have been so often treated in ways that verge on objectification. It would seem that for many years the question was virtually never raised:

'What is it like actually to be experiencing a dementing illness?' Even members of the family seem very rarely to have asked it, if we are to judge by the majority of bio-graphical accounts. Perhaps the question was too threatening, too destabilizing of a fragile *status quo*. More radically, the question might even have been unthinkable by those who were deeply alienated from their own subjective life. It is only on the ground of our subjectivity, and an appreciation of that of another person, that what Buber calls true 'meeting' can take place. 'The primary word I–Thou can only be spoken with the whole being.'

Relatedness

This is the third guiding theme. Again, this goes sharply against one of the main ideas of the present time, which is to see human beings as separate and separated, coming together primarily to 'do deals' of some kind or other, rather like the supposedly rational agents who feature in conventional economic theory. Personhood, however, is constituted differently. It requires a living relationship with at least one other, where there is a felt bond or tie. Without this as a minimum the human psyche disintegrates, except in the most exceptional cases. It is also necessary for an individual to have some place of significance within a human grouping, bound together on the basis of family, friendship, occupation, religion, neighbourhood or whatever. It is as if the group comes to exist within the individual, as well as the individual within the group. We easily forget that human beings emerged as highly social beings, living out their lives in fairly small face-to-face groups, where the confirmation of their being was continually bestowed by others, and the presence of interpersonal bonds was more assured. This is the kind of psychological milieu which is natural to our species. Neither the pursuit of self-determination nor existence in a nameless crowd can ever provide us with an authentic human existence.

It is one of the great failures of dementia care, in the patterns we have inherited, that the theme of relatedness has been so largely forgotten. Recent work, interpreting some of the distress of those who have dementia in terms of Bowlby's attachment theory, is a very important corrective (Miesen, 1992). For in the traditional institution people often lived out their lives in a kind of collective loneliness, desperately anxious in their isolation. Even today, some forms of intervention seem to have the nature of short-term fixes, without regard for lasting attachments. At the very point, then, where social being needed to be enhanced because of the lack of inner stabilizers or buffers, people with dementia often found that what remained of their social being was taken away. In contrast to this we might see a good care environment as a place of enhanced sociability, bearing in mind that this will have different forms for those whose dispositions tend to be more extraverted or introverted. In a sense this sociabil-ity is a kind of 'coming home'; for this is the habitat to which our nature is truly adapted.

Reconsidering 'normality'

In this chapter I have characterized the essence of personhood, relating it to the original concept of caring. I have also tried to sketch out a broad historical picture, describing how we have arrived at the present turning-point and the possibilities that lie ahead of us now. In relation to dementia our knowledge of what we ought to do has advanced tremendously over the last ten years or so. Despite the difficulties, there is much to urge us on our way.

If, however, we take a standpoint as searching as that which I have taken here, it is clear that we are dealing with much more than the specific issue of the care of those who have dementia. In a sense we are questioning the standard assumptions and practices of everyday life; we are challenging what commonly passes as 'normality'. Our social world, so easily taken for granted, might be regarded as bizarre, sub-human, pathological in many respects. The problems we face in relation to dementia care are part of something much larger. Whatever damaging influences there are in a society, they are likely to emerge most powerfully in what is done to those who are most vulnerable and needy. Conversely, if we make some vital rediscoveries about the meaning of personhood in this type of context, and are able to sustain these in new patterns of practice, this is a very hopeful sign for society as a whole.

So – does this emphasis on personhood really mean some kind of normalization: that is, bringing people with dementia back into our ordinary ways of relating? In one sense the answer is 'yes', because the concept certainly implies that each individual should be treated in the same way as all others; there is to be no 'us–them' divide. But in another sense the answer is 'no', because treating human beings consistently as persons is so rare in everyday life. The concept of personhood presents a huge challenge to our ideas of what normality means.

References

Bell, J. and McGregor, I. (1994) 'Breaking free from the myths that restrain us'. *Dementia Care* 2 (4): 14–15.

Bowlby, J. (1979) *The Making and Breaking of Affectional Bonds*, London: Tavistock.

Buber, M. (1937) *I and Thou*, English translation by R. Gregor Smith (first German edition, 1923), Edinburgh: Clark.

——(1970) *I and You*, English translation by W. Kaufmann, (first German edition, 1923), New York: Scribner.

Eysenck, H. (1985) *The Decline and Fall of the Freudian Empire*, Harmondsworth: Penguin.

Foucault, M. (1967) *Madness and Civilization*, English translation by Richard Howard (first French edition, 1961), London: Tavistock.

Gay, P. (1988) *Freud: A Life For Our Time*, London: Dent.

Harré, R. (ed.) (1976) *Personality*, Oxford: Blackwell.

Hobson, R. E. (1985) *Forms of Feeling*, London: Tavistock.

Kitwood, T. (1990) 'The dialectics of dementia: with particular reference to Alzheimer's disease', *Ageing and Society* 9: 1–15.

——(1993) 'Person and process in dementia', *International Journal of Geriatric Psychiatry* 8: 541–545.

Laing, R. D. (1961) *Self and Others*, Harmondsworth: Penguin.

Lomas, P. (1992) *The Psychotherapy of Everyday Life*, Oxford: Oxford University Press.

Miesen, B. (1992) 'Attachment theory and dementia', in G. M. M. Jones and B. M. L. Miesen (eds) *Care-Giving in Dementia: Research and Applications*, vol. 1, London/New York: Tavistock/Routledge.

Murphy, E. (1991) *After the Asylums*, London: Faber.

Sartre, J.-P. (1971) *Sketch for a Theory of the Emotions*, English translation by P. Mairet, (first French edition, 1939), London: Methuen.

Smail, D. (1993) *The Origins of Unhappiness*, London: HarperCollins.

Tournier, P. (1957) *The Meaning of Persons*, London: SCM Press.

3.4

Personhood, dementia and dementia care (1997)

As the twentieth century draws towards its close, the industrialised societies of the western world find themselves in an extraordinary and paradoxical predicament. It is becoming clear that the system of liberal democracy, the economic life of which is grounded in the pursuit of profit, is incapable of delivering a secure and prosperous way of life for all its citizens. In many nation states 'welfare capitalism' is virtually at an end. And yet, even while old expectations have been breaking down, a new culture of caring has been gaining ground; more strongly committed, more psychologically aware, more practical and more pragmatic than anything that has gone before. The care of people with dementia has been radically affected by this new humanism. And yet, among all social issues, this is the one that is most deeply caught up in the contradictions, because the need is so intense and the size of the problem is so vast.

How matters will be resolved, in the long term, is impossible to know. There can be no doubt, however, that many profoundly positive changes have been taking place. Around 1980 the prevailing view of the conditions known as 'primary degenerative dementia' was that they presented a hopeless picture. Care for those who were affected was seen mainly as a matter of giving attention to basic physical needs while the process of degeneration in nerve tissue took its inexorable course. Generally it was believed that very little could be done in a truly therapeutic way through direct human intervention. No radical changes would be brought about until medical science had elucidated the underlying biochemistry and emerged with treatments that would arrest or prevent the pathological process. In effect, the *person* with dementia did not exist; 'going senile' was a sentence to radical exclusion.

Now, however, the whole situation looks very different. There is a growing awareness of how much can be done to enable people who have dementia to retain their well-being, and even many of their abilities, simply through better care practice and provision. At the same time we are coming to terms with the sobering fact that the achievements of biomedical research thus far have been very limited, despite a pro-digious expenditure of effort, talent and financial resources. The biggest improvements in quality of life have not come from medical breakthroughs, but from the recognition of personhood in those who have dementia, and its many practical applications.

...∪ ∪...ergence of the person in dementia care

The old culture of 'care' for those suffering from mental distress, formed and re-formed over 400 years ago or so, was deeply dehumanising, as many historical studies have shown (e.g. Foucault 1967; Ussher 1991). Dementia became a major feature in this scene only during the 20th century, as a result of the great demographic changes that created, on average, a much older population. Those who were put in the institutions tended to receive the very worst forms of care, and working in psychogeriatric settings was widely considered to bring little professional interest or personal reward. For many years, none of the main professions that were involved did anything strategic to improve the quality of care, and the personhood of those who had dementia was generally not considered.

The first real glimmer of hope came from the practice known as Reality Orientation. The origins of this lay in the rehabilitation of men who had been traumatised by war; it was an attempt to help restore them to the stability of civilian life. When Reality Orientation was taken into work with confused older people its good effects, in the form of renewed vitality and hopefulness, were clearly visible (Taulbee and Folsom 1966). Later research confirmed its beneficial effects, at least in some contexts (Holden and Woods 1995). It was all too easy, of course, to apply Reality Orientation in crude, crass and insensitive ways, and even to turn it into an instrument of oppression – an attempt to conform people to a 'reality' that was not their own. Nevertheless, Reality Orientation was the first sustained attempt to recognise the personhood of people with dementia, expressing the belief that they were not to be written off; it was worth taking the trouble to try to bring them back into a 'normal' way of life.

A few years after Reality Orientation had taken hold, another positive approach was developed, termed Validation Therapy (Feil 1982, 1993). Here there was a dramatic move away from the prevailing emphasis on cognition towards the realm of feelings and emotions, where dementia often brings far less impairment. This marked a big step forward in the care of people with dementia; above all it expressed a belief that their experience is to be taken with the utmost seriousness – and not dismissed, or 'corrected', as was so common in care practice. This humanitarian belief was taken even further in the approach known as Resolution Therapy, with its emphasis on developing empathy and communication (Stokes and Goudie 1989).

Another major contribution was the development of reminiscence work, along with the assimilation of biographical information into care practice (Gibson 1991, 1994). The crucial recognition here was that people with dementia, like the rest of us, are historical beings, whose identity is inextricably linked to their personal 'narrative'. The value of reminiscence lies partly in the sense of orientation and stability that it provides; it can be very reassuring – for some at least – to renew contact with the memories of people, places and activities from former times. As reminiscence work developed it became clear, too, that the past can provide metaphorical resources for people to talk about their present situation (Cheston 1996; Sutton 1995).

After the evident success of practices such as these, many ways of enriching the lives of people with dementia were explored: for example, music, dance, drama and graphic art (Jones and Miesen 1993, 1995). One of the most recent additions to this array is the use of various methods to provide pleasurable stimulation to the senses, bypassing cognition almost entirely (Benson 1994). Each of these forms of intervention, at its best, embodies a fuller recognition of those who have dementia as sentient beings, still capable of communicating their desires and feelings, and of living in a world of relationships. More details concerning these and other practices are to be found in Chapter 10 of this volume.

Around ten years ago it was virtually inconceivable that psychotherapy might be possible with people who have dementia. The common assumption was that they had no insight, and that, lacking the retentive power of memory, they would not be able to consolidate any of the changes that did take place (Kitwood 1990a). Now, however, several forms of therapeutic work are being explored: with individuals, with couples and with groups. In innovations such as these, a further dimension is added to the reinstatement of people with dementia; for the possibility is being considered that some form of 'personal growth' can occur, even in the face of cognitive decline.

In several countries there have been moves to design new patterns of group living, where people with dementia largely fend for themselves, but with a small background input of care. One of the best known of these is the Domus Project in Britain. Unlike some new schemes, this one has been evaluated, and the evidence is promising. There is a greater level of interaction, a decrease in depression and a lower rate of general decline, as compared with more traditional settings (Murphy, Lindesay and Dean 1994). New work is currently underway in sheltered housing, again suggesting that when attention is given to the meeting of psychological needs, this form of accommodation is far better suited to people with dementia than was previously believed (Petre 1995, 1996).

This is only a small fragment of the story of the transformation of attitudes and practices in dementia care. A detailed review, together with an appraisal of some of the relevant research, is given by Holden and Woods (1995). The cumulative weight of experience and systematic inquiry points overwhelmingly to two conclusions. The first is that people with dementia are far more resourceful, in virtually every aspect of life, than they were once assumed to be. They can learn new skills, if given sufficient time; they can give support to each other; they have much to tell us, if only we will listen – as Chapter 7 by Goldsmith makes clear. The second conclusion is that the course of a primary degenerative dementia is far less fixed than was formerly believed; it is open to change as a result of purely human intervention. Powerful evidence on this topic is to be found in the current series on person-centred care in the *Journal of Dementia Care* (see Kitwood 1995a). Surprisingly, however, in most of the positive initiatives to which I have referred above, very little attempt was made to give a systematic explication of the concept of personhood itself. Indeed, in some cases the theory that accompanied a particular form of practice was clearly inadequate. Reality Orientation, for example, was unjustified in seeing the person primarily as a cognitive being; Validation Therapy had a tendency to see problems overmuch as lying in the past rather than the present, and within the individual rather than in the social milieu (Kitwood 1994). From the period when care was beginning to improve there is, however, one statement that stands out above all others. This is the document, *Living Well into Old Age*, published by the King's Fund in 1986. Here it is plainly stated that people with dementia are individuals, and that they have the same value, the same needs and the same rights as everyone else. This was the first time – in Britain at least – that the ethical issues were clearly exposed, and that people with dementia were explicitly brought into the arena of moral concern.

The concept of personhood

It is vitally important to fill the theoretical void concerning personhood in dementia, if the many people committed to good practice are to gain in confidence and find a voice. The concept itself lies at the meeting point between two different kinds of discourse, the one ethical and the other social-psychological (Kitwood 1990b). Roughly speaking, the ethical discourse is concerned with what we ought to do, while the social-psychological discourse is concerned with how to do it. If we take this view, the term 'personhood' means a standing or status, bestowed on one individual by others; and there are empirical grounds for knowing whether or not personhood is being maintained. Some philosophers have tended to take the concept mainly as a component of moral theory (Quinton 1973). There are also theorists who have taken personhood simply as a psychological category. Tobin (1991), for example, makes it roughly equivalent to the idea of psychological resilience, in the face of much that might undermine a person in old age. However, it is when the concept of personhood retains both its ethical and its social-psychological meaning that it serves its proper function. At the heart of the ethic that underpins the concept of personhood lies the Kantian principle that each person should be treated as an end and never as a means to some other end (Mackie 1977). Kant attempted to provide a purely humanistic justification for this principle, taking rational argument to its outer limits; a similar doctrine, however, is to be found in the highest ethical teaching of each of the main religions and spiritual paths. The principle still leaves open the question of who is to be taken as a person, and on what basis. If autonomy and the fully developed use of reason are taken as criteria – as has often been the case in popular thinking – then people with dementia (like others with severe mental disabilities) are not worthy of inclusion. Here is the perfect rationalisation for 'uncare'. If, however, emotion, feeling and relational capability are taken as the key criteria, those who have dementia are undoubtedly to be viewed as persons. This view has recently been set out with great eloquence by Post (1995), who suggests an additional principle, that of moral solidarity: essentially that we should stand by people who have dementia, and never exclude them because of the failing of their mental powers.

At the social-psychological level, I would like to suggest that a model or theory of personhood suited to our purpose should meet the following criteria. First, it must be reflexive: that is, the categories that are used to describe or explain one group of people (in this case, those who have dementia) must be applicable in principle to the 'professionals' who use them (Little 1972). This is not only a methodological, but also a moral requirement. Second, it must view the person as a social being, not as a monad as has so often been the case in clinical work and in reductionistic theory (Burkitt 1993). That is why a moral theory that speaks of persons and obligations is more powerful than one which merely speaks of individuals and their 'rights'. Third, it must be developmental, showing how people can change – for good or ill – throughout the span of life. Fourth, it must bring out some of the most relevant psychological differences between people: doing what the blander forms of psychometric work simply cannot do (Harré 1976). Fifth, it must be compatible with what neuroscience tells us about how the brain develops and functions, both in health and in disease. Sixth, it must shed light on the psychological predicament of people who have dementia and suggest what they might need. Finally, it should be able to tell us something about the nature and meaning of good dementia care.

The psychology of personal being

It is a difficult and daunting task to create a model of the person which meets all seven criteria, and it can be done in several different ways. What follows here is no more than a sketch, building on some of my own earlier work (Kitwood 1987, 1989, 1990c, 1993, 1996). In effect, the model that I have developed brings together the frameworks of symbolic interactionism and depth psychology: the former dealing with the manifest aspects of social life, and the latter with processes that are said to be 'unconscious'.

The developmental study of infancy and childhood gives us a rich picture of the emergence of the psychological self, the sense of 'I'. There are many stages on the journey: the forming of attachments, the acquisition of a sense of agency (an ability to 'make things happen'), the realisation that many people exist in the world, the acceptance of experience that involves both pleasure and pain. One of the biggest steps is the acquisition of language, for when that is acquired there is not simply a self, but also a self-concept: a 'Me' as well as an 'I'.

There are vast differences in the quality of early relational experience, depending on the extent to which the key figures in a child's life are responsive, available, consistent and resourceful. It does not appear that perfection is required – simply a form of care-giving that is 'good enough' (Winnicott 1973). The tragedy is that for many children even this modest standard is not met; there is an excessive amount of privation and uncertainty, and in some cases outright cruelty and oppression. Whatever may be the case, each child, sooner or later, has to come to terms with a world that is often harsh, competitive and hypocritical, and to find a way of surviving within it. Here is the origin of what has been called the 'false self': formed not in joy, trust and creativity, but in adaption and survival. When virtually all of a child's development is around the false self there is an extreme of alienation and isolation, sometimes described as a schizoid state (Fairbairn 1952).

The idea of two types of 'self', two main patterns of development, runs right through those psychologies that are concerned with the promotion of personal 'growth' and positive change. In Jung's work it appears primarily as a distinction between ego and Self, but also as that between persona and shadow. The ego is formed through taking on some of the variety of roles that are provided, ready made, by society. On the basis of ego each person gives life a direction and finds a niche. Problems arise if living according to ego is too restrictive, if too much potential remains unexplored and undeveloped. According to Jung that is why some people have existential crises in mid-life; the prime task of later years is to move away from ego to develop a greater wholeness and completeness; this is the movement towards the Self (Jung 1933).

Parallels to these ideas are to be found in the work of several of the humanistic psychologists. For Rogers the issue was one of congruence: of there being a match between what a person is actually undergoing, what they are experiencing, and what they are presenting to others (Rogers 1961). In Transactional Analysis it comes in a more elaborated form, but the key issue is the distinction between the 'ego states' of the adapted child and the free child. The adapted child arises as a result of conformity to others' expectations, and particularly to pressures from critical or controlling parents; in some cases, too, from the attempt to avoid abuse or violence. The free child state, in contrast, expresses a condition where a person is able to be spontaneous, sensuous and intimate, and where the prime activity is play (Stewart and Joines 1987).

There are difficulties if the disjuncture is forced too far, and especially if a radical divide is posited between a false self and one which is somehow 'true', existing outside any real social context. (Whatever one might assume at a metaphysical level is a different matter). We can, however, legitimately use the terms 'adapted self' and 'experiential self'. The former refers to the person as highly and tightly socialised, particularly in relation to the performing of given roles. Sometimes, but not always, adaption involves both falsehood and estrangement. The experiential self, in contrast, arises from being with others in conditions of equality, mutual attention and mutual respect: what I have described elsewhere as 'moral space' (Kitwood 1990b). There is a famous distinction between two fundamentally different types of relationship: I–It and I–Thou (Buber 1922). Part, but by no means all, of the adapted self might be seen as a reaction to being treated as an 'it', an object. The experiential self is formed and nourished in the context of I–Thou relating.

We can use these ideas to explore some of the ways in which each person is unique. There are differences between individuals in their patterns of adaption, according to their social circumstances. Some of these patterns are relatively benign, especially where roles give scope for personal expression and moral commitment. This, however, is not always the case; some roles are degrading and dehumanising in themselves, and many kinds of stress arise from the different forms of role conflict. There are also great differences in the extent to which the experiential self develops. One key source of evidence here is the vast amount of reflection that has taken place on the experience of counselling and psychotherapy. Rogers (1961), for example, has described a continuum of 'personal growth'. At one end is a stage in which there is virtually no ability to experience or communicate on the feeling level, while at the other feelings are experienced in their richness and variety, are freely expressed and are used as a source of learning about the self. Furthermore, there are differences in the manner in which the experiential and adapted selves are related; the development of one does not necessarily imply the development of the other. An individual might, for example, have a highly elaborated 'front', or persona, and yet have an extraordinarily impoverished inner life.

At a very general level this model is applicable to all people, regardless of age, sex, class or society, although the categories which supply the content will vary from one culture to another. While the model is certainly one which professionals such as doctors, nurses and social workers can use in trying to understand their clients, it is also one which they can apply instructively to themselves. The model makes sense in neurological terms, if we accept the assumption of ontological monism: that there is only one (exceedingly complex) reality, which we attempt to describe in a number of different discourses. The brain is now recognised as a highly adaptive organ; interneuronal circuits are being continually formed and re-formed in response to the new learning that the organism requires (Damasio 1995). Each time that a new role is learned, for example, brain structures are established to enable the tasks to be performed efficiently; and when a role is ended these structures are slowly dismantled. Similarly, there is a neuronal counterpart to the experiential self; and as a person's experiential frame is enlarged, there are corresponding changes in brain structure. Presumably, also, those processes that are termed 'ego defence' (repression, denial, rationalisation, displacement etc.) are instantiated at a neurological level; in some cases through the deactivation of those proto-structures through which certain events or conflicts might have been consciously experienced.

We can use the model also to illustrate how each person develops through the life course. The adapted self is elaborated in many ways, but primarily through the taking on of new roles. Thus it proliferates throughout childhood and adolescence, with each step in the enlargement of skill, opportunity and social life. The process continues into adulthood, as a person enters the world of work (or unemployment), and perhaps takes on new responsibilities such as a committed relationship, parenting or the running of a home. With many people, it seems to be the case that the adapted self reaches its highest level of elaboration in the age period around 40–60, when roles and responsibilities are being added faster than they are being lost. Later life, for many people, brings a dismantling of the adapted self. Some major roles, such as that of parent or employee, are relinquished; a lowered income or problems of ill-health may cause a further diminution. The theorists of disengagement saw this as part of the natural progression of life. There is much evidence, however, to support a contrary view. Many people who make a success of their old age have managed to maintain a high level of engagement, perhaps taking on new but less demanding roles (Stevenson 1989).

The story of the experiential self is, to a large extent, that of the person in contexts of I–Thou relating, for it is here that it becomes possible to develop a subtle, sensitive and responsive way of being with others, and an 'inner discourse' of feeling and emotion (Hobson 1985). Where the experiential self does not develop well, this is in part a consequence of a person being subjected to oppression, conflict, rejection and exploitation – and, more rarely, actual trauma. The human organism is too sensitive to be able to bear these things in isolation, and so processes of defence exist to ward off an excess of anxiety or pain. The experiential self, however, is presented with many opportunities for development throughout life, particularly through love, friendship and spiritual commitment; a small minority find help through some form of therapy or counselling. There is no fundamental reason why the experiential self should not continue to grow in the later years and even, as clearly happens in some cases, during the course of a terminal illness. Much, however, in the process of ageing (as it has been constructed in contemporary industrial societies, at least), tends to hinder growth and to engender defensiveness, apathy or depression.

This model of personal being, which could be elaborated in much greater depth and detail, seems to meet the first five of the criteria which I suggested would be necessary for conceptualising personhood in the context of dementia care. It is reflex-ive, social and developmental; it reveals interpersonal differences; and it is compatible with neuroscientific knowledge. The last two criteria were that it should be directly relevant to the predicament of people who have dementia, and that it should be capable of shedding light on the meaning of good care. These are the two topics to which we shall now turn.

The agenda for dementia care

The concepts of experiential and adapted self can tell us much about the predicament of people who have dementia. Almost always, during the years before any cognitive deficits became noticeable, there have been losses in the adapted self. This can be illustrated by the example of two women from my psychobiographical research (Kitwood 1990c). For the first, the loss happened in several small stages; one bereave-ment succeeded another, and her life gradually closed in due to a decline in her general health. For the second, it happened through a single dramatic transition. She had spent almost all of her adult life in Southern Rhodesia, where she ran a hotel. When she returned to Britain, around the time of Independence, she lost her entire way of life, and found herself in what was virtually a foreign country. From a purely psychological point of view, both women were in a highly vulnerable position; their social connectedness, via the adapted self, had been greatly weakened. With the onset of dementia the adapted self almost always undergoes a further reduction, largely because of the inability or unwillingness of other people to support existing roles (Sabat and Harré 1992). If a person goes into residential care there is likely to be a further diminution. In the old-style institutional regimes many of the last vestiges of the adapted self were taken away and a single new role was created – that of inmate. If the inmate was also 'senile', virtually all was lost (Meacher 1972).

The experiential self, too, is imperilled through the process of dementia. There is a little evidence to suggest that people in whom it is only poorly developed may actually be at risk of developing dementia (for example, Oakley 1965). As cognitive impairment advances, the experiential frame is profoundly disturbed. Failures of memory and judgement are alarming in themselves, but they may also bring second-ary consequences such as delusions (essentially a misattribution of causes). Desperate needs for comfort and security come to the surface. Those who remain walled off by defences are protected for a while, but when the defences eventually break down there may be a powerful invasion of emotion which they have no capacity to understand. A small proportion of people also have to endure hallucinations, and here their isolation is profound.

The aim of dementia care, in the broadest sense, is to maintain personhood in the face of advancing cognitive impairment. Through the concepts of experiential self and adapted self it is possible to see what this means in a little more detail. The principles that underlie the points that follow apply across all contexts of care, because they relate primarily to the existential plight of the person with dementia. However, some of the realities are more complex and difficult when care-giving has taken over from a relationship of another, and more mutual, kind; for here both parties have already made deep psychological investments.

Taking care of the adapted self means, essentially, enabling a person to continue, as far as possible and for as long as possible, in familiar roles. Each role provides, so to speak, a 'beaten track', where a way of being and doing has been deeply learned. Each role, also, is an arena where a person is recognised, acknowledged and integrated into a form of life that is shared with others. When a person with dementia is living at home it is possible for some roles, such as grandparent, host, shopper and gardener, to continue to some degree. Imaginative help may be needed to provide parts of the action that a person cannot now carry out alone; and in some instances the problems lie with the sequencing, not with the actions themselves. As cognitive impairment advances it is inevitable that some roles will have to be relinquished (driver or domestic accountant, for example), and here it is vital to help the person with dementia to maintain a sense of self-worth and significance in the face of loss. Very similar issues arise in the contexts of formal care, where people with dementia often want to contribute something, rather then just be passive receivers. It is not uncommon, for example, for a person to frame attendance at a day centre as 'going to work', and in some cases at least, there is work that they can do, particularly in helping to care for others. All too often the needs of the adapted self have been ignored, perhaps because care-givers are too insistent on their own projects or too committed to order and control.

The more joyous and fulfilling aspects of dementia care, however, both for receiver and giver, are likely to be on the basis of the experiential self. The central point here is that a person with dementia still has an emotional and relational life, even though without the stabilisation and compensation that cognitions ordinarily provide. One kind of interaction in dementia care is 'holding': providing a safe space where it is possible to experience psychological pain without being overwhelmed. A person might, for example, be subject to terrifying hallucinations, but these are just bearable if he or she is in actual physical contact with a carer who is known and trusted. Another type of interaction is validation; not in the sense of a total 'therapy', but simply acknowledging the subjective truth of a person's experience, without an obsessional concern with 'cognitive rectification'. Yet another type of interaction might be termed 'timulation': a neologism which means providing pleasurable stimulation to the senses, but in a way that respects a person's boundaries and values. Here there is the opportunity for simple sensuous enjoyment without the demands of thought or the restrictions imposed by a harsh and critical moralism. A further example is 'celebration': simply sharing in the beauty, the fun and the joy of living, where the free child is welcomed and encouraged. Strikingly, it is often in episodes of celebration, such as parties, outings and dances, that people who have dementia behave most 'normally', and the us–them barriers dissolve away to nothing.

As yet we do not know the full range of possibilities for the experiential self, when the care is of a very supportive and empowering kind. The first glimpses are now appearing of a different long-term pattern of dementia, in which people do not inevitably decline into vegetation. Some, at least, may actually be enabled to undergo a form of personal growth which even surprises and delights their relatives: becoming less obsessive, more trustful, or emerging from depression into a state of acceptance and tranquillity (Kitwood 1995b). The overall pattern cannot be described at present; that will only be possible after a large body of evidence has been collected.

Finally, this brief exploration of personhood gives us small glimpses of the skills and sensitivities that are required in those who are involved in care-giving. A good careworker must, of course, be thoroughly competent in all the standard tasks which the job entails, and in that sense be well adapted to the role; the same applies, although in a less formal sense, to a family member or a friend who has become a carer. But beyond that, effective care-giving requires a well-developed experiential self. This involves being familiar with the world of feeling and emotion; being willing to bear the burden that arises from attachment; being comfortable with an intimacy that needs no words; and being capable of play. In counselling and psychotherapy the central quality required of a practitioner is sometimes described as that of giving 'free attention'. This is not learned as mere technique, but arises through real development. A person becomes more insightful and self-accepting, less distracted by inner conflict and anxiety; and hence more able to set his or her own issues on one side for the sake of another. A similar quality is needed, and to a high degree, in dementia care. One encouraging sign is that some family carers are able to move in this direction if they are well supported, even while they are enduring so much suffering and stress (Coates 1995).

Looking to the future

There can be no doubt about the tremendous progress that has been made in recent years, as a new culture of dementia care has gradually come into being. Each chapter of this book demonstrates this in some way. If good care, in all its aspects, is seen as a kind of mosaic, it seems likely that many of the individual pieces have already been found (Kitwood 1995a). One of the tasks that lies ahead is fitting them all together to create the whole rich pattern, and here a clear conception of personhood is essential. Beyond that, there is the problem of actually setting up the services that embody what we know, with all the training and personal development which that implies. This is a difficult and daunting task, not least because there are so many countervailing forces: negative traditions in care practice, the severe lack of public funding, and the many corrupting pressures of the market. There is also a huge research task in investigating the consequences of new practices and, in contrast to much biomedical work, this holds the promise of immediate benefits.

Among the historically new features of our time, none is more significant than the widespread presence of people with dementia. If we fail them at this point, it will not be because of a lack of knowledge, but because our social, educational, political and economic arrangements are inadequate to the task. If we succeed, it will be one of the most hopeful signs that it is yet possible to build a society in which compassion and integrity prevail.

References

Benson, S. (1994) 'Sniff and doze therapy.' *Journal of Dementia Care 2*, 1, 11–15.

Buber, M. (1922) *I and Thou*. English translation by Ronald Gregor Smith (1937). Edinburgh: Clark.

Burkitt, I. (1993) *Social Selves*. London: Sage.

Cheston, R. (1996) 'Stories and metaphors: talking about the past in a psychotherapy group for persons with dementia.' *Ageing and Society 16*, 579–602.

Coates, D. (1995) 'The process of learning in dementia-carer support programmes: some preliminary observations.' *Journal of Advanced Nursing 21*, 41–46.

Damasio, A.R. (1995) *Descartes' Error*. London: Picador.

Fairbairn, W.R.D. (1952) *Psychoanalytic Studies of the Family*. London: Routledge and Kegan Paul. (See, especially, Chapter 1).

Feil, N. (1982) *Validation: the Feil Method*. Cleveland: Edward Feil Productions.

Feil, N. (1993) *The Validation Breakthrough*. Baltimore: Health Promotions Press.

Foucault, M. (1967) *Madness and Civilization*. London: Tavistock.

Gibson, F. (1991) *A Positive Approach to Dementia*. Jordanstown: University of Ulster.

Gibson, F. (1994) *Reminiscence and Recall*. London: Ace Books.

Harré, R. (ed) (1976) *Personality*. Oxford: Blackwell.

Hobson, R.E. (1985) *Forms of Feeling*. London: Tavistock.

Holden, U. and Woods, R. (1995) *Positive Approaches to Dementia Care*. Edinburgh: Churchill Livingstone.

Jones, G.M.M. and Miesen, B.M.L. (1993) *Caregiving in Dementia*. London: Routledge.

Jones, G.M.M. and Miesen, B.M.L. (eds) (1995) *Caregiving in Dementia*. Volume II. London: Routledge.

Jung, C.G. (1993) *Modern Man in Search of Soul*. London: Routledge and Kegan Paul. (See, especially, Chapter 5.)

King's Fund (1986) *Living Well into Old Age: Applying Principles of Good Practice to Services for Elderly People with Severe Mental Impairments*. London: The King's Fund.

Kitwood, T.M. (1987) 'Dementia and its pathology: in brain, mind or society?' *Free Associations 8*, 81–93.

Kitwood, T.M. (1989) 'Brain, mind and dementia: with particular reference to Alzheimer's disease.' *Ageing and Society 9*, 1–15.

Kitwood, T.M. (1990a) 'Psychotherapy and dementia.' *Psychotherapy Section Newsletter 8*, 40–56.

Kitwood, T.M. (1990b) *Concern for Others*. London: Methuen.

Kitwood, T.M. (1990c) 'Understanding senile dementia: a psychobiographical approach.' *Free Associations 19*, 60–76.

Kitwood, T.M. (1993) 'Towards a theory of dementia care: the interpersonal process.' *Ageing and Society 13*, 15–67.

Kitwood, T.M. (1994) 'Review of *The Validation Breakthrough* (by Naomi Feil).' *Journal of Dementia Care 2*, 6, 29–30.

Kitwood, T.M. (1995a) 'Building up the mosaic of good practice: introducing a new series in person-centred care.' *Journal of Dementia Care 3*, 5, 12–13.

Kitwood, T.M. (1995b) 'Positive long term changes in dementia: some preliminary observations.' *Journal of Mental Health 4*, 133–144.

Kitwood, T.M. (1996) 'The concept of personhood and its implications for the care of those who have dementia.' In G.M.M. Jones and B.M.L. Miesen (eds) *Caregiving in Dementia*. Volume II. London: Routledge.

Little, B.R. (1972) 'Psychological man as humanist scientist and specialist.' *Journal of Experimental Research in Psychiatry 6*, 95–118.

Mackie, J.L. (1977) *Ethics*. Harmondsworth: Penguin.

Meacher, M. (1972) *Taken for a Ride*. London: Longmans.

Murphy, E., Lindesay, J. and Dean, M. (1994) *The Domus Project*. London: The Sainsbury Centre.

Oakley, D.P. (1965) 'Senile dementia – some aetiological factors.' *British Journal of Psychiatry 111*, 414–419.

Petre, T. (1995) 'Dementia and sheltered housing.' In T. Kitwood, S. Buckland and T. Petre (eds) *Brighter Futures: A Report on Research into Provision for Persons with Dementia in Residential Homes, Nursing Homes and Sheltered Housing*. Anchor Housing Association (in collaboration with Methodist Homes for the Aged).

Petre, T. (1996) 'Back into the swing of her sociable life.' *Journal of Dementia Care 4*, 1, 24–25.

Post, S. (1995) *The Moral Challenge of Alzheimer's Disease*. Baltimore: Johns Hopkins Press.

Quinton, A. (1973) *The Nature of Things*. London: Routledge.

Rogers, C.R. (1961) *On Becoming a Person*. Boston: Houghton Mifflin.

Sabat, S. and Harré, R. (1992) 'The construction and deconstruction of self in Alzheimer's disease.' *Ageing and Society 12*, 443–461.

Stevenson, O. (1989) *Age and Vulnerability*. London: Edward Arnold.

Stewart, I and Joines, V. (1987) *TA Today*. Nottingham: Lifespace Publications.

Stokes, G. and Goudie, F. (1989) *Working With Dementia*. Bicester: Winslow.

Sutton, L. (1995) *Whose memory is it anyway?* Unpublished PhD thesis, University of Southampton.

Taulbee, L.R. and Folsom, J.C. (1966) 'Reality orientation for geriatric patients.' *Hospital and Community Psychiatry 17*, 133–135.

Tobin, S.S. (1991) *Personhood in Advanced Old Age*. New York: Springer.

Ussher, J.M. (1991) *Women's Madness: Misogyny or Mental Illness?* London: Harvester.

Winnicott, D.W. (1973) *The Child, The Family and the Outside World*. Harmondsworth: Penguin.

3.5

On being a person (1997)

A few months before this book was completed, a day centre was approached by an agency concerned to promote awareness about Alzheimer's disease and similar conditions. Could the day centre provide some photographs of clients, to be used for publicity purposes? Permission was sought and granted; the photographs were duly taken and sent. The agency, however, rejected them, on the ground that the clients did not show the disturbed and agonized characteristics that people with dementia 'ought' to show, and which would be expected to arouse public concern. The failure of the photographic exercise, from the standpoint of the agency, was a measure of the success of the day centre from the standpoint of the clients. Here was a place where men and women with dementia were continuing to live in the world of persons, and not being downgraded into the carriers of an organic brain disease.

Alzheimer victims, dements, elderly mentally infirm – these and similar descriptions devalue the person, and make a unique and sensitive human being into an instance of some category devised for convenience or control. Imagine an old-fashioned weighing scale. Put aspects of personal being into one pan, and aspects of pathology and impairment into the other. In almost all of the conventional thinking that we have inherited, the balance comes down heavily on the latter side. There is no logical ground for this, nor is it an inference drawn from a comprehensive range of empirical data. It is simply a reflection of the values that have prevailed, and of the priorities that were traditionally set in assessment, care practice and research. The time has come to bring the balance down decisively on the other side, and to recognize men and women who have dementia in their full humanity. Our frame of reference should no longer be $_{person}$-with-DEMENTIA, but PERSON-with-$_{dementia}$.

This chapter, then, is concerned with personhood: the category itself, the centrality of relationship, the uniqueness of persons, the fact of our embodiment. Rather than emphasize the differences that dementia brings, we will first celebrate our common ground.

The concept of personhood

The term personhood, together with its synonyms and parallels, can be found in three main types of discourse: those of transcendence, those of ethics and those of social psychology. The functions of the term are different in these three contexts, but there is a core of meaning that provides a basic conceptual unity.

Discourses of transcendence make their appeal to a very powerful sense, held in almost every cultural setting, that being-in-itself is sacred, and that life is to be revered. Theistic religions capture something of this in their doctrines of divine creation; in eastern traditions of Christianity, for example, there is the idea that each human being is an 'ikon of God'. Some forms of Buddhism, and other non-theistic spiritual paths, believe in an essential, inner nature: always present, always perfect, and waiting to be discovered through enlightenment. Secular humanism makes no metaphysical assumptions about the essence of our nature, but still often asserts, on the basis of direct experience, that 'the ultimate is personal'.

In the main ethical discourses of western philosophy one primary theme has been the idea that each person has absolute value. We thus have an obligation to treat each other with deep respect; as ends, and never as means towards some other end. The principle of respect for persons, it was argued by Kant and those who followed in his footsteps, requires no theological justification; it is the only assumption on which our life as social beings makes sense. There are parallels to this kind of thinking in the doctrine of human rights, and this has been used rhetorically in many different contexts, including that of dementia (King's Fund 1986). One problem here, however, is that in declarations of rights the person is framed primarily as a separate individual; there is a failure to see human life as interdependent and interconnected.

In social psychology the term personhood has had a rather flexible and varied use. Its primary associations are with self-esteem and its basis; with the place of an individual in a social group; with the performance of given roles; and with the integrity, continuity and stability of the sense of self. Themes such as these have been explored, for example, by Tobin (1991) in his work on later life, and by Barham and Hayward (1991) in their study of ex-mental patients living in the community. Social psychology, as an empirical discipline, seeks to ground its discourses in evidence, even while recognizing that some of this may consist of pointers and allusions. Robust measures such as those valued by the traditional natural sciences usually cannot be obtained, even if an illusion is created that they can.

Thus we arrive at a definition of personhood, as I shall use the term in this book. It is a standing or status that is bestowed upon one human being, by others, in the context of relationship and social being. It implies recognition, respect and trust. Both the according of personhood, and the failure to do so, have consequences that are empirically testable.

The issue of inclusion

As soon as personhood is made into a central category, some crucial questions arise. Who is to be viewed and treated as a person? What are the grounds for inclusion and exclusion, since 'person' is clearly not a mere synonym for 'human being'? Is the concept of personhood absolute, or can it be attenuated?

Such questions have been examined many times, particularly in western moral philosophy. In one of the best-known discussions Quinton (1973) suggests five criteria. The first is consciousness, whose normal accompaniment is consciousness of self. The second is rationality, which in its most developed form includes the capacity for abstract reasoning. The third is agency: being able to form intentions, to consider alternatives, and to direct action accordingly. The fourth is morality, which in its strongest form means living according to principle, and being accountable for one's actions. The fifth is the capacity to form and hold relationships; essential here is the ability to understand and identify with the interests, desires and needs of others. Quinton suggests that each criterion can be taken in a stronger or a weaker sense. We can make the distinction, for example, between someone who has all the capabilities of a moral agent, and someone who does not, but who is nevertheless the proper subject for moral concern.

With the arrival of computers and the creation of systems with artificial intelligence, doubts began to be raised about whether the concept of personhood is still valid (Dennett 1975). The central argument is as follows. In computers we have machines which mimic certain aspects of human mental function. We can (and often do) describe and explain the 'behaviour' of computers as if they were intentional beings, with thoughts, wishes, plans and so on. However, there is no necessity to do this; it is simply an anthropomorphism – a convenient short cut. In fact the behaviour of computers can be completely described and explained in physical terms. It is then argued that the same is possible, in principle, with human beings, although the details are more complex. Thus an intentional frame is not strictly necessary; and the category of personhood, to which it is so strongly tied, becomes redundant.

Behind such debates a vague shadow can be discerned. It is that of the liberal academic of former times: kind, considerate, honest, fair, and above all else an intellectual. Emotion and feeling have only a minor part in the scheme of things; autonomy is given supremacy over relationship and commitment; passion has no place at all. Moreover the problems seem to centre on how to describe and explain, which already presupposes an existential stance of detachment. So long as we stay on this ground the category of personhood is indeed in danger of being undermined, and with it the moral recognition of people with mental impairments. At a popularistic level, matters are more simple. Under the influence of the extreme individualism that has dominated western societies in recent years, criteria such as those set out by Quinton have been reduced to two: autonomy and rationality. Now the shadowy figure in the background is the devotee of 'business culture'. Once this move is made, there is a perfect justification for excluding people with serious disabilities from the 'personhood club'.

Both the mainstream philosophical debate and its popularistic reductions have been radically questioned by Stephen Post, in his book *The Moral Challenge of Alzheimer's Disease* (1995). Here he argues that it has been a grave error to place such great emphasis on autonomy and rational capability; this is part of the imbalance of our cultural tradition. Personhood, he suggests, should be linked far more strongly to feeling, emotion and the ability to live in relationships, and here people with dementia are often highly competent – sometimes more so than their carers.

Post also suggests a principle of *moral solidarity*: a recognition of the essential unity of all human beings, despite whatever differences there may be in their mental capabilities as conventionally determined. Thus we are all, so to speak, in the same boat; and there can be no empirically determined point at which it is justifiable to throw some people into the sea. The radical broadening of moral awareness that Post commends has many applications in the context of dementia: for example to how diagnostic information is handled, to the negotiation of issues such as driving or self-care, and ultimately to the most difficult questions of all, concerning the preservation of life.

Personhood and relationship

There is another approach to the question of what it means to be a person, which gives priority to experience, and relegates analytic discussion to a very minor place. One of its principal exponents was Martin Buber, whose small book *Ich und Du* was first published in 1922, and later appeared in an English translation, with the title *I and Thou*, in 1937. It is significant that this work was written during that very period when the forces of modernization had caused enormous turmoil throughout the world, and in the aftermath of the horrific brutalities of the First World War.

Buber's work centres on a contrast between two ways of being in the world; two ways of living in relationship. The first he terms I–It, and the second I–Thou. In his treatment of Thou he has abstracted one of many meanings; making it so to speak, into a jewel. In older usage it is clear that a person could be addressed as Thou in many forms of 'strong recognition': command, accusation, insult and threat, as well as the special form of intimacy that Buber portrays. Relating in the I–It mode implies coolness, detachment, instrumentality. It is a way of maintaining a safe distance, of avoiding risks; there is no danger of vulnerabilities being exposed. The I–Thou mode, on the other hand, implies going out towards the other; self-disclosure, spontaneity – a journey into uncharted territory. Relationships of the I–It kind can never rise beyond the banal and trivial. Daring to relate to another as Thou may involve anxiety or even suffering, but Buber sees it also as the path to fulfilment and joy. 'The primary word I–Thou can only be spoken with the whole being. The primary word I–It can never be spoken with the whole being' (1937: 2).

Buber's starting point then, is different from that of western individualism. He does not assume the existence of ready-made monads, and then inquire into their attributes. His central assertion is that relationship is primary; to be a person is to be addressed as Thou. There is no implication here that there are two different kinds of objects in the world: Thous and Its. The difference lies in the manner of relating. Thus it is possible (and, sad to say, all too common) for one human being to engage with another in the I–It mode. Also it is possible, at least to some degree, to engage with a non-human being as Thou. We might think, for example, of a woman in her 80s whose dog is her constant and beloved companion, or of a Japanese man who faithfully attends his bonsai tree each day.

In the English language we have now almost lost the word Thou. Once it was part of everyday speech, corresponding to the life of face-to-face communities. Its traces remain in just a few places still; for example in North country dialects, and in old folk songs such as one about welcoming a guest, which has the heart-warming refrain:

Draw chair raight up to t'table;
Stay as long as Thou art able;
I'm always glad to see a man like Thee.

Among minority groups in Britain, the Quakers were the last to give up the use of Thou in daily conversation, and they did so with regret. Their sense of the sacredness of every person was embedded in their traditional form of speech.

One of the most famous of all Buber's sayings is 'All real living is meeting' (1937: 11). Clearly it is not a matter of committees or business meetings, or even a meeting to plan the management of care. It is not the meeting of one intellectual with another, exchanging their ideas but revealing almost nothing of their feelings. It is not the meeting between a rescuer and a victim, the one intent on helping or 'saving' the other. It is not necessarily the meeting that occurs during a sexual embrace. In the meeting of which Buber speaks there is no ulterior purpose, no hidden agenda. The ideas to be associated with this are openness, tenderness, presence (present-ness), awareness. More than any of these, the word that captures the essence of such meeting is *grace*. Grace implies something not sought or bought, not earned or deserved. It is simply that life has mysteriously revealed itself in the manner of a gift.

For Buber, to become a person also implies the possibility of freedom. 'So long as the heaven of Thou is spread out over me, the wind of causality cowers at my heels, and the whirlwind of fate stays its course' (1937: 9). Here, in poetic language, is a challenge to all determinism, all mechanical theories of action. In that meeting where there is full acceptance, with no attempt to manipulate or utilize, there is a sense of expansiveness and new possibility, as if all chains have been removed. Some might claim that this is simply an illusion, and that no human being can escape from the power of heredity and conditioning. Buber, however, challenges the assumption that there is no freedom by making a direct appeal to the experience of the deepest form of relating. It is here that we gain intuitions of our ability to determine who we are, and to choose the path that we will take. This experience is to be taken far more seriously than any theory that extinguishes the idea of freedom.

Buber's work provides a link between the three types of discourse in which the concept of personhood is found: transcendental, ethical and social-psychological. His account is transcendental, in that he portrays human relationship as the only valid route to what some would describe as an encounter with the divine. His account is ethical, in that it emphasizes so strongly the value of persons. It is not, however, a contribution to analytic debate. For Buber cuts through all argumentation conducted from a detached and intellectualized standpoint, and gives absolute priority to engagement and commitment. Against those who might undermine the concept of personhood through analogies from artificial intelligence, Buber might simply assert that no one has yet engaged with a computer as Thou.

In relation to social psychology, we have here the foundation for an empirical inquiry in which the human being is taken as a person rather than as an object. There is, of course, no way of proving – either through observation or experiment – whether

Buber's fundamental assertions are true or false. Any attempt to do so would make them trivial, and statements that appeal through their poetic power would lose their meaning. (It would be equally foolish, for example, to set about verifying the statement 'My love is like a red, red rose, that's newly sprung in June'.) The key point is this. Before any kind of inquiry can get under way in a discipline that draws on evidence, assumptions have to be made. Popper (1959) likened these to stakes, driven into a swamp, so that a stable building can be constructed. These assumptions are metaphysical, beyond the possibility of testing. Thus, in creating a social psychology, we can choose (or not) to accept these particular assumptions, according to whether they help to make sense of everyday experience and whether they correspond to our moral convictions (Kitwood and Bredin 1992a).

To see personhood in relational terms is, I suggest, essential if we are to understand dementia. Even when cognitive impairment is very severe, an I–Thou form of meeting and relating is often possible. There is, however, a very sombre point to consider about contemporary practice. It is that a man or woman could be given the most accurate diagnosis, subjected to the most thorough assessment, provided with a highly detailed care plan and given a place in the most pleasant surroundings – without any meeting of the I–Thou kind ever having taken place.

The psychodynamics of exclusion

Many cultures have shown a tendency to depersonalize those who have some form of serious disability, whether of a physical or a psychological kind. A consensus is created, established in tradition and embedded in social practices, that those affected are not real persons. The rationalizations follow on. If people show bizarre behaviour 'they are possessed by devils'; 'they are being punished for the sins of a former life'; 'the head is rotten'; 'there is a mental disorder whose symptoms are exactly described in the new diagnostic manual'.

Several factors come together to cause this dehumanization. In part, no doubt, it corresponds to characteristics of the culture as a whole; where personhood is widely disregarded, those who are powerless are liable to be particularly devalued. Many societies, including our own, are permeated by an ageism which categorizes older people as incompetent, ugly and burdensome, and which discriminates against them at both a personal and a structural level (Bytheway 1995). Those who have dementia are often subjected to ageism in its most extreme form; and, paradoxically, even people who are affected at a relatively young age are often treated as if they were 'senile'. In financial terms, far too few resources have been allocated to the provision of the necessary services. There is also the fact that very little attention has been given to developing the attitudes and skills that are necessary for good psychological care. In the case of dementia, until very recently this was not even recognized as an issue, with the consequence that many people working in this field have had no proper preparation for their work.

Behind these more obvious reasons, there may be another dynamic which excludes those who have dementia from the world of persons. There seems to be something special about the dementing conditions – almost as if they attract to themselves a particular kind of inhumanity: a social psychology that is malignant in its effects, even when it proceeds from people who are kind and well-intentioned (Kitwood 1990a). This might be seen as a defensive reaction, a response to anxieties held in part at an unconscious level.

The anxieties seem to be of two main kinds. First, and naturally enough, every human being is afraid of becoming frail and highly dependent; these fears are liable to be particularly strong in any society where the sense of community is weak or non-existent. Added to that, there is the fear of a long drawn-out process of dying, and of death itself. Contact with those who are elderly, weak and vulnerable is liable to activate these fears, and threaten our basic sense of security (Stevenson 1989). Second, we carry fears about mental instability. The thought of being insane, deranged, lost forever in confusion, is terrifying. Many people have come close to this at some point, perhaps in times of great stress, or grief, or personal catastrophe, or while suffering from a disease that has affected mental functioning. At the most dreadful end of these experiences lies the realm of 'unbeing', where even the sense of self is undermined.

Dementia in another person has the power to activate fears of both kinds: those concerned with dependence and frailty, and those concerned with going insane. Moreover, there is no real consolation in saying 'It won't happen to me', which can be done with many other anxiety-provoking conditions. Dementia is present in almost every street, and discussed repeatedly in the media. We know also that people from all kinds of background are affected, and that among those over 80 the proportion may be as high as one in five. So in being close to a person with dementia we may be seeing some terrifying anticipation of how we might become.

It is not surprising, then, if sensitivity has caused many people to shrink from such a prospect. Some way has to be found for making the anxieties bearable. The highly defensive tactic is to turn those who have dementia into a different species, not persons in the full sense. The principal problem, then, is not that of changing people with dementia, or of 'managing' their behaviour; it is that of moving beyond our own anxieties and defences, so that true meeting can occur, and life-giving relationships can grow.

The uniqueness of persons

At a commonsensical level it is obvious that each person is profoundly different from all others. It is easy to list some of the dimensions of that difference: culture, gender, temperament, social class, lifestyle, outlook, beliefs, values, commitments, tastes, interests – and so on. Added to this is the matter of personal history. Each person has come to be who they are by a route that is uniquely their own; every stage of the journey has left its mark.

In most of the contexts of everyday life, perhaps this kind of perception will suffice. There are times, however, when it is essential to penetrate the veil of common sense and use theory to develop a deeper understanding. It is not that theory is important in itself, but that it can challenge popular misconceptions; and it helps to generate sensitivity to areas of need, giving caring actions a clearer direction (Kitwood 1997a).

Within conventional psychology the main attempt to make sense of the differences between persons has been through the concept of personality, which may roughly be defined as 'a set of widely generalised dispositions to act in certain kinds of way' (Alston 1976). The concept of personality, in itself, is rich enough to provide many therapeutic insights. However, by far the greatest amount of effort in psychology has been spent in attempts to 'measure' it in terms of a few dimensions (extraversion, neuroticism, and so on), using standard questionnaires – personality inventories, as they are often called. The questions tend to be simplistic and are usually answered through self-report. This approach does have some value, perhaps, in helping to create a general picture, and it has been used in this way in the context of dementia. The main use of personality measurement, however, has been in classifying and selecting people for purposes that were not their own. Psychometric methodology is, essentially, a servant of the I–It mode.

There is another approach within psychology, whose central assumption is that each person is a meaning-maker and an originating source of action (Harré and Secord 1972, Harré 1993). Because of its special interest in everyday life it is sometimes described as being ethogenic, by analogy with the ethological study of animals in their natural habitats. Social life can be considered to consist of a series of episodes, each with certain overriding characteristics (buying a pot plant, sharing a meal, and so on). In each episode the participants make their 'definitions of the situation', usually at a level just below conscious awareness, and then bring more or less ready-made action schemata into play. Interaction occurs as each interprets the meaning of the others' actions. Personality here is viewed as an individual's stock of learned resources for action. It is recognized that one person may have a richer set of resources than another, and in that sense have a more highly developed personality. A full 'personality inventory' would consist of the complete list of such resources, together with the types of situation in which each item is typically deployed.

This view can be taken further by assimilating to it some ideas that are central to depth psychology and psychotherapeutic work. The resources are of two main kinds, which we might term *adaptive* and *experiential*. The first of these consists of learned ways of responding 'appropriately' to other people's demands (both hidden and explicit), to social situations, and to the requirements of given roles. The process of learning is relatively straightforward, and is sometimes portrayed as involving imitation, identification and internalization (Danziger 1978). The second kind of resource relates to a person's capacity to experience what he or she is actually undergoing. Development here occurs primarily when there is an abundance of comfort, pleasure, security and freedom. In Jungian theory the adaptive resources correspond roughly to the ego, and the experiential resources to the Self (Jung 1934). The term that I shall use for the latter is 'experiential self'.

In an ideal world, both kinds of personal resource would grow together. The consequence would be an adult who was highly competent in many areas of life, and who had a well-developed subjectivity. He or she would be 'congruent', in the sense used by Rogers (1961): that is, there would be a close correspondence between what the person was undergoing, experiencing, and communicating to others. In fact, however, this is very rarely the case. The development of adaptive resources is often blocked by lack of opportunity, by the requirements of survival, and sometimes by the naked imposition of power. The growth of an experiential self is impeded where there is cruelty or a lack of love, or where the demands of others are overwhelming. Many people have been subjected to some form of childhood abuse: physical, sexual, emotional, commercial, spiritual. Areas of pain and inner conflict are hidden away, and the accompanying anxiety is sealed off by psychological defences. According to the theorists of Transactional Analysis, this is the context in which each person acquires a 'script' – a way of 'getting by' that makes it possible to function in difficult circumstances (Stewart and Joines 1987). As a result of extreme overadaptation, so Winnicott suggested, a person acquires a 'false self', a 'front' that is radically out of touch with experience and masks an inner chaos (Davis and Wallbridge 1981).

These ideas, which I have sketched here in only the barest outline, can be developed into a many-sided view or model of personal being. As we shall see, it can shed much light on the predicament of men and women who have dementia. Where resources have been lost, we might ask some very searching questions about what has happened and why. If personhood appears to have been undermined, is any of that a consequence of the ineptitude of others, who have all their cognitive powers intact? If uniqueness has faded into a grey oblivion, how far is it because those around have not developed the empathy that is necessary, or their ability to relate in a truly personal way? Thus we are invited to look carefully at ourselves, and ponder on how we have developed as persons; where we are indeed strong and capable, but also where we are damaged and deficient. In particular, we might reflect on whether our own experiential resources are sufficiently well developed for us to be able to help other people in their need.

Personhood and embodiment

Thus far in this chapter we have looked at issues related to personhood almost totally from the standpoint of the human sciences. The study of dementia, however, has been dominated by work in such disciplines as anatomy, physiology, biochemistry, pathology and genetics. If our account of personhood is to be complete, then, we must find a way of bringing the discourses of the human and natural sciences together.

There is a long-standing debate within philosophy concerning the problem of how the mind is related to the body, and to matter itself. The debate first took on a clear form with the work of Descartes in the seventeenth century, and since that time several distinct positions have emerged. I am going to set out one of these, drawing to some extent on the work of the philosopher Donald Davidson (1970), and the brain scientists Steven Rose (1984) and Antonio Damasio (1995). The starting point is to reject the assumption with which Descartes began: that there are two fundamentally different substances, matter and mind. Instead, we postulate a single (exceedingly complex) reality; it can be termed 'material', so long as it is clear that 'matter' does not consist of the little solid particles that atoms were once taken to be.

We can never grasp this reality, as it really is, because of the limitations of our nervous system, but we can talk about it in several different ways. Often we use an intentional kind of language, with phrases such as 'I feel happy', 'I believe that you are telling the truth', 'I ought to go and visit my aunt'. Through this kind of language we can describe our feelings, draw up plans, ask people to give reasons for their actions, and so on. Often when we speak and think along these lines we have a sense of freedom, as if we are genuinely making choices, taking decisions, and making things happen in the world.

The natural sciences operate on very different lines. Here the aim is to be rigorously objective, using systematic observation and experiment. Within any one science regularities are discovered, and processes are seen in terms of causal relationships. People who work as scientists sometimes have a sense of absolute determinism. The determinism is actually built in from the start; it is part of the 'grammar'. We know no other way of doing the thing called natural science.

Each type of discourse has its particular uses. One of the greatest and commonest mistakes is to take the descriptions and explanations given in language as if these were the reality itself. Once that is done, many false problems arise; for example, whether or not we really have free will, whether the mind is inside the brain, whether the emotions are merely biochemical, and so on. There are strong reasons for believing that the reality itself, whatever it may be, is far too complex to be caught fully in any of our human nets of language.

Moving on now to the topic of mind and brain, the basic assumption is that any psychological event (such as deciding to go for a walk) or state (such as feeling hungry) is also a brain event or state. It is not that the psychological experience (ψ) is causing the brain activity ($\mathbf{b}$) or vice versa; it is simply that some aspect of the true reality is being described in two different ways.

Hence in any individual, $\psi \equiv \mathbf{b}$

The 'equation' simply serves to emphasize the assumption that psychology and neurology are, in truth, inseparable.

It is not known how far experiences which two different individuals describe in the same way have parallel counterparts in brain function; scanning methods which look at brain metabolism do, however, suggest broad similarities (Fischbach 1992).

Now the brain events or states occur within an 'apparatus' that has a structure, an architecture. The key functioning part is a system of around ten thousand million (10^{10}) neurones, with their myriads of branches and connections, or synapses. A synapse is the point at which a 'message' can pass from one neurone to another, thus creating the possibility of very complex 'circuits'. So far as is known, the basic elements of this system, some general features of its development, and most of the 'deeper' forms of circuitry (older in evolutionary terms), are genetically 'given'. On the other hand the elaboration of the whole structure, and particularly the cerebral cortex, is unique to each individual and not pregiven. The elaboration, then, is epigenetic: subject to processes of learning that occur after the genes have had their say. Each human face is unique; so also is each human brain.

It is probable that there are at least two basic types of learning: explicit and implicit (Kandel and Hawkins 1992). The former involves, for example, remembering faces and places, facts and theories. The latter involves acquiring skills that have a strong physical component; for example learning to walk, to swim or to play the piano. In both cases, learning is thought to proceed by stages. First, over a period of minutes or hours, existing neurone circuits are modified, by the strengthening and weakening of synaptic connections that already exist. Then, and much more slowly – over days, weeks and months – new synaptic connections are formed.

> The design of brain circuits continues to change. The circuits are not only receptive to the results of first experiences, but repeatedly pliable and modifiable by continued experience. Some circuits are remodelled over and over throughout the life span, according to the changes that the organism undergoes.
>
> (Damasio 1995: 112)

The brain is a 'plastic' organ. The continuing developmental aspect of its structure can be symbolized as B^d.

In dementia there is usually a loss of neurones and synaptic connections, making it impossible for the brain to carry out its full set of functions (Terry 1992). Some of this occurs slowly, and is a 'normal' part of ageing. It probably arises from the accumulation of errors in the reproduction of biological materials over a long period, and chemical processes such as oxidation. The more serious and rapid losses, however, appear to be the consequence of disease or degenerative processes, and these may be symbolized as B_p (brain pathology). So, very crudely, the situation within an individual can be represented thus:

$$\frac{\psi \equiv \mathbf{b}}{(B^d, B_p)}$$

(Any psychological event or state is also a brain event or state, 'carried' by a brain whose structure has been determined by both developmental and pathological factors.)

If this view is correct in principle, it shows how the issues related to personhood are also those of brain and body. Here, there is one particularly important point to note. It is that the developmental, epigenetic aspects of brain structure have been grossly neglected in recent biomedical research on dementia; moreover, there is scarcely a hint of interest in this topic in contemporary psychiatry and clinical psychology. Yet neuroscience now suggests that there may be very great differences between human beings in the degree to which nerve architecture has developed as a result of learning and experience. It follows that individuals may vary considerably in the extent to which they are able to withstand processes in the brain that destroy synapses, and hence in their resistance to dementia.

In this kind of way we move towards a 'neurology of personhood'. All events in human interaction – great and small – have their counterpart at a neurological level. The sense of freedom which Buber associates with I–Thou relating may correspond to a biochemical environment that is particularly conducive to nerve growth. A malignant social psychology may actually be damaging to nerve tissue. Dementia may be induced in part, by the stresses of life. Thus anyone who envisages the effects of care as being 'purely psychological', independent of what is happening in the nervous system, is perpetuating the error of Descartes in trying to separate mind from body. Maintaining personhood is both a psychological and a neurological task.

Part 4

ORGANIZATIONAL CULTURE AND ITS TRANSFORMATION

Organizational culture and its transformation

Readings

Kitwood, T. (1990) On organizations: their imperatives and constraints. In *Concern for Others: A new psychology of conscience and morality*. London: Routledge.

Bredin, K., Kitwood, T. and Wattis, J. (1995) Decline in quality of life for patients with severe dementia following a ward merger, *International Journal of Geriatric Psychiatry*, 10(11): 967–973.

Kitwood, T. (1995) Cultures of care: tradition and change. In Kitwood, T. and Benson, S. (eds) *The New Culture of Dementia Care*. London: Hawker.

Kitwood, T. (1997) Some notes on personhood and deformation. In Fletcher, C.L. (ed.) *Values in Adult Education*. Wolverhampton: University of Wolverhampton.

Kitwood, T. (1998) Professional and moral development for care work: some observations on the process, *Journal of Moral Education*, 27(3): 401–411.

Critical commentary

At some point during or after diagnosis the majority of people with dementia will find themselves, at least temporarily, in a formal care setting of some kind. This may or may not be as a direct result of dementia (the person may, for example, need to be admitted to hospital as the result of a physical illness or injury) and the range of possible care settings is diverse, including hospital assessment or psychiatric units; general and acute hospital wards; residential or nursing care, and day care facilities. In many cases, a person with dementia will experience a number of different care settings in a relatively short period of time and at each transition he or she will face the challenges of adapting to an unfamiliar environment and people, while simultaneously experiencing the loss of the familiar. This is the kind of situation in which we all tend to feel anxious, but for a person with dementia, who is particularly vulnerable as a result of existing confusion and disorientation, such moves can be particularly traumatic. The fear and distress that can result will inevitably be exacerbated if the staff are inexperienced or dismissive, too overworked to provide the help and support the person needs, or if the care regime of the organization in question is task- rather than person-oriented. In such situations it is not unusual for dementia to appear to progress with untypical speed. Kitwood (1997a: 36) notes that:

Even over a few months a person can deteriorate from a state of coping almost normally to being drastically 'demented'. The adverse changes that often follow hospitalization or going into residential care are well known. Clearly, more than simple neuropathology is needed to explain these changes.

The kind of downward (or 'involutionary') spiral that can result from repeated changes of environment, insensitive care practice, and stigmatization of the person with dementia is what Kitwood means by the 'dialectics of dementia'. The person is perceived as having become more 'severely demented', often presaging another move to a yet more controlling environment where the 'symptoms' of dementia will be further exacerbated. A specific example of this kind of 'vicious circle' (relating to Margaret B) is given in Kitwood (1997a: 52) and the involutionary spiral is discussed in detail in Part 1 of this Reader. Empirical evidence to support this view comes from a study by Bredin et al. (1995) *Decline in Quality of Life for Patients with Severe Dementia Following a Ward Merger*, in which it was found that a merger between two existing long-stay wards had drastic effects on staff morale and on the quality of care they provided. This study used Dementia Care Mapping (DCM) to collect observational data on the patients before and after the ward merger took place. The DCM measures indicated a significant deterioration in quality of life of the patients with dementia following the ward merger which the authors explain as follows:

> There was a general background insecurity and unsettlement among staff, who had worked hard under difficult conditions and felt that new changes were being forced through for managerial reasons. Their morale was already low and they were highly vulnerable to pressures of any kind ... The response of staff was to perform their duties in a less personal way and to abstain from the kind of 'psychological care work' that goes beyond practical nursing ... The reactions of staff to their new situation in turn led to an increased depersonalization of the patients. Some patients went into a state of almost complete vegetative withdrawal, others manifested their distress through an increase in 'problem behaviours'. (1995: 972/302–303)

The deterioration noted in these patients occurred much more rapidly than would normally be expected in the course of dementia, suggesting that this was actually the result of the care (or indeed 'uncare') provided on the merged ward. Also, it is implied, the anxieties and resentments that the staff themselves experience can exacerbate the situation so that a 'cycle of demoralization and depersonalization [is] set into effect, the needs of both patients and staff being drastically unmet' (1995: 972/303). This sits well with the more recent findings of, for example, Balfour (2006) who describes staff on a busy hospital unit as being 'irradiated with distress'. 'Without containment and support,' Balfour argues, 'they can find themselves acting in ways that echo the difficulties of their patients. In this way the emotional world of older people with dementia can "infect" those around them, creating a parallel emotional process that ... may be mirrored and enacted by staff' (2006: 341).

In institutional contexts in general, Kitwood believed the existing care regime is often one that is likely to increase anxiety, confusion, apathy and behaviour that staff find it difficult to deal with. It becomes clear, then, that in order to develop our under-standing of dementia it is important to look at what is happening in the places where dementia care is provided, and at the characteristics of care settings that may help or hinder the meeting of the psychological needs of people with dementia. Kitwood's exploration of organizational culture is extremely valuable in that it helps to bring aspects of the caring organization, which may have been simply part of a 'taken-for-granted reality', much more clearly into the foreground. Some aspects of care practice within organizations are deeply embedded and very resistant to change, and in exploring these Kitwood drew on the concept of 'organizational defence', suggesting that in group working situations there can be a process of unconscious collusion in which responsibil-ity is handed over to the organization. In this way a collective denial of the nature of problems, or threats to personal integrity, can be maintained:

> In many organizations it is as if the members have made agreements together, at an unconscious level, about what must be hidden from awareness . . . When people are bound together in this kind of way, part of their individual psyche has, so to speak, been lost – 'made over' to the organization. (1997a: 113–114)

In this part of the Reader, we will first outline the origins of Kitwood's ideas on culture and organizational change in relation to dementia care. We will also consider his identification of the characteristics of 'old' and 'new' cultures of dementia care (Kitwood 1995a) and some of the difficulties that are raised by this dichotomization. We will then go on to look in more detail at Kitwood's application of the theory of organizational defence and his proposals regarding the transformation of organizational culture, with particular reference to education. In conclusion, we will consider some of the more problematic aspects of Kitwood's work on culture change and the challenges they raise for future explorations in this area.

Origins of Kitwood's thinking on organizational culture

Kitwood's main work on organizational culture in dementia care dates from the mid-1990s. As such it is a relatively late development in his thinking and an area that was still comparatively new at the time of his death, although its roots can be traced in much of the earlier work. Here, we consider some of the main strands in this development, from the ideas put forward in some of his publications unrelated to dementia care – which deserve detailed consideration – to the impact of his work in implementing Dementia Care Mapping (DCM).

First then, we turn to two articles that do not relate specifically to dementia care. Kitwood's book, *Concern for Others* (1990c) includes a particularly relevant chapter, 'On organizations: their imperatives and constraints', in which he comments that:

> Formal organizations of a hierarchical kind have taken over to a very considerable degree, the major functions of society, pushing informal action to the margins. They are remarkably effective in moulding people, harnessing their motives, defusing their discontents, drowning out the voice of criticism, dismantling the social movements that would cast the system into disarray. (1990c: 156/278)

And later in the same chapter:

> Some organizations have real goals that are, in moral terms, indefensible. Yet many individuals, with the most acute and sensitive moral capabilities, have little option but to work within them; even in some of the most affluent societies, the alternative is to be in danger of homelessness and near-starvation. (1990c: 163/282)

Here, Kitwood takes a very strong line on the power of organizations at best to mould, and at worst to oppress and corrupt, those within them. In this and his other publications – including those related to organizational culture in dementia care – it is, however, sometimes difficult to know whether Kitwood is referring to organizations at the macro level – for example in the sense of the 'ideological state apparatuses' described by Althusser (1970) – or at the more local level of individual businesses and small companies. This is an important distinction, as we will go on to see, because many of the organizations providing dementia care are, themselves, at the mercy of external forces over which they have little, if any, control, and there are clearly significant differences between the factors that impinge on those working within the National Health Service or social services, and those who are employed to work in voluntary or independent sector care settings.

In a later article, *Some Notes on Personhood and Deformation*, Kitwood (1997e) summarizes what he takes to be the prevailing climate of the 'business culture':

> Now it is not only 'Do not give any employee a training beyond the operational requirements of the work role', but also 'Do not give any employee a rate of pay or a form of job security that places more than minimal demands upon the organisation'. Tragically, this even applies in many areas of care work. Employees have little option but to become cynical and self-protective in their attempt to minimize the process of personal deformation, perhaps reserving trust and commitment only for the arena of private life. (Kitwood, 1997e: 49/318)

The problems Kitwood highlighted in this article are certainly endemic in the field of dementia care. While these problems will be all too familiar to readers working in this field today, it is noticeable, however, that the employment rights, rates of pay, and job security of dementia care workers were never major themes in Kitwood's writing on dementia (1997e).

Kitwood suggests that there are two methodological routes to explore the processes of personal deformation. The first is an overtly historicist approach. Kitwood cites Fromm (1941) and Reich (1946) as key proponents of this approach, noting that the intense and class-based deformations brought about by capitalism were merely a 'latter-day instantiation' of the earlier divisions brought about by patriarchy and property ownership. The alternative approach is, he says, 'rather less ambitious, and involves looking at aspects of individual development in a particular period. *This will be my model here*' (1997e: 47/36, emphasis added). In other words, Kitwood is allying himself with a kind of mid-range approach which will admit the social while avoiding any engagement with deep-rooted and longstanding social divisions. Thus he does not go on to engage specifically with poverty, gender, discrimination or exploitation as aspects of social injustice, but returns to the arena of individual psychology. Stress, low pay and temporary contracts are, for example, discussed in terms of their deformative effects on the individual psyche, rather than in terms of the material constraints they impose on disadvantaged groups in society.

This article highlights a frequent difficulty in Kitwood's work – that of creating an argument having rhetorical impact rather than empirical or theoretical coherence. In order to *minimize* personal deformation, Kitwood suggests, employees become 'cynical and self-protective . . . perhaps reserving trust and commitment only for the arena of private life' (p. 49/318). We may then ask, in what personal deformation consists if not cynicism and self-protection? And how can we explain a form of unconscious and deep-rooted personal deformation that affects the work arena but does not also affect the arena of private life? How is someone who is already 'personally deformed' still able to be trusting and committed at all? Apart from widespread psychotherapy, Kitwood does not appear to see a solution to this problem. Here we can also find examples of the difficult to resolve 'best of times, worst of times' flavour about much of his writing.

> If we look at the 'state of the world' . . . the picture is a gloomy one indeed. One part of the globe after another is being overtaken by the advance of a rapacious capitalism which wrecks culture and creates poverty on a massive scale.

While later, on the same page:

> Perhaps we are now seeing the very first signs of a reversal . . . as the personhood of children is recognised more strongly, and as the injustices of gender, class ethnicity and ageism are beginning to be corrected . . . It is possible that, compared to their parents and grandparents, a far greater number have essentially sound psychological foundations. (1997e: 50/319)

Here we sense a somewhat awkward shifting of position between philanthropy and misanthropy, optimism and pessimism, distal and proximal influences, rather than a consistent world view from which a model of social and organizational change might be mounted.

What is clear, however, from extracts such as these is that Kitwood was familiar with sociological perspectives that problematize social organization and hierarchical power relationships, rather than attributing the sources of human misery to the personal and intersubjective domain. This sociological perspective was, however, somewhat marginalized in his work on dementia.

A second trend in the development of Kitwood's thinking on organizational culture is his development of the concept of an *interpersonal* culture in dementia care, which goes beyond the dyadic, carer/cared for interchange that had dominated his earlier publications on dementia. In a 1993 article, for example, Kitwood outlined a 'culture of dementia' characterized by positive and supportive relationships *between* people who have dementia and suggested that this may happen 'when a person-centred approach to care has been used consistently over an extended period. Individuals have received a more or less enduring facilitation and their personal resources are no longer dwindling' (Kitwood 1993d: 64/219). Here, Kitwood recognizes that the experience of formal dementia care is part of a social milieu in which relationships within and between the client group and the staff team are also important to quality of life. This marked the beginning of a move away from the sometimes rather punitive focus on the individual care worker in his earlier work. If the problem of dementia cannot be located 'inside' the individual as part of his or her diagnosis, that is to say, neither can it, coherently, be located 'inside' the caregiver; a person-centred approach should consider the person-hood of all those involved in the process of providing care.

Finally, it is inevitable (although not explicit within his published work) that Kitwood's thinking on the importance of organizational factors in either promoting or hindering the improvement of care practice evolved through his personal experience of negotiating with care organizations and groups of staff around the implementation of DCM and from other direct interfaces with the practice field. The difficulties of trying to change a situation from within, and to avoid hypocrisy or collusion while still maintaining amicable working relationships, are significant and Kitwood was acutely aware of the psychological complexities of this kind of work. When DCM began to be used developmentally (i.e. as part of a repeated cycle of mapping, staff development and remapping) it seemed that a number of patterns were beginning to emerge. For example, organizations were, not infrequently, resistant to the findings – managers might suggest, for example, that an evaluation indicating a relatively poor quality of care was unjustified because staffing levels were particularly low on the day of the evaluation. During feedback on the evaluation, members of the care staff would sometimes deny that something recorded by the observers had actually happened. In addition, preparation for DCM evaluations and feedback on the results often revealed much about the nature of hierarchies and power relationships within the organization. Managers sometimes insisted that they should receive the results of the evaluation themselves before deciding what, if anything, they were prepared to pass on to staff. On occasions, there were attempts to use DCM data for purposes for which they had never been intended – for example, to support the view that a particular resident's behaviour was so extreme that he or she should be moved to a different kind of care setting. Such responses may be taken to indicate that there are high levels of defensive avoidance within the care setting (see the discussion of organizational defence later).

A note on malignant social psychology: individual or collective responsibility?

The shift in Kitwood's thinking towards a more cultural perspective on care practice can be traced through refinements in his concept of 'malignant social psychology' (MSP) over time. In early editions of the DCM manual Kitwood introduced the term MSP simply to describe a range of different categories of negative care practice that he had observed in care practice. Both here and in the prototype list of examples of 'bad practice' given in Person to Person (Kitwood and Bredin 1992b), it is evident that the perpetrator of the bad practice or malignant social psychology is taken to be the individual caregiver. While there is no imputation of deliberate malice, it is the *individual* who is responsible for changing his or her practice:

> Poor care hardly ever comes from deliberate cruelty or heartlessness . . . we may find ourselves reacting without thinking and losing touch with what is really needed.

It is best to forgive ourselves our failings, accept that we're not perfect and learn to do better. (Kitwood and Bredin 1992b: 21)

In the seventh edition of the DCM manual (current at the time of Kitwood's death) the concept of malignant social psychology appears, however, to have been extended to the care environment as a whole. The 17 categories of negative care practice that had been identified were now named 'personal detractions' (see Part 2 Box 2.3) and it was suggested that high levels of personal detraction towards people with dementia by care staff were an indication of malignant social psychology inherent within the whole atmos-phere of the care setting. 'The strong word malignant signifies something very harmful, symptomatic of a *care environment* that is deeply damaging to personhood.' (Kitwood 1997a: 46, emphasis added). Here, there appears to have been a shift from viewing malignant social psychology as an act or series of acts, perpetrated by individuals, to an organizational culture within which poor care practice is condoned or allowed to pass unnoticed. There is only a subtle distinction between these two positions (and Kitwood is far from consistent on this point in his later publications), but this does tend to indicate that his concept of malignant social psychology was becoming rather more social and collective at the point where his work came to its premature end.

'Old' and 'new' cultures

Probably Kitwood's most widely known work on organizational culture is the chapter 'Cultures of Care: Tradition and change' from *The New Culture of Dementia Care* (1995a). Here, Kitwood makes the important point that 'the power of a culture stems from the fact that when people are immersed in it, the framework that it provides seems self-evident. What nature is to creatures whose lives are governed by instinct, culture is to human beings' (1995a: 7/306). Much of the dementia care practice that is now coming to be recognized as inappropriate, insensitive or inhumane – this is to say, was not considered to be so in the past, because it was simply the accepted way of doing things within the organization or workplace in question.

Kitwood goes on to present 10 key points of contrast between the old and the new cultures of dementia care. For example, in relation to Point 4: 'Emphasis for research', he contrasts the 'old culture' view that little can be done for the person with dementia until medical breakthroughs arrive and thus much more biomedical research should be done, with the 'new culture' belief that there is much that can be done for the person with dementia in the here and now, by researching better ways of caring (1995a: 9/308).

Drawing on the work of Williams (1976) Kitwood identifies three components of a culture: institutions, norms and beliefs. He does not, however, elaborate on these in relation to the characteristics of the old and new cultures. Davis and Nutley (2000: 115) have presented a slightly more elaborate model of a three-level organizational culture as follows:

1   *assumptions*: 'taken-for-granted' views of the world and how it is possible to under-stand and intervene in it
2   *values*: foundations for making judgements and distinguishing between what is 'right' and what is 'wrong'

3 *artefacts*: physical and behavioural manifestations of culture, including dress codes, rituals, recording practices etc.

Kitwood's 10 key points of difference between the old and new cultures contain examples of all three levels identified by Davis and Nutley. For example, in Point 2: 'General view of dementia' the old culture view that 'the primary degenerative dementias are devastating diseases of the central nervous system, in which person-ality and identity are progressively destroyed' (1995a: 8/307) is an *assumption* that many people (including many who are deeply committed to person-centred care) have held and still hold to be a fact – so unquestionably obvious that it is impossible to think otherwise. The 'new culture' alternative is, however, Kitwood suggests, that we see dementing illnesses 'primarily as forms of disability. How a person is affected depends crucially on the quality of care . . . The focus is on enabling and empower-ing, through the provision of what is necessary to compensate for disability, and on recognising the unique way in which each person deals with his or her damaged world' (1995a: 8/307). In Point 8: 'Problem behaviours' (1995a: 10/310), the new culture commitment to viewing so-called problem behaviours as attempts at com-munication corresponds to Davis and Nutley's definition of a *value*. We can also find within Kitwood's discussion of the old culture, examples of what Davis and Nutley describe as *artefacts*. In Point 5: 'Us and them' (1995a: 9/309), for example, we find the old culture insistence on staff wearing uniform and having separate meal-times and toilets.

From a didactic point of view, Kitwood's characterization of the old and new cultures of dementia care using a binary (either/or) model is a helpful tactic, since it unquestion-ably makes the material memorable and easy to grasp. It has also been extremely successful in helping to popularize his ideas. By the same token, this is a rather crude and simplistic distinction. The likelihood is that any real world care setting will share indicators of both cultures rather than belonging to one or the other, and that any change which is brought about will be gradual and contingent, dependent on a multiplicity of variables, many of which are unpredictable. As a contemporary reviewer of *The New Culture of Dementia Care* noted: 'The notion that there is, indeed, a "new culture" of dementia care is one that confuses many . . . whether one regards dementia care as entering a radically new culture, or as subject to a gradual shift in emphasis (Cheston 1996: 37). Kitwood's forced distinction between old and new cultures also contrasts oddly with the prefatory sections of the chapter in which he draws on the work of Foucault. As Kitwood has noted elsewhere, it was Foucault who advised us to "abandon the convenience of terminal truths" (1967: xi) and Foucault himself belonged to the poststructuralist school of philosophy in which binary thinking is viewed as part of the problem rather than part of the solution.

Kitwood (1995a: 11/312) himself draws attention to the 'very great' contrast between the old and new cultures he is proposing and adds: 'Sometimes when I make comparisons in this kind of way I wonder if I am exaggerating. It is all too easy to set up a straw man and then demolish it in order to score points.' He resolves these doubts by referring to an (unreferenced) article entitled *Alzheimer's – No Cure, No Help, No Hope*, which relates the depressing story of a man with early onset dementia and the burden this placed on his family. 'This account offered not a ray of hope at the human level, but ended with an invitation to donate to a particular fund for neuroscientific research' (1995a: 11/312).

In offering this article as a demonstration of the existence of the old culture however, Kitwood creates an unacknowledged ambiguity. The old culture, as he presents it here, incorporates not only the culture of therapeutic nihilism (i.e. 'no cure, no help, no hope') but also, by implication, the newer 'smart' culture of neuroscientific progress, with its emphasis on drug treatments, genome research and neuroimaging techniques. While the values enshrined in the culture of therapeutic nihilism are recognizably 'old' in the historical sense that they go back to a time when the institutional sedation and 'warehousing' of those with dementia were believed to constitute an acceptable standard of care, the culture of scientific progress and advance is always by definition 'new', no matter how deceptive its promises may sometimes turn out to be. This research culture – which could equally be described as a 'new culture' opposed to therapeutic nihilism – inevitably impacts on care settings from the outside, influencing expectations, hopes and attitudes within them. As an example here, we might draw on the case of the cognitive enhancer drugs which were widely believed in the mid-1990s to offer a panacea that would transform the nature of dementia care work once and for all; or as one care home manager remarked circa 1997: 'Once we get them all on Aricept, we'll be laughing.' This may appear to be a rather hollow claim today.

If the important dimensions of difference in culture are, in fact, merely oldness and newness – out-of-dateness and novelty – neuroscience cannot conveniently be relegated to the 'old' culture as Kitwood appears to suggest. Moreover, in presenting his own alternative person-centred culture as 'new' Kitwood suggests an unfortunate division between past and present, where past = bad, and present/future = good. While Kitwood is arguing here for the implementation of forms of dementia care practice that are certainly kinder, more humane, and more sensitive than has ever been *the norm*, there is little basis in evidence for thinking that individuals were more lacking in these qualities in the past than they are today. And some, of course, might argue that in the past people were kinder and more caring, families more committed to looking after each other and communities more closely knit than they are today.

In his later book *Dementia Reconsidered* (1997a), Kitwood retained the old culture/new culture distinction but applied this to what he now termed Type A and Type B organizational cultures – Type A being unsuited to dementia care, and Type B being highly suited. Acknowledging that there was no systematic research base for his analysis, Kitwood noted that his method had been to create 'slightly abstract ideal types' based on his own observations, 'consultation with several people who have had extensive experience [and] data gathered during training courses where participants share their experiences of good and bad organizational practices' (1997a: 104). Later in the same chapter he acknowledges that those consulted found it much easier to come up with examples of 'bad' (Type A) organizations, so it is important to bear in mind that the characteristics of Type B organizations mentioned in Kitwood's analysis are his own and others' ideal view rather than a representation of any actually existing person-centred care organization.

So we find, not surprisingly, that, on the one hand, Type A organizational cultures are hierarchical and top down in their management structure, characterized by strictly regimented divisions, bureaucratically fetishistic about paperwork and insensitive towards the feelings of staff. Type B organizations, on the other hand, are characterized by a facilitative style of management, respect and trust between colleagues, a lack of status divisions and effective channels of communication. While few would disagree with Kitwood's vision of the ideal care organization, it is difficult to read this material without being aware of both its utopianism and its perfectionism. We read of Type B organizations, for example, that: 'The whole staff group thrives on cooperation and sharing'; and that 'there is a rich body of knowledge that is held within the living culture' (1997a: 105). At times this material almost seems to take on the language of advertising or to be couched in terms that might be adopted by an ambitious home manager intent on promoting his or her establishment regardless of the underlying realities.

As we will go on to discuss in the next section, the tendency to avoid unpleasant realities and give an overly favourable account of the quality of care is, in itself, an aspect of what Kitwood describes as 'organizational defence'. As Kitwood notes (1997a: 115): 'Most organizations involved with dementia care wish to be seen as giving excellent care; it is certainly what their "customers" desire. The challenge is to get organizations actually to do it, rather than simply maintain a façade.' It has become axiomatic in recent years that person-centred care is far more widely talked about than it is implemented (for example, Sheard 2004), so it is unfortunate that one of the consequences of Kitwood's rhetorical creation of old and new cultures has been a tendency for care organizations to wish to claim that they are already part of the new culture. This is, however, unsurprising because the stark contrast Kitwood presents between the two is so extreme that no one could wish to be associated with the grossly impersonal and dehumanizing picture he presents of the old culture. In a sense, then, Kitwood's own rhetoric can at times become inimical to the kind of reflection that is needed in order to make the more modest, gradual, and sustainable changes in practice that are needed.

Organizational defence

In putting forward his theory of organizational defence in dementia care practice Kitwood (1997a) draws on 'depth psychology' (a term he frequently uses to refer to psycho-analytic or psychotherapeutic approaches in general) in order to explain why both individuals and organizations may be unable to engage in conscious reflective assessment of the true state of affairs in their provision of dementia care. Depth psychology, in all its variants, is characterized by the view that our true motivations for acting in a given way are inaccessible to us because they are unconscious; that is, they lie outside the realm of day-to-day awareness. Often this is because they are too threatening or uncomfortable to be admitted to the conscious mind. At the individual level this is usually held to be the result of a repressed fear or trauma; for example having lost a close relative with dementia or the unacknowledged dread that we may develop dementia ourselves. At an organizational level these individual fears can be multiplied, Kitwood suggests, and they may both be held in place, and exacerbated, by regimented care practices and routines.

Drawing on work by Menzies (1972), Kitwood discusses the impact on caregivers of emotional demands for which they are often provided with little support. Menzies had noticed that although the nurses involved in her study were subjected to highly stressful working conditions they employed coping mechanisms that appeared analogous to individual defence mechanisms. For example, they maintained an emotional distance between themselves and their patients and tended to focus on tasks rather than providing more psychological forms of care. As Nichol and Raye (2001: 2) have pointed out, this sometimes went to extremes that seem bizarre: for example nurses would wake patients up in order to give them sleeping pills so that they could demonstrate that they had carried out the tasks allocated to them to the letter.

While such work practices may protect caregivers from their initial anxieties, in the longer term they often becomes the source of new ones, as the caregivers' own value system has to be repressed in order to comply with the demands of organizational routine:

> When defences are entrenched it is likely that an organization will be severely impaired in its ability to provide good care. The discourses of everyday life will be too trivial; too much feeling will go unexpressed; members of staff will have lost too much of themselves in the collective defences. (Kitwood 1997a: 114)

Kitwood saw such psychological defences as being a huge obstacle to organizational change and he suggested that they might be overcome at an individual level by either psychotherapy or meditation (1997a: 131). Although it might be argued that the time and resource implications of this kind of intensive approach to individual staff development make it rather unrealistic in practice, Kitwood also suggests a variety of more pragmatic ways of bringing about organizational change, including staff supervision and induction, in-service training and staff development programmes, effective quality assurance and arrangements for accrediting and promoting highly committed staff (1997a: 109–112) He suggests that identifying one or two people within the organization to participate in externally validated programmes of education may act as a means of creating role models and equipping them with the skills to act as mentors and tutors within the organization:

> If individual accreditation is to become an established practice, it will probably involve one or two members of the senior care team themselves becoming qualified as assessors, tutors or mentors, in addition to their ordinary role in supervision. Indirectly the heightened level of activity will improve the quality of care. Also, as more opportunities are provided for staff members to gain qualifications specifically related to dementia care, the general status of this work is likely to rise. (1997a: 111)

Increasingly, then, towards the end of his life Kitwood was coming to see formal academic courses of education as the route to organizational change. This period coincides, of course, with the development of Bradford Dementia Group's academic portfolio and the University of Bradford's accreditation – under Kitwood's leadership – of the first dementia-specific modules and courses to be offered in higher education in the UK. In the next section we will summarize Kitwood's thinking about the role of education in organizational change.

Cultural transformation: the role of education

From the early days of his work on dementia Kitwood was actively involved in teaching about the person-centred approach to dementia care, both through Dementia Care Mapping (DCM) courses and on shorter one-day courses provided for organizations wishing to introduce the basic concepts to their staff. He also devised the *Depth Psychology of Dementia Course*, which drew on psychotherapeutic principles and techniques. By comparison, however, he wrote relatively little about the role of education in cultural change until late in his dementia career. In some of the earlier publications, the need for education in order to develop care practice seemed, indeed, to have been rather overlooked. In a 1993 article, for example, Kitwood commented on the potential benefits and drawbacks of therapeutic approaches such as validation therapy, reminiscence work and resolution therapy. While sceptical about the claimed therapeutic potential of such approaches, he accepted that 'when practised with skill and kindness they do undoubtedly provide some basis for a real meeting between the dementia sufferer and the Other' (1993d: 53/210). Kitwood did not, however, at this time appear to reflect that many care workers would be unaware that such approaches even existed, let alone have the skill or confidence to put them into practice. Without a commitment from management to their learning such skills – and the theory and principles behind them – it was impossible that these interventions could have been put into practice at all.

There had, then, been a strong tendency in Kitwood's early work to imply that the transformative input capable of enhancing the well-being of the person with dementia would come solely from 'the Other' (the direct care giver) in a fundamentally dyadic relationship. What the Other might need, however, in order to be able to bring this about was given far less consideration. It is true that in any interpersonal act of communication it is possible to be positive or negative, sensitive or insensitive, respectful or derisory. In the broader context of dementia care delivery, however, staffing levels, time pressures, organizational imperatives and priorities, including (in some cases) maximization of profit, all impact on the quality of interpersonal relationships. Moreover, there are many versions of the 'us–them' divide in the field of dementia care, and in some of them it is direct care staff themselves who occupy the status of the derided 'them'.

By 1995 Kitwood had begun to acknowledge that 'the maintenance and enhancement of another's personhood is something that requires very delicate sensitivities, very highly developed skills, *and hence new forms of preparation*' (1995a: 9, 309, emphasis added) and, in *Dementia Reconsidered*, his awareness of the lack of appropriate dementia specific education in the preparation of staff working in this field was becoming increasingly evident:

> In Britain the recognition is slowly dawning that there is a vast training and educational deficit, and that none of the existing forms of professional preparation properly address the issues arising in dementia care. In recent years there have been many small and piecemeal training initiatives; at least this is a beginning. In strategic terms my own estimate is that in the UK we urgently need around 2000 people who have the capacity to train home care assistants and staff in

formal care settings, and a similar number of people who are capable of organizing and delivering a programme of carers' support. (1997a: 143)

This theme was developed further in two articles published posthumously in the *Journal of Nursing Care* (Capstick and Kitwood 1999; Kitwood and Capstick 1999). These articles draw particular attention to the lack of dementia-specific content in nurse education. While the availability of the ENB N11 module on care of the older person with mental health problems (which was not dementia specific and has since been withdrawn, following the demise of the English Nursing Board) was acknowledged as a step forward:

> There is still a tendency, however, for these basic inputs of training to centre on a diluted version of the 'medical model', with its emphasis on diagnostic categories and the underlying neuropathology. While these are important topics they do not form the core of what nurses need to know for good practice. (Kitwood and Capstick 1999: 12)

The second of these two articles went on to outline aspects of a core curriculum for dementia care education, including the reframing of 'problem behaviour' as meaningful action, understanding the 'version of reality' of a person with dementia, and the maintenance and enhancement of physical health. This article also points to the importance of adopting a student-centred model of learning to match the person-centred approach to care:

> This is based on the philosophy that each student's personal experience of working with people with dementia is his or her best resource for learning. By encouraging students to reflect on their experience, to draw new insights from it and to value it, we hope to enable them to becomes skilled, resourceful and confident 'reflective practitioners'. (Capstick and Kitwood 1999: 6)

In one of his last published articles *Professional and Moral Development for Care Work: Some observations on the process* Kitwood (1998a) explains in more detail how this approach to reflection based on the learner's own experience might work. He offers three experiential learning exercises designed for use with dementia care workers taking part in courses on person-centred care: a case study analysis; the preparation of a life history and a role play exercise. Kitwood goes on to explain in detail what these exercises consist of, and what main learning outcomes arise from them. For example, following the life history exercise:

> The resident is seen as a real person, perhaps for the first time ever. Up to the point of preparing a life history, the careworker may have responded with kindness and sincerity, but in many respects this was done blindly; stereotypes and superficial banter had often been used to fill the empty spaces in their knowledge. A relationship that had been largely instrumental now becomes personal. (Kitwood 1998a: 405–406/325)

Exercises of this nature were perhaps rarer in 1998 than they are today, but Kitwood makes a sound case for the benefits of experiential and reflective learning in dementia care. His suggestion that care staff are in need of moral development is, however, more problematic. 'It is remarkable', he writes:

> How little attention has been given as yet to the topic of providing a moral education for those who will work, or are already working, in the so-called caring professions: for example, nurses, social workers, occupational therapists and staff at all grades in residential settings (significantly the majority of these people are women) . . . Many people enter these professions very poorly prepared *in moral terms*, for the tasks that they will face; often nursing assistants and care assistants have had *no preparation at all*. (1998a: 401/322, emphasis added).

Kitwood is no doubt using the term 'moral development' here to indicate the need for care workers to conform to his own cultural value base, rather than as a suggestion that they are morally deficient in the broader sense of the term. Even so, the associations he implies between lack of formal education and lack of moral values, and between being female and being in need of moral development, are insensitive to say the least. Beyond this, they may be taken to indicate something about taken-for-granted assumptions of Kitwood's own that are unintentionally revealed here and this late article again raises troubling questions about his attribution of responsibility for the quality of dementia care.

Conclusion

Kitwood's work on organizational culture raises many important empirical questions that still deserve further consideration and contextualization. The importance he was coming to attach to this area of work can be seen in the fact that the whole of the last four chapters of his major text *Dementia Reconsidered* are devoted in one way or another to the question of how to bring about organizational change. Much of this content was, however, relatively new and had perhaps not been subjected to the same kind of maturational process as his work on the interpersonal aspects of dementia care. In view of this, it would be unfair to upbraid Kitwood for not having pursued subjects that he may well have gone on to follow up had his work not come to such a premature end. In spite of its internal ambiguities, then, this work should be seen as a welcome move towards putting dementia and dementia care practice within a broader social and cultural context.

What is, perhaps, a more serious consideration is that Kitwood's work has had such a profound influence on the dementia care field that it seems almost to have set the agenda for the decade since his death, in a way that has, perhaps, as we will argue later, led to some narrowing of perspectives on the topic under inquiry. It might be argued that to some extent the field is still suffering from what Bloom (1973), in his theory of poetry, referred to as the 'anxiety of influence' – the way that poets are hindered in the creative process by their ambiguous relationship with precursor poets, so that they become derivative and fail to develop their own voice. While we would argue that a detailed engagement with Kitwood's work is vital for anyone studying, practising or researching in the field of dementia care, it should not be allowed to determine the parameters of our thinking. For all we owe to Kitwood's work (and the debt is considerable) it may, in some ways, be time to come out from his shadow. In conclusion to this section, we will, therefore, suggest three key areas in which Kitwood's work on organizational culture deserves further critique and development.

First, while the relative absence of sociological theorizing on dementia care is now beginning to be addressed in a number of areas, (see, for example, Innes et al. 2004) there are still noticeable aporia and Kitwood's own emphasis on the psychological domain may be at least in part responsible for this. As we have emphasized throughout this Reader, Kitwood's concept of the personal was predominantly psychological; that is, it was fundamentally concerned with enquiry into the individual mind, whether that of the person with dementia or that of the caregiver. Kitwood's psychology was, admittedly, always 'social' to the extent that he was, from the outset, concerned with the ways that social factors impinge on the formation of identity and personality, but his work on dementia paid little attention to concepts drawn from sociological theory *per se* (i.e. theories about the nature of human groups and societies). This was clearly not the result – as would often be the case in academia – of early specialization in psychology as a specific discipline. Kitwood's postgraduate study had been in the fields of both psychology and sociology and he taught in an interdisciplinary university department where both were core subjects. His work on dementia makes, however, very little reference to what were central issues in sociological theory at the time he was developing his ideas about dementia care. Issues such as ideology, social control, ethnicity, gender, sexuality and the role of the media are, for example, given little consideration in Kitwood's work on organizational culture in dementia care, nor did he draw to any significant degree on work from parallel fields such as gerontology, mental health or disability studies.

Second, Kitwood is often reticent on the subject of where organizational hierarchies and their associated distortions of human experience originate, and as a result his model of organizational culture in dementia care sometimes appears to create a 'chicken and egg' problem, where it is not clear what needs to come first – better individual caregivers or better organizations for them to work within. In seeking to explain organizational culture, Kitwood places emphasis on the inertia and lack of insight that result from an agglomeration of the psychological defence processes of individuals working within the organization. His perspective on organizational culture takes little account of the higher level influences that are brought to bear on care providers as a result of government policy, the advance of the 'audit culture' or economic constraints. In choosing, for this purpose, to treat dementia care organizations as though they are effectively hermetically sealed institutions separate from the rest of the social world and its economic agendas and priorities, Kitwood may significantly overestimate the potential for change at the organizational level. In order to bring about real change in dementia care it may be necessary for this field to become more proactively oriented towards rights rather than needs and and – as in the case of women's, black and gay rights before it – to learn that 'the personal is political'.

Finally, Kitwood was clearly aware of, and to some extent persuaded by, bodies of critical theory such as postmodernism and deconstructionism but he chose to apply these only very selectively in his work on dementia. For example, as Adams (1996) points out, Kitwood's work 'may be seen as a deconstruction of the medical model of dementia: a technique developed most fully by the French philosopher Derrida . . . who draws his reader's attention to the way in which seemingly consistent systems of thought contain anomalies which undermine them' (Adams 1996: 951). This is an astute observation, but it should be noted that Kitwood did not choose to describe his work in this way or to present it within the context of Derrida's philosophical approach. Further, in his occasional references to Foucault, Kitwood failed to note the irony of quoting this anti-humanist philosopher to support his own overtly humanist position. We can only speculate about the relationship between Kitwood's work on dementia and his uneasy position in relation to theorists such Derrida and Foucault, although an article published in 1990 indicates something of his ambivalence in relation to post-modernism: '[This] is the era of postmodernism. The accepted verities that underlay the long cherished belief in progress have all been called in question: a chaos is revealed . . . and no clear direction forward can be discerned' (Kitwood 1990d: 3).

Later in this article Kitwood comments that his *own* ideas on psychotherapy have not been 'eroded by the acids of postmodern criticism' (1990d: 4). There is no substantive reason, however, to believe that dementia care is a subject that should be exempt from analysis from a postmodernist or decontructionist perspective. On the contrary, dementia is such a fascinating phenomenon in itself that it is surprising that this has not happened to a greater extent already. Explorations of the construction and deconstruction of dementia care and of the 'grand narratives' within which it has historically been enmeshed may have much to offer the development of such bodies of theory themselves, as well as offering alternative ways of seeing dementia. We should, thus, we would argue, resist the temptation to keep the study of dementia and its social contexts a bland and homogenized field of work in which the integration of biomedical and psychosocial models is seen as being as far as theory needs to go.

4.1

On organizations: their imperatives and constraints (1990)

When dealing with the effect of 'socio-moral atmosphere' on people's judgements and behaviour, Higgins, Power, and Kohlberg write:

> In the massacre at My Lai during the Vietnam War, individual American soldiers murdered non-combatant women and children. They did so, not primarily because their moral judgment that such action was morally right was immature, or because, as individuals, they were 'sick' in some sense, but because they participated in what was essentially a group action taken on the basis of group norms. The moral choice made by each indiviual soldier who pulled the trigger was embedded in the larger institutional context of the army and its decision-making procedures. The decisions were dependent in large part on a collectively shared definition of the situation and of what should be done about it. In short, the My Lai massacre was more a function of the group 'moral atmosphere' that prevailed in that place at that time than of the stage of moral development of the individual present.
>
> (Higgins, Power, and Kohlberg 1984: 75)

This passage raises some fundamental, yet curiously neglected, moral issues. For we are social beings, and the greater part of most people's lives takes place in relation to collectives of some kind. Thus it is relatively rare for people to act purely as separate individuals, and the psychology of morality would make a great mistake if it failed to take the special dynamics of collectives into account. The behaviour of organizations, their internal social relations, the psychological effects they have on their members, and the part they play both in the nation state and the world system, all are valid subjects for consideration. The My Lai example points to one crucial aspect: that some of the greatest atrocities are committed under the imperatives of the collective. But possibly of greater significance, and nearer home, is the fact that many organizations, *qua* organizations, are blind to moral issues, and quietly and persistently commit acts of violence both on their own members and outside. A sea is devastated by pollution; a rain forest is decimated in order to grow pineapples for the affluent; a Third World city is massacred through a chemical disaster; a settled community is wiped out because production is found to be more 'economic' in another part of the globe; confused and helpless people are subjected to cruel or even violent treatment in institutions. Perhaps such events take place, not because those involved are especially wicked, but because in some way the organization has incapacitated them as moral beings. It is necessary, then, to look carefully at the way in which collectives operate. One of the most searching questions for humankind, at this point in history, is this: are there ways of carrying out large-scale tasks 'efficiently', but under a social-psychological dynamic that is healthy and creative, as judged in moral terms?

In social science there has been a tendency to look at behaviour in collectives using some form of image of the 'rational cognitive actor' (see page 65). The individual might be an instrumental goal-seeker, a maximizer of approval, a Goffman-esque performer, or whatever. However, if we are to develop a satisfactory account of collective behaviour, we need also to draw on depth psychology, and explore how unconscious motives and psychic defences are called into play. There is ground for supposing that, in evolutionary terms, it was the human or proto-human group that long antedated any clear sense of individuality, and that conscious awareness is a late offspring of a psyche whose complex workings were oriented to a group existence; its operative realm would now be classed as the unconscious. Moreover, the highly individual 'ego experience' which is prevalent among people in contemporary industrial societies is only a few centuries old. Some of that experience is painful and anxiety-ridden, because it speaks so strongly of isolation and mortality; naturally enough, there is a continuing tendency to try to escape from it, to be submerged again into a group.[1] Thus the collectives of today may be regarded not simply as aggregates of individuals, but as a re-constitution of something that is archaic. Of course, some organizational forms are historically new, and the individuals who are bound together in collectives today do not have the same kind of psychic structure as their remote forebears. In contemporary organizations, then, it may well be the case that social-psychological processes age-old and of great power are in operation, despite a veneer of rationality and control. It must be remembered that the development of moral insight over and against the imperatives of oppressive collectives was a slow process, and hard won. Not surprisingly, it is all too easily extinguished.

Organizations and society

One feature of the collectives that developed with modern society is immediately apparent. Those organizations which have the most social effect, and produce the most highly co-ordinated actions, have a common basic form: they are pyramidal, hierarchical, with a chain of command. Through many variations, their fundamental design is such that orders flow downwards, and information upwards. The simplest of such structures merely have two levels; and the most complex, involving several thousand people, might have ten. Collectives of this kind have often been called bureaucracies, drawing attention, in a double sense, to the existence of an office. There is a position within the structure with precisely defined responsibilities and rewards; and there is a physical place, separate from home, where duties are carried out and documents are kept.

The hierarchical kind of formal organization is of great antiquity. It was a feature, for example, of the imperial rule of Assyria, Persia, and China, and later that of Rome. The Catholic church, and some of the groupings within it such as monastic orders, operated on similar lines, often securing amazing loyalty and self-sacrifice from their members. However, it is only very recently, within the last two centuries, that the hierarchical organization has come to occupy the centre of the stage in working life. Around 1800, in nations such as England or France, by far the greater part of work was carried out informally; only some 10–20 per cent of the working population were employed in formal organizations: in government, the army, the church – and, to a very small extent, the factory. With the growth of capitalist enterprise in industry, the urge towards 'efficiency' in administration and law, and the exigencies of technological war, the hierarchical structure gradually came into pre-eminence in virtually all areas of public life. Now, it has been estimated, some 90 per cent of the working population in contemporary industrial societies are employed in hierarchical organizations,[2] and there are trends in a similar direction in those nations that are now undergoing industrialization. In addition, it is necessary to take account of the 'clients' (pupils at school, patients in hospital, old people in rest-homes, and others) who are subject to imperatives corresponding to those of the employees. Clearly, behaviour in formal organizations is no marginal question; it is certainly something that moral psychology cannot afford to ignore.

One of the main traditions in sociology, that of structural-functionalism, has been particularly effective in putting organizations into a broader context.[3] Every social system is viewed as having four main 'problems', and hence tasks. The first is that of guaranteeing continuity, by making individuals into effective members, and ensuring their long-term commitment. The second is that of adaptation to the social and natural environment in which the system is placed. The third is that of defining overall purposes and goals, and deploying human resources accordingly. The fourth is that of maintaining solidarity and co-operation between members, including carrying out the repair work when social breakdown has occurred. Viewed at this high level of abstraction these problems (commonly termed 'pattern-maintenance', 'adaptation', 'goal-attainment', and 'integration') are claimed to be common to all human groups, whether family, club, church, or nation state; also to all societies, whether 'primitive' or 'modern'.

Within a primal society, such as a band of hunter-gatherers, sub-groupings related to these four functions may be scarcely discernible, although there is, in an obvious sense, some division of labour. A feature of highly industrialized societies, however, is that there are very many collectives, more or less discrete. Each contributes, to some extent, to all four functions, but most of them relate primarily to one. 'Pattern-maintenance' clearly involves families, schools, medical services, recreational facilities, and the media. Adaptation involves, primarily, those organizations that produce goods, and facilities such as roads or electricity; also armed forces and diplomatic services. Goal-attainment is the task of central and regional government, trade unions, and public administration. The function of integration is fulfilled by many kinds of organization; clubs, neighbourhood groups, churches, and the apparatus of law all have a major part. Gross disintegration is ultimately prevented by police and prisons.

Put in this way, there is much that might seem banal. Also, sociology in the structural-functionalist tradition is often markedly uncritical, and can easily provide a bland apologia for western industrial capitalism, using a dense pseudo-scientific jargon. But one feature does stand out from this kind of analysis, so much a part of the taken-for-granted world that it is easy to overlook it. Formal organizations of a hierarchical kind have taken over, to a very considerable degree, the major functions of society, pushing informal action to the margins. They are remarkably effective in moulding people, harnessing their motives, defusing their discontents, drowning out the voice of criticism, dismantling the social movements that would cast the system into disarray. Structural-functionalism does not imply that fundamental social change is impossible, but does suggest that the systemic resistance to it is extremely strong. There is now a vast 'intermediate zone', which stands between individuals, with their close personal ties, on the one hand, and the state on the other.[4] Its presence is, historically, a very recent phenomenon; and in moral terms, this is an extremely problematic way of bringing human beings together.

Another point must be mentioned, and it is one to which attention is hardly ever drawn by organizational theorists. The 'intermediate zone' is overwhelmingly dominated by men. The simplest empirical test of this is to draw a graph showing the distribution of social positions according to status (and hence power) against the frequency of occupation by individuals, both for males and females. In virtually all the major formal organizations of western society, whether of industry, politics, law, medicine, or education, the graph has roughly the form shown in Figure 6.1.

In such a distribution the presence of a few female exceptions of high status, such as a chief constable, a senior executive, a judge, or even a prime minister, does not invalidate the general point that the intermediate zone is one dominated by men. Also, for a woman to reach a high position, it is very likely that she will have taken on many of the features of a masculine culture.

In the growth of the intermediate zone, then, we are witnessing much more than part of the process of the 'rationalization' of society: its deliverance from older forms of tradition and the ties of neighbourhood and kinship. In another sense, it is the entrenchment of that social order which had been coming into existence since the sixteenth century: that of the bourgeois class, and specifically of the males within it. The hierarchical mode of organization, which had already proved conspicuously successful in securing compliance in religious and military organizations, and also to

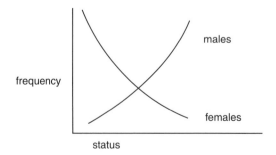

Figure 6.1

some extent in the manufactory, gradually became accepted as the norm; and with it a subtle, yet exceedingly effective, mode of domination.

The study of 'moral atmosphere'

Within the psychology of morality, as it presently exists, formal organizations have been given only very scant attention. However, some promising beginnings in this area have been made by Kohlberg and his co-workers, from about 1970 onwards. Here, in attempting to take Piaget's work fully into account, they began to assimilate some of the key ideas of Durkheim; not an easy task, since Kohlberg's approach was strongly liberal and individualistic, whereas Durkheim had given such primacy to understanding how collectives fashion the way in which people both think and act. Thus far, psychological work has focused on two main types of organization: schools and prisons.

One of the early studies was that of Kohlberg, Scharf, and Hickey (1972), working with prison inmates. The prisoners expressed their relationship to the staff primarily in stage 1 terms, focusing on such issues as coercion and punishment; and they tended to see one another largely in terms of stage 2, securing their self-interest mutually, but without any genuine respect for persons. It seemed that the prison was affecting their general outlook, moulding them into a morality that was below their 'private' best. From this and other studies Scharf also showed that organizations might have different types of 'justice structure', more or less independent of the personal morality of the members. The 'lowest' structure would be one where coercion was the norm; and the 'highest', one where a principled morality was, so to speak, built in – roughly corresponding to Rawls' idea of a just society (see page 32). In further work Scharf related different modes of prison treatment to the idea of justice structure; those that used behaviour modification seemed to be of type 2 (instrumental exchange); and those that used some form of psychotherapy approximated to stage 3, in which norms were informally created, and accepted with good will.

Perhaps rather better known than the prison studies is the work of the Kohlberg group on alternatives in schooling.[5] In 1974 a small school, designed to operate as a just community, was set up within the larger framework of an old-established high school in Cambridge, Massachusetts. This was named the Cluster School. Issues within the school were to be settled, not by authority, but by a community meeting in which all could participate and each member, both staff and students, had one vote. Within this experimental project it was possible to observe the gradual growth of a sense of community, and the development of social mores very different from those prevailing in a typical state high school. In due course further alternative schools were set up, based upon similar principles.

In their formal research on alternatives in schooling, Kohlberg and his associates focused specifically upon the emergence of new collective norms, to use a phrase from Durkheim. It was possible to identify, tentatively, both the moral 'stage' of the norm, and the degree to which it had been accepted.[6] For example, during the first year of the Cambridge Cluster School stealing was widespread; by the second year patterns of trust and shared responsibility were clearly developing; during the subsequent three years no episodes of stealing were reported, and evidently most students believed that stealing had been extinguished. It is interesting to note that in this school no norm against drug abuse developed; merely one against being found out. In another alternative school, however, drug abuse was strongly sanctioned. From their studies the researchers tentatively sketched out a developmental process in the formation of new collective norms, from the point where they were first voiced to that at which they were strongly enforced by social control. Also, they marked out the stages in the transformation of a mere organizational aggregate, meeting for instrumental purposes, into what might properly be regarded as a community of persons.

A more detailed methodology for examining 'moral atmosphere' was later developed by Higgins, Power, and Kohlberg (1984). In one study four groups – two from regular schools and two from alternative schools – were compared. It was found that students from the alternative schools showed a closer correspondence between their hypothetical and practical judgements, made more judgements of responsibility, and showed a much greater degree of community valuing. Also, whereas collective norms based on concern for others were clearly held in the alternative schools, this feature was strinkingly absent in the regular schools. In educational settings, then, there is some convincing evidence of the importance of 'moral atmosphere'. And the Kohlberg group is surely correct in drawing the Durkheimian implication, that any sound programme of moral education must be concerned about the form of social life in which pupils are involved, not merely with pedagogic methods that focus upon giving theoretical knowledge to individuals.

Research of this kind is but a token of a much-needed shift in moral psychology, away from the extreme individualism and the concern with private choices that have dominated the field in recent years. It might be argued that within the whole subject area, a much more sociological emphasis is required. For example, the focus of the work we have been examining has been on only two out of a large array of organizations, serving different functions in society. Schools and prisons do, of course, have features that are deeply disturbing to anyone with moral sensitivity, and they also have some potential for promoting a genuine respect for persons. There are, however, other organizations that are far more problematic, and perhaps of wider social influence. But there is a more important point. Concepts such as 'justice structure' and 'moral atmosphere' are too vague, and are uncritically grounded in a general liberal humanism. They do not enable us to get to grips with a great deal of what is happening in formal organizations. Moral psychology requires a more incisive analytical frame; one that allows us to speak clearly about differences of power, about class structure and its relation to the broader social structure, about ideology, and about unconscious motivation. This is a vast project; what follows in this chapter is no more than the briefest sketch of how it might proceed.

The anatomy and physiology of formal organizations

In moving from the sociological to the psychological level of analysis, five features of formal organizations are particularly relevant. To use an analogy: in studying a living organism, we might first look at the large-scale arrangement of the bones, muscles, and organs, and gain some idea of how their functions interrelate; then we might look in more detail at the cellular metabolism.

Structure

Every formal organization provides a set of social positions: managing director, store-keeper, salesperson, and so on. To each position is attached a status, expectations, and rewards. How, precisely, do these positions cohere together? The 'ideal' structure is shown in official documents, plans, and flow-charts, indicating the chain of command as a naïve senior manager might suppose or desire it to be. The 'actual', or 'extant', structure, as related to the formal tasks, is always somewhat different; intermediaries may be bypassed, individuals may take on responsibilities that lie outside the official requirements, and so on. The real state of affairs is constantly changing, and can only be discovered through detailed empiricial enquiry. In addition, members are connected to one another by many ties that do not derive strictly from the organizational task: based on ethnicity, religion, leisure pursuits, areas of residence, and those relationships of friendship and love which arose initially from contact in the workplace. This 'informal' structure is a flexible web of human bonds that crosses over the formal anatomy of the organization at many points. Skilled operators know how to use it. The groundwork for new resource allocation is laid at dinner parties; major industrial disputes have been settled on the golf course.[7]

Weber depicted a pure form of bureaucracy, in which all functions are specialized, all procedures formalized, and all authority centralized; perhaps his real-life model here was the Prussian state. Detailed empiricial study of organizations shows that there is, however, a wide structural variety, even though the hierarchical principle is maintained.[8] Those which involve the co-ordination of many different tasks (such as large-scale manufacturing corporations) tend to be fairly decentralized; scientists and innovative engineers, especially, are often allowed wide scope for their personal initiative and creativity. Many organizations, such as small banks, breweries, and bus companies, have a fairly loose and light-weight authority structure, where formal and informal aspects tend to merge.

The structure of an organization, whether 'ideal', 'extant', or 'informal', is never a totally internal matter. For each member also belongs to society at large, and has a social class position within it: embodied in patterns of ownership, activity, and consumption, and grounded in personal wealth and security. In the organization there is always a reflection of social class, though never a precise replication; and the tensions between different social classes, which are mitigated in times of prosperity but accentuated in times of economic depression, are always present to some degree. One example is that of schooling, which a long tradition of research has shown clearly is primarily a middle-class affair for and by middle-class people.[9] It is a weakness of the Kohlberg work in this field that it never seems to have come to terms with the sociology of education.

Goals

Although there is a strict sense in which only individuals may be said to construct their action in an intentional way, it does make sense to talk about the goals of an organization. Primarily, these are to be inferred by an examination of what the organization actually does, rather than from public apologias; or glossy brochures; or

comments made by individual members, who may not understand the true significance of what they are doing. Indeed, a major sociologist has gone so far as to assert,
'One of the advantages of specialization-and-coordination is that it is not necessary
for all the participants in a plan of cooperation to have an exact idea of the common
goal' (Johnson 1961: 281). To some extent there is an analogy with psychoanalysis. A
person may be self-deceived, or have powerful but repressed desires, and mask his or
her true intentions by a specious rationalization; it is only when the sense of threat has
been vastly lowered that an honest avowal of intention can be made.

One of the crucial examples here is that of technical innovation. The prevailing
rationalization is that this is the way that industry meets existing human needs more
effectively, brings forth a new range of needs, and creates a more benign and efficient
working environment. Like all rationalizations, this has a sufficient basis for it to be
plausible. In the 'analytic hour', however, the truth emerges, and it is both crystal clear
and chilling. Capitalist industry has two overriding goals, barely meeting even the
lowest criteria of morality: survival in a cut-throat world, and the maximizing of
profitability. Beyond this, virtually everything is *ad hoc* and unprincipled.

> The challenge, then, is not only one of innovation, but of *managing technological
> innovation for profit* ... The only justification for devoting scarce financial
> resources to research and development is the belief that they will generate innova-
> tions which will contribute to the company's survival and continued profitability.
> Furthermore, it must lead to the attainment of these objectives more cheaply than
> if the money were spent in some other way.
>
> (Twiss 1980: 2; author's own italics)

Evidence that this is the truth abounds in the history of innovation. For example,
corporations such as Boeing, General Dynamics, and Chrysler gave massive attention
to relatively 'safe' military innovations (such as the cruise missile and the supertank)
when they began to face a major crisis of profitability in the 1960s.[10] Lucas rejected
a carefully researched plan from its own shop stewards to develop a new range of
socially useful products, and remained committed to its heavy involvement with
weaponry – purely on grounds of profitability.[11] In the field of innovation, then,
any product is acceptable, even though wasteful, shoddy, dangerous, or polluting,
provided that a sufficiently lucrative market can be found.

The case of capitalist industry is a striking one, but it illustrates a general point.
Some organizations have real goals that are, in moral terms, indefensible. Yet many
individuals, with the most acute and sensitive moral capabilities, have little option but
to work within them; even in some of the most affluent societies, the alternative is to be
in danger of homelessness and near-starvation.

Culture

Broadly speaking, the culture of a social group may be regarded as its shared way of
viewing the world, its definitions of what is real and true, of what is important and
worth pursuing; its sense of history; its ideas of those personal qualities that are to be
esteemed. There is a sense in which a collective (by the classifications it provides, the

stories it tells, the records it keeps, and so on), may even be said to 'perceive', to 'remember', and to 'forget'.[12] An individual can only survive, psychologically, within the collective by accepting its shared representations.

Those who occupy high social positions are sometimes inclined to believe that their organization has a single culture, rather like that of a great 'happy family': a culture that is clearly related to the overall goals. The truth usually seems to be that there are several cultures, fairly easy to distinguish from one another. Each one is grounded in the actual conditions of life experienced by its members. Thus, for example, it is often the case that the culture of manual workers is one that involves a good deal of solidarity and co-operation, and with sanctions against anyone who tries to co-operate too much with management or to secure an individual advantage; it has arisen in part as protest and resistance, a way of retaining a sense of personhood over and against the demands of these with power, which would often turn human beings into mere appendages of machines.

The crucial point is that the culture envelops, and even defines, the individual; often there is no place for moral considerations. Again, the case of technical innovation is instructive. Once a person is within the innovator's culture, a whole range of exceedingly complex and fascinating considerations come into the foreground, related to the lived practice of research and development. These include the uncertainty of radical innovations, the difficulty of knowing how far the present state of the art must be surpassed; the prediction of the life-course of products that are already on the market, and those about to be launched; the construction of a sound 'portfolio of innovations', so that those which are risky can be balanced by those which are safe and predictable; and so on. This culture provides great challenges to human creativity; its participants are lured by what is 'technically sweet; anyone who raised moral considerations as valid for technical decision-making would be discounted, ridiculed, or dismissed'.[13] With all the major innovations that have shaped the industrialized societies of today – the automobile, chemicalized agriculture, computers, nuclear power, and so on – it is clear that moral thinking had no part in the innovator's decisions. In the case of the Lucas shop stewards, to which we have already referred, where there was a serious proposal to relate innovation in a moral way to human need, the leader soon afterwards lost his job (see notes 11 and 13).

If a person is to sustain a credible identity within an organization, it is absolutely necessary to participate in the culture appropriate to his or her social position. Of course, there is abundant scope for individuality at a first-order level; an analytical chemist might have a perverse preference for NMR above all other techniques, or a psychiatrist might have an aversion to administering ECT. There is, however, no place for deviance at a second-order level. A chemist cannot continue in research while challenging the fundamental epistemology of natural science; a psychiatrist who disbelieved in the existence of mental illness would soon have no professional standing. Those who place themselves outside the culture are, in the literal sense, idiots, utterly alone; and from the standpoint of the cultural adherents they may well be regarded as wicked or insane.

Social control

This refers to some of the more obvious ways in which organizations encapsulate and constrain their members, binding them by near-religious ties. For those on the path of upward mobility there is, first of all, a selection process, in which a few who appear to have the right aptitudes and personalities are chosen. Once within the organization, a new member's actions and attitudes are moulded suitably through training and supervision. Perhaps here social learning theory is an entirely appropriate theoretical frame; an employee first learns certain behaviours by imitation, and then gradually comes to feel that they are his or her own. Records on performance are kept by superior authority, and provide the basis for consideration for promotion; often the details are kept secret. Desirable behaviour is encouraged by the incentive of privileges and salary increases. Standards are maintained by the threat of various kinds of sanction: the prospect of being passed over for promotion, or relegated to work of low prestige. Ironically, it seems that the highest levels of commitment are achieved when social control operates by means that are apparently gentle and democratic: when people are consulted, when they do not feel coerced or forced into competitive relations with others, when they are given considerable freedom to be creative. There are cases where social control extends even into private life. It has been observed that some corporations, in selecting a male executive, consider his wife's suitability as a social asset; and that some increase the productivity of their employees by putting subtle pressure on their spouses.[14]

At its crudest, social control in the workplace is exercised by the imposition of technology: the assembly line, automation, the programmed lathe, the continual monitoring of productivity by computer. At its most liberal, social control operates by little more than insinuation: that a doctor's knowledge is out of date, that an academic has failed to produce a sufficient number of research papers. Often it is those organizations which are morally most dubious that have to undertake the largest task of deconstruction and reconstruction. A young army or navy officer, for example, is subjected to a thorough re-definition of the world; his self-esteem is first damaged, then recreated; his identity destroyed, and then re-founded; his motives cauterized, and then reorganized towards his 'service' career.[15] There is a sense in which the organization is almost bound to win over the individual. The only effective way of resisting, while remaining within it, is through forming a new collective, such as a trade union. It is a notable feature of the present time that union activity is often seen, from the standpoint of the managerial culture, as dangerous or immoral.

Roles

Anatomically, organizations provide social positions. Physiologically, they provide roles, or patterns of acceptable performance. Roles always exist in the context of what people are requiring from one another, and never in isolation. A nurse expects practical co-operation, but not necessarily emotional support, from other nurses; anticipates certain (mainly technical) instructions from doctors; and assumes that some low-level tasks will be carried out by cleaners or trainees. Often roles are conceptualized in terms of positive and negative prescriptions, related to the various 'role-senders'; but it is also possible to see a role as some kind of definition of the boundary within which organizational behaviour must be constrained. Many roles involve a good deal of contradiction and stress, and activate anxieties that might otherwise lie dormant. From the organization's point of view the crucial thing is that action must be structured in such a way that the overall goals are achieved. Without role-definition the organization would lose direction, and might very soon collapse into a chaos of conflicting desires and fears.

Some aspects of role performance

For some purposes there is no objection to referring to organizations almost as if they were human beings, with desires, goals, unconscious motivations, and defences. It need hardly be said that this should not be taken in a literal sense. For organizations consist of individual persons, and ultimately it is their actions which are to be explained. These actions, however, are not precisely similar to those of individuals in their private life, to which moral psychology has given most of its attention. Actions within and for organizations are usually carried out within imposed boundaries, under constraint. The key concept here is that of role.

Role is, of course, no more than a metaphor derived from the theatre, although its application to everyday life has profound significance, and its ancestry is of long standing. Correctly used in social theory, it certainly implies that there is a part to be played; but there is no suggestion that everything is completely pre-set, word for word, gesture for gesture. Even theatrical performance allows considerable scope for individual interpretation of a role, according to the actor's personality and emotional experience. In the most general way the concept of role signifies the existence of patterns of acceptable action, which have some kind of enduring quality, in response to others' expectations. There is a sense in which even breast-feeding, gossiping, or making dinner are examples of role performance. In this broad sense role carries no implication of insincerity, artifice, or self-distancing. The important thing is the wholeness, the flow, and the skilled nature of mutual interaction. When a role has been learned and practised a little, action can proceed with a sense of spontaneity, and attention can be directed towards other matters. Role performance thus defined may be an aid rather than a hindrance to morality. Knowing, in a broad sense, how to behave, a person might be freer to attend to the needs and interests of others. In other words, the presence of a role boundary can, at times, facilitate the creation of moral space. A reciprocal role relationship, then, might be illustrated as in Figure 6.2,[16] using again the idea of the individual's 'total field of experience' as developed in Chapter 3 (especially page 82). The crucial point is that the role boundary, the definition of what is appropriate, does not in itself contribute to individual alienation; and (as in the case of psychotherapy), can even provide conditions in which alienation may, in part, be overcome.

In relation to formal organizations, however, role often has more precise, and less benign, connotations. The crucial point now is that the occupant of a social position is rather firmly 'locked in' to a framework of given expectations, by virtue of the organization's structure, goals, culture, and social control. Here the genuinely interpersonal tends to be curtailed or distorted because of more overarching requirements, and

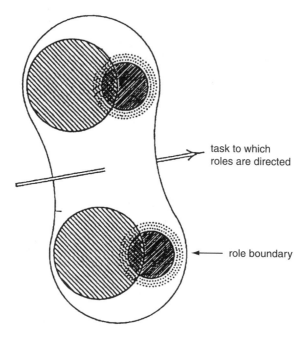

task to which
roles are directed

role boundary

Figure 6.2

some of these are backed by severe sanctions. Ultimately, if the actor will not play the part, he or she must leave the stage. It is role performance in this sense that is so problematic from a moral point of view. In a similar manner to Figure 6.2, the position may be represented as shown in Figure 6.3 on page 169.

The point now is that the constraints embodied in the role relationship are such as to enhance the fragmentation of the psyche, and that role performance by an individual must necessarily involve him or her in a high degree of alienation. The extent to which this is the case depends, of course, on how tightly the role boundary is drawn in real life.

Sometimes it is suggested that formal roles can 'take over' those who occupy them. A classic case in the literature is the prison simulation experiment devised by Haney, Banks, and Zimbardo (1973). Twenty-one male volunteers took part, who had been judged, on the basis of earlier tests, to be stable, mature, and socially well-developed. At the start, they were strangers to one another. By random allocation ten were given the part of prisoners, and eleven that of guards. A realistic prison environment was created in the basement of a building in Stanford University, with cells 6 feet by 9 feet. The experiments went on continuously, day and night, with the guards doing their duty in shifts. The guards had uniforms, and the prisoners a rough tunic; interpersonal differences were thus minimized.

At the start of the experiment the prisoners were realistically 'arrested' by the police, and were taken through the standard procedures at the police station. Each one was then stripped, sprayed with a delousing preparation, made to stand naked in the prison yard, photographed, assigned a number, and incarcerated. As the experiment

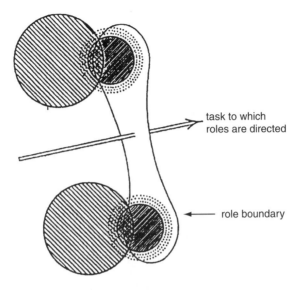

task to which
roles are directed

role boundary

Figure 6.3

went forward, it appeared that all participants began to find the situation 'real'. The guards were meticulous in coming to work, and some stayed on duty long after their shift had come to an end. They became increasingly aggressive and authoritarian; for example, in carrying out extremely lengthy 'counts' at which they tested prisoners on their knowledge of the rules. The prisoners, on the other hand, tended to become passive, and to some extent depersonalized. Five had to be released due to acute stress reactions, and eventually the whole experiment was called off, prematurely, after six days. The prisoners expressed delight and relief; on the other hand, some of the guards seemed to be distressed by the decision.

An experiment such as this is open to several methodological criticisms. For example, the environment was no more than a very crude caricature. In a real prison both guards and prisoners have a continuing culture, and it is generally the case that some kind of working consensus develops between them, humanizing the milieu to at least a small degree.[17] In other words, the role boundaries in the experiment were probably tighter than those of real life. But this and similar experiments show remarkably clearly not just that roles take over, but that existing alienation can be dramatically enhanced. Once familiarized to their roles, the participants seem to have lost contact with the greater part of their everyday selves.

At this point we seem to be close to one of the most alarming features of organizational atrocity. It is often the case that people believe that they are doing their duty, even when involved in the most appalling acts. Primo Levi describes this behaviour in Auschwitz, as another batch of Jewish men was being marked out for the gas chambers.

The officer, followed by the doctor, walks around in silence, nonchalantly, between the bunks. . . . Now he is looking at Schmulek; he brings out the book, checks the number of the bed and the number of the tattoo. I see it all clearly from above: he has drawn a cross besides Schmulek's number. Then he moves on. . . . In this discreet and composed manner, without display or anger, massacre moves through the huts of Ka-Be every day.

(Levi 1987: 59)

Such acts are rational, in the logical sense of being related to a pro-attitude and a belief; but psychologically, they are most readily explicable as being the consequence of an extreme alienation.

From a managerial standpoint, role performance in an organization is often seen as the easy fitting of individuals into a collective, rather as well-machined cogs into a smoothly running machine. This is part of the ideology that supports the organization's goals, and it is derived from the experience of power. The truth for most individuals and especially, perhaps, for those who are in middle positions (such as foremen or chief clerks) is that role performance is usually a matter of handling contradictions; of achieving a compromise between conflicting demands, and of realizing at some level that no solution is fully satisfactory. Organizational stress may be understood in part as the response of the body to the presence of these contradictions, while they remain largely in the field of 'unacknowledged experience' (cf. page 83).

Theorists often make the point that elements of the role requirement are often unclear, or mutually incompatible. For example, a given 'role-sender' may expect 'good' performance as judged by criteria that cannot be reconciled, such as speed and accuracy. Also, the various role-senders may have different expectations – or at least that is how the occupant of the role perceives it. The academic senses pressure from students for good teaching; from peers for good research; from management for sound administration. The nurse is torn between the needs of the patient for close personal care and attention; the doctors' requirement of technical efficiency; and the demand of the hospital authorities for order, cleanliness, punctuality, and accurate record-keeping. Furthermore, most people occupy several roles, perhaps in different organizations – and to maintain them all convincingly may require considerable skill. To give a typical example from the North of England. A man in his twenties is developing his career in sales for the Electricity Board; here he has to be smooth and deferential to customers. He is also a member of the Rugby League team, which requires extreme machismo, and heavy spending on a Saturday night. He is already married, and becoming a 'traditional' husband and father. Each week he visits his eighty-three-year-old grandmother, now in residential care, to whom he is still a little boy. Across such strongly contrasting roles, he somehow has to 'get his act together'.

There are many conflicts, then, in the area of the role requirements. In addition, the performance of a role may simply be in conflict with desire. Historically, the inculcation of a work orientation that feels 'natural' was no easy matter, and this is still the case in countries that have not had the full impact of industrialization. Finally, there are times when role prescriptions come into direct clash with personally held convictions. A doctor, strongly committed to the task of promoting good medical care, takes on the job of 'unit general manager' in the British National Health Service. Under new policies the role requires the bringing about of major cuts and closures, for which salary incentives are offered. If he refuses to do this, he has failed in the role; if he complies, he has violated his own medical and moral principles.[18]

It is clear, then, that role performance is very far from the straightforward matter that it is often taken to be, especially by managerial theorists and by psychologists with a markedly individualistic orientation. From a moral standpoint that is grounded in depth psychology, there seem to be two crucial problems. One is that the role tends to promote or enhance the condition of alienation; the other that the occupancy of a role almost certainly involves conflict, and that of several kinds. Not surprisingly, successful role performance has been described, in quasi-Freudian terms, as an 'ego achievement'.[19] The Freudian ego had to cope essentially with conflict, and hence anxiety, from 'within'. The organizational member has that, but also a great deal more.

Collusive defence in organizations

Formal organizations of a hierarchical kind seem to have the potential to arouse four rather different kinds of anxiety. The first is engendered by the structure of authority itself, from the fact that most members are at the behest of one or more figures who are 'superior'. If depth psychology has some truth here, it would imply that for some people, at least, there will be a shadowy recollection of other authority situations, especially those of early life. In other words, however the situation is defined in consciousness, it may also be defined pre-consciously in relation to the predicament of the child, who had neither power nor adequate understanding. The second kind of anxiety derives from the fact of responsibility, of having a task to carry out which it may not be possible to fulfil; there are always uncertainties, not least those deriving from the behaviour of others. The third is related to the task itself. Some organizational tasks are physically dangerous – as, for example, armed combat, traditional mining work, or extracting oil from sources beneath rough seas. Some tasks involve the continual taking of life, like work in poultry farms or abattoirs. Some, like technical innovation, involve the hazards of the unknown. Some require a person to be in close contact with frightening and disturbing human predicaments, such as severe illness, extreme frailty, insanity, and dying. The fourth type of anxiety arises from the several kinds of conflict that may be present in the role situation, such as those touched on in earlier pages of this chapter.

Considering the many grounds for anxiety, it is remarkable how much organizational work is carried out with apparent efficiency. Many soldiers, so it seems, go cheerfully into battle; many executives carry very heavy responsibilities and yet, apparently, leave them aside when their working day is over; many nurses go through long periods of contact with great suffering, and yet, apparently, are undisturbed. One possible explanation, which has been widely taken up by those concerned with the psychoanalysis of organizations,[20] is that besides individual defences against anxiety, there are collusive defences 'built in' to the organizational culture. The suggestion is that there is a kind of tacit, pre-conscious agreement between members, that if they do their work in a particular kind of way, and view the task and themselves from a particular perspective, they will be more secure. Certain facts which are too difficult to bear consciously will be blanked out, and in the sharing of a common, if extremely limited, outlook, there will be a feeling of mutual support. One case that has been studied in some detail is that of nurses. Their routine is such that the division of labour, the shift system, the attitudes inculcated during training, and the prevailingly technical emphasis of hospital care, all serve to prevent a more personal and painful engagement with patients. It seems likely that some of the new approaches, providing a more continuing contact between particular nurses and patients, will in themselves do only little to amend this situation. Without the collusive defences, and psychologically prepared as they now are, many nurses might find the demands of life on the ward impossible to bear.[21]

It seems, then, that Figure 6.3, suggesting a consciously understood role boundary which binds members of an organization together in pursuit of their common task, is very far from the whole story. The truth, for many roles, may be as shown in Figure 6.4.

This diagram attempts, very crudely, to suggest that when the collusive defence is high, the individuals are bound together in ways they do not consciously apprehend. It was to something of this kind that Freud was pointing in his monograph on mass psychology of 1922; within his frame, the hypothesis was that individuals 'make over' their superego to an authority figure, thus having something of a collective identity, but at the cost of having lost part of what is truly themselves.

Presumably the collusive defences are highly functional to organizations in achieving their goals. However, they may, over an extended period, have a damaging effect on the individuals involved; so much of what they are undergoing remains unacknowledged. Before coal mining was mechanized, many miners were invalided out with the strange condition known as nystagmus, with its accompaniment of vertigo and psychological malaise; soldiers fall victim to shell-shock or combat neurosis; social workers, apparently without prediction, have episodes of burn-out; executives develop pains in the chest and somehow, unaccountably, find they can no longer go

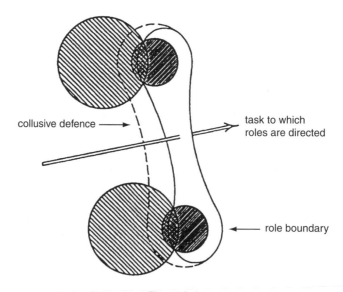

Figure 6.4

to work. Perhaps these are the individuals for whom collusion no longer provides the additional support needed to contain their anxiety. They are the victims. But the 'intermediate zone' remains in working order by generally keeping the collusive defences intact.

When the conditions for an organization are relatively easy (a secure government bureaucracy, perhaps, or an industrial producer with high profit margins) work within it comes to resemble, to some extent, that of a 'good' traditional family, with a generous and benign patriarch at its head. Anxiety is lowered, and members can carry out sophisticated tasks, with some balance between competition and co-operation, and the sense that senior management is on their side. Perhaps the paradigm case here is the research laboratory, engaged on prestige projects with abundant funding. Such conditions do not necessarily make for personal or moral development, although they may be conducive to highly creative work. Broad (1985) provides a graphic description of some of the young scientists involved in the basic research for the Strategic Defense Initiative. In many respects they are still high-school boys: intellectually precocious as they work on the 'weapons of life', but often emotionally insecure and immature. As one of them described himself, and his involvement with science:

> I loved it. It was a treat. I had emotional problems at home with my family life and mother. Science was a world that was pure and that no longer had emotions. It would never go away and would never leave you. And it was always correct. There was always a right answer. So it had a strong attraction for me emotionally. On top of that I had a knack for it.
>
> (ibid.: 38)

This gives an indication of the way in which science, with its intense objectivity, can form part of the apparatus of collusive defence.

When an organization is under pressure, however, matters are very different. Perhaps there are deep structural changes, with rationalization, closure, and redundancy looming large. In the extreme, the organization's goals are reduced to the single one of naked survival, at virtually any cost to persons. Now the well-established collusive defences may no longer be sufficient, even for the majority. The organization takes on the aspect of an angry, hostile, or vindictive parent, and all manner of archaic anxieties in individuals are aroused. As some Kleinians might put it, 'bad objects' latent in the psyche are revived, and then perhaps externalized, projected on to some seemingly malignant authority figure. There is a disastrous loss of capacity to work creatively, to co-operate with others. Eventually, as new conditions become consolidated, fresh forms of collusive defence are established, and some form of 'efficiency' is restored.

This account of organizational defence has been somewhat sketchy, and it is not well supported by empirical evidence; as yet there has not been much research from this point of view. But if there is some truth here, it may point to a basic reason why so many formal organizations are morally unsatisfactory. Following the argument of page 96, the position seems to be this. For 'moral space' to exist those involved must, of necessity, have free attention available. This is not primarily a matter of time and conscious concentration, but of lowered psychic defences. Organizational roles, however, work powerfully against this. Not only do they bring pressing demands to the conscious self (which are, in principle, not incompatible with the presence of moral space), but they also often create anxieties which must be dealt with by additional defences. Paradoxically, this may be as much the case in some 'caring' roles as in those that are obviously materialistic. If an organizational member were, by some means, to lower his or her defences, there might be a flooding of the psyche with new anxieties; and with no opportunity to 'work them through' (that is, assimilate them into conscious experience with the support of others), role performance might become impossible. If problems of this kind exist in hierarchies, there is no reason to suppose that they would disappear overnight in organizations of a more co-operative kind. There people have to face another set of anxieties, related to mutual trust. But it does seem probable that some of the psychological difficulties, especially those associated with authority, and carrying responsibility in a highly individual way, could be largely avoided.

The morality of organizations

The account given in this chapter might, at first, seem a long way removed from the psychology of morality, especially considering the way this topic has been construed during the last twenty years or so, with its emphasis on the private ought. There is, however, a long tradition of thought, going back at least to Aristotle, which suggests that morality is first and foremost to do with the form of social life, because it is here that individuals acquire their personal way of being. The problem of formal organizations, then, is but part of a very large agenda.

Perhaps the first aspect which requires scrutiny is that of the goals of an organization: not its legitimating ideology, nor its official codes of practice (interesting as these are), but what it actually does in the world, the ends to which its collective action truly points. There is an analogy with the study of the individual; it is his or her lived morality, rather than theoretical statements about what ought to be done, that is the more important. In the case of organizations it is easy to be seduced by commonsensical views about what they are doing, and it may be the case that this has occurred with the Kohlberg group, in their studies of prisons and schools. Sociology, however, invites us to look beyond and behind the 'obvious' to discover more of what is really happening: the latent, as well as the manifest function. Prisons do not simply restrain and rehabilitate offenders. They are part of a social order with great structural injustices, an appendage of a legal system which is subtly biased towards property and privilege. Schools do not simply bring forth the abilities of their pupils. They divert resources and attention to a minority of high achievers, and actually inhibit the development of many. Schooling subtly replicates society, and prepares individuals to accept their place within it with resignation.

When seen in a sociological light, virtually every major organization of contemporary society is highly problematic. Both the latent and the manifest functions can be examined from a moral standpoint. In the case of any organization we may ask two questions. In what way does it, or does it not, meet human need? In what way does it, or does it not, make for social justice? With some organizations, most notably the large industrial corporations, the implications are global. Of course, the identification of human needs and the finding of criteria for social justice, in a way that engages with the contemporary predicament, are major tasks of moral theory, not psychology *per se*. Beyond their external goals, and the effects upon their 'clients', organizations may be evaluated morally with respect to the social relations experienced by their members: in particular, whether or not persons are truly respected within the organizational frame. It was this, primarily, that came under Marx's moral censure, when he saw industrial labourers as deeply alienated and exploited, unable to express their humanity in the workplace, and often condemned to an exceedingly impoverished existence outside it. Those who are forced to sell their labour power as a commodity, waiting to be bought like cattle in a market-place, are bound to be, to some extent, depersonalized. Now, a century later, this is still a major issue, considering the exploitation of industrial labour on a global scale.

The question of the social relations of an organization, however, raises many further issues. Probably some degree of alienation is present in virtually all work within formal organizations. Also, they tend to impose a heteronomous morality; their 'justice structure' is typically that of instrumental exchange. But organizations are never static, and their justice structure fluctuates. When times are good, when there is little external threat, they can ascend to a stage where members can be like 'good' children, trying to please a benevolent parent; when times are bad they rapidly degenerate to something like Hobbes' state of nature, where the prime motivations embodied in the structure are purely selfish, centred on the avoidance of punishment. Perhaps it is significant that Weber, the great theorist of bureaucracy, considered only two main motives for organizational work: status-seeking and conformity.

This, however, is by no means the whole story of the internal morality of organizations; we have simply considered what is strictly required by the hierarchical form. There is another aspect, related more to the informal structure. That is, what place does the organization 'accidentally' provide for the life of its members as sentient beings, and for the growth of a morality of mutual respect, when its strict role requirements have been fulfilled? The truth, surely, is that moral space is continually being created, despite the organizational constraints. Sometimes there are even small enclaves, or groups of workers tied by special bonds, approximating to the idea of moral community. These are potentially subversive of hierarchy, but may well serve to make organizational membership more tolerable in the short term.

Organizations vary greatly in the moral space that they provide. The clearest example of where it was virtually non-existent is that of the concentration camp, where Jews awaited the gas chamber. Here the prisoners were so devastatingly deprived, so monstrously threatened, that all that remained of a common morality was an extreme egocentrism.[22] The people who were generally admired were those who had enough strength and resourcefulness to avoid starvation and illness, to stay their execution for a few more weeks; any signs of altruism were taken as weakness. Only a very few quite exceptional persons could retain a concern for others under such conditions. Towards the other extreme are those organizations which are relatively unpressured, and sufficiently well resourced, for role requirements to be broad, and for the informal structure to pose no obstacle to the overall goals. Privileged universities are a good example, as also are hospitals backed by generous provision. Genuine co-operatives are very much more rare, especially in the area of production. It is here, much more fundamentally, that the hierarchical principle is challenged. A 'liberal' and 'democratic' society is not significantly threatened by the presence of a few alternative organizations; indeed, they provide token evidence of tolerance and pluralism. If, however, organizations which were based on respect for persons, while also having clear social goals, began to flourish, the whole 'intermediate zone' would fall into disarray, and with that the social structure to which it is so strongly connected. The advocates of hierarchy, faced with this possibility, fear that the result might be chaos, or a new hierarchy in which, as in *Animal Farm*, the former subordinates become the bosses. But the co-operative principle, widely applied in organizations, might prove to be one of the harbingers of a different, and in moral terms, much better kind of society, in which the very experience of personhood was different.

We need to consider, finally, the long-term effect of organizational membership on personality or, in moral terms, on character. From a purely cognitive-developmental point of view, those who have had to equilibrate over a long period to a low-level justice structure for the greater part of the day are likely to carry its effects in their whole moral outlook; one who has to be authoritarian at work will probably be authoritarian at home and at play. Depth psychology takes this matter much further. The typical organizational role, with its defensiveness, its selective inattention, its avoidance of responsibility, is the activation of a part-self; it is likely that a person who occupies such a role for a long period will enhance the division and fragmentation of his or her psyche. Perhaps this will especially be the case for one also identifies strongly with the role. The formal organizations of contemporary industrial society, then, create an enormous psychological problem for their members. The years of retirement, restricted in other ways as they are for very many people, do not always make for recovery.

All this implies a vast moral project; it stares us in the face, and yet it is generally ignored. Moral development cannot merely be a matter for individuals, in their private lives. If, as human beings, we do have such strong tendencies to form bonds and associations, to fit in with others' expectations, the crucial task is that of creating collectives that are conducive to moral being, while also fulfilling their instrumental goals. This, however, cannot validly be conceived in isolation from deep changes in the structure of society as a whole; and also, by implication, the world-system, with its vast North-South inequities. In the short term, at least one possibility is to increase and cultivate the moral space actually within the hierarchical system. But there is no clear ground, other than prejudice and tradition, for supposing that formal hierarchy provides 'the one best way'.

Notes

1   There is a point which Fromm reiterated in his many writings. He deals with it in great detail in *The Fear of Freedom* (1942).
2   See Jacques' introduction to this topic, in his *General Theory of Bureaucracy* (1976).
3   A good example of the whole approach, and clear in its treatment of organizations, is the text by Johnson (1961).

4 The term 'intermediate zone' was coined, or at least brought into common use, by Jacques; and as he used it, it referred in part to the way in which unconscious motives are harnessed. Sociologically, Jacques' work tends to side with a rather uncritical structural-functionalism.

5 See, for example, the account by Wasserman (1976).

6 Some of this work is reported by Power and Reimer (1978) see also Power (1988).

7 The latter point was made to me personally by a former trade union official, who felt aggrieved at the deal that had been struck at a high level between his union and management.

8 One valuable empirical study is that of Pugh and Hickson (1968). Although the details have dated now, their principal finding stands.

9 The sociology of education provides alarming news for well-intentioned liberals. See, for example, the collection of articles edited by Dale, Esland, and McDonald (1976).

10 This particular point comes from the economic study by Perlo (1963).

11 The Lucas shop stewards actually produced an alternative corporate plan. For the plan, and its implications for the trade-union movement, see Wainwright and Elliot (1982).

12 For an illuminating recent discussion, see Mary Douglas' book *How Institutions Think* (1987). Here she draws heavily both on Durkheim and the theory of science produced by Otto Fleck, whose ideas were published a long time before the better-known work of Kuhn.

13 This point comes, primarily, from Mike Cooley, one of the main designers of the Lucas Alternative Plan. It is also based in part on my own direct experience, having been involved for a short time in work with those planning and managing technical innovation. See also Davidov (1986).

14 The classic account of this kind of activity is Whyte's *The Organization Man* (1960).

15 A vivid description of this is given by Dornbusch (1958).

16 Here I draw a little on Jacques' ideas, but adapt them considerably. He envisaged the interpersonal as always within the role boundary.

17 This point comes out clearly in the study by Mouledos (1964).

18 The doctor in question found the managerial role extremely stressful, and in fact resigned from his post, returning to his work as a consultant.

19 See the article by Levinson (1959). This was one of the most fruitful of the early attempts to bring about *rapprochement* between psychology and sociology in understanding organizational behaviour. Levinson, however, had no concept of 'collusive defence'.

20 See de Board (1978).

21 The collusive defence of nurses is examined by Menzies (1970). I touch on this, in relation to dementia, in my paper of 1987.

22 This comes out very strongly in the account given by Primo Levi (1987). Altruism in such contexts, though well documented, is exceedingly rare.

4.2

Decline in quality of life for patients with severe dementia following a ward merger (1995)

Summary

The effect of a ward merger on the quality of life of patients with severe dementia in a mental hospital was investigated by means of the observational method of Dementia Care Mapping (DCM). Nineteen patients in two long-stay wards were included in the study prior to the merger. Fourteen of these were observed in the merged ward, together with five newly admitted patients. Key DCM indicators showed that the quality of life of patients included in both phases of the study had declined significantly. This may be explained, in part at least, in terms of a 'cycle of demoralization and depersonalization' in the interaction of staff and patients. Further research is required into the dynamics of this cycle.

KEY WORDS—patients with dementia; quality of life; ward merger; dementia care mapping

Changes in Government policy related to long-term care have led to a general reduction in the number of long-stay beds in NHS hospitals, including provision for patients with dementia. As a result, many patients have been relocated, and serious questions have been raised about the effects of the relocation process on their well-being. There is particular cause for concern in the case of those who have dementia, because their need for security is very great (Miesen, 1992) and their ability to make sense of what is happening to them is very limited.

An important, although crude index of the effect of relocation is patient mortality. A review by Borup (1983) of 28 relocation studies found evidence of increased mortality in 21 out of 28 instances, and a more recent study by Robertson et al. (1993) of the relocation of patients with dementia found increased mortality among those whose lives were most disrupted. Evidence related more directly to quality of life has, however, been remarkably lacking. The method of dementia care mapping (DCM) is well suited to the study of relocation, since it provides a reliable way of assessing patients' quality of life through direct observation (Wilkinson, 1993). The study reported here is the first substantial piece of research based on DCM to be published. It shows very clearly how the relocation process can have strongly negative effects where it is not sufficiently guided and controlled.

Background to the study

The two wards involved in this research (let us call them A and B) were in a large Victorian mental hospital; both contained only women patients. A merger was proposed as a cost-effective way of implementing new policy, bearing in mind the incomplete occupancy (ward A had 10 beds occupied and ward B nine beds out of the total of 24 in each case). The merger was carried out by transferring seven patients from ward B to ward A and by retaining seven of the patients already on ward A. In addition, five new patients were admitted to the merged ward to bring the total up to 19. Thus before-and-after data were obtained for 14 of the original 19 patients. The data for the five 'leavers' and the five 'newcomers' provided valuable supporting evidence concerning the consequences of the relocation in this case.

Eight of the staff on the merged ward came from ward A and seven from ward B; four new staff were introduced and two new student nurses replaced the two who had previously been present on ward B. The ratio of trained to untrained staff increased slightly as a result of the merger (from 1:1.4 to 1:1.0), while the mean patient-to-staff ratio during the daytime observation periods also increased to a small extent (from 4.4:1 to 5.5:1). Before the merger the two wards together had a total of 24 full-time and 14 part-time staff; after the merger there were 10 full-time and 11 part-time staff, excluding student nurses.

For each phase of the study dementia care mapping was carried out over virtually the whole of two successive days, ie from the time the first patients entered the day room through to the late evening. This gave a mean period of 21 hours of continuous observation for each ward. Phase 1 of the study took place during the week preceding the merger. Phase 2 took place some 3½ months later, by which time short-term disruptive effects had probably subsided and a new steady state had been attained.

Dementia Care Mapping: a new observational method

The original purpose for which DCM was designed was the 'developmental evaluation' of dementia care settings: that is, the provision of information in a very direct way so that care staff and managers could bring about improvements in the quality of life of those whom they were looking after (Kitwood and Bredin, 1992a). It very quickly became apparent that DCM was highly suitable for quality assurance also (Kitwood, 1992), and it has in fact been fully incorporated into at least one such framework (Dingleton Hospital, 1993). In both of the contexts above, rough-and-ready data are sufficient, without the use of standard statistics, for the prime aims are immediate communication and change. Surprisingly, however, DCM has also begun to be used in research. Although in certain respects it violates the canons of 'object-ive', 'value-free' inquiry, strong claims can be made about both its reliability and its validity, and it compares favourably with well-known research methods in the same general domain (Brooker, 1995).

The method has its theoretical grounding in the ethogenic approach in social psychology (Sabat and Harré, 1992; Harré, 1993). Here, in contrast to behaviourism, persons are viewed as agents who operate within a framework of shared meanings; for those who have dementia, however, meanings may be confused, partial or labile

(Kitwood, 1993). The ethogenic approach has analogies with ethology, which studies the behaviour of species other than humans, in their natural settings, and seeks to discover the patterns of their life in adaptation to particular environments. The main reason for developing an observational method was simply that those with even moderate dementia cannot make the kind of cumulative value judgements that are involved in giving an opinion about whether or not a service has met their needs and expectations.

The DCM method codes the everyday life of persons with dementia in two parallel ways. The first, named behaviour category coding (BCC), keeps a record of what has principally been happening to each person being observed, in successive time frames of 5 minutes. A letter indicates the type of activity or inactivity that has predominated during the 5-minute period (for example, sleeping, walking, playing a game); there are 22 such categories in all. Also the concomitant state of well-being or ill-being is denoted by a number (−5, −3, −1, +1, +3, +5); in effect, this is a six-point scale, and the numbers have come to be known as 'care values'. The second coding frame keeps a record of 'personal detractions' (PDs), episodes in which an individual is demeaned or discounted in some way; often these episodes are so short-lived that they would be lost from the BCC frame, and yet they are powerful indicators of the quality of the care environment. In all, 46 types of personal detraction have been operationalized, in five grades of severity. Technically (Hutt and Hutt, 1970), the PD frame uses simple event recording, whereas the BCC frame adopts a compromise between time sampling and event recording; this has been given the name 'event summation'. Many detailed rules are involved in the application of the method and these are set out in a lengthy manual which is now in its sixth edition (Kitwood and Bredin, 1994). The method has been progressively refined through repeated use and this has added greatly to its present efficacy as a research tool.

Dementia care mapping is extremely labour-intensive, involving long periods of observation and often requiring considerable resourcefulness on the part of observers, who are typically expected to 'follow' five persons simultaneously. The positive side of this is that the method yields a far richer body of data than most observational methods in general use, for example studies of engagement (McFayden, 1984), or the seven-category system used by Bowie and Mountain (1993). The raw data can be processed in a variety of ways to yield both quantitative and qualitative indicators. In the former category two of the most important are the individual care score (ICS) and the group care score (GCS), derived by the aggregating of relevant care values; in the latter category the most important is the behaviour category profile, which summarizes the kind of activities and inactivities that have taken place. The main quantitative data are amenable to non-parametric statistics, of which one main example is used in this study.

The inter-observer reliability of DCM has been repeatedly tested, with concordances lying typically in the range 0.75–0.95 and kappa coefficients marginally lower. In preparation for the research reported here the two main observers found a concordance of 0.95; the third observer had already established concordances consistently above 0.8 with one of these two; the fourth observer, who was far less experienced, had attained concordances above 0.7 with the same person. Thus far, reliability has only been established through inter-observer checks. Test–retest reliability is far more problematic for a method such as this; it is a research question in itself to ascertain the bounds of 'natural variation', and hence the framework within which test–retest measures would be feasible.

The method has strong face validity since the measures are so directly tied to the phenomena under investigation. The construct validity of DCM is based on a careful theorizing of the social psychology of the dementia care environment (Kitwood, 1990; Kitwood and Bredin, 1992b). In relation to the use of DCM in any study, content validity depends on the extent to which sampling is involved, both of persons and of time. In the research reported here all persons on the wards were observed, and for virtually two whole days in each phase of the study. On all grounds, then, this research may be judged to have high validity.

Results

The individual care scores for all patients involved in the study are shown in Table 1 and the mean ICSs are shown in Table 2. The findings are also shown graphically in Figs 1 and 2. For 13 of the 14 patients involved in both phases, there was a lowering in ICS. In 10 cases this was more than 0.5 points on the scale, which is a large decline when the highly condensed nature of the data is taken into account. It is also noteworthy that five of the ICSs in phase 2 were negative (including the score for one 'newcomer'). This is a strong indicator of poor-quality care; DCM is very lenient in that even very short-lived positive interactions are sufficient for a care value of +1 to be allocated. Negative ICSs, then, if relating to an extended period of observation, indicate problems in urgent need of attention. Taking the ICSs for the 14 patients on whom before-and-after data were obtained, the decline is statistically significant (Mann–Whitney test: $U = 75$, $p = 0.0016$). This is the central finding of the study.

An indicator of the quality of a care environment that is often used in developmental evaluation work with DCM is the 'dementia care quotient' (DCQ). This not only takes into account the care values, which are aggregated as the group care score (GCS), but also the patient-to-staff ratio (r). The DCQ thus enables rough-and-ready comparisons to be made between care environments, taking the staffing levels into account. It is derived as follows:

$$DCQ = GCS \times \frac{(r+5)}{2} \times 10$$

(In this formula the 5 acts as a 'stabilizer', reducing the sensitivity to r, and the 10 simply brings the DCQ into a convenient range. Thus if the GCS were 2 (which would indicate care of moderately high quality) and r were 5 (which is typical of dementia care), the DCQ would be $2 \times (5 + 5)/2 \times 10 = 100$.)

The GCSs and DCQs were worked out for both wards in phase 1 (including all patients) and for the merged ward in phase 2 (including the 'newcomers'). The results are shown in Table 3. Here, as with the ICSs, the data suggest a dramatic decline in patient well-being; and hence, by implication, in the quality of care.

Table 1 Individual care scores for all patients

	Phase 1	Phase 2
	Patients originally on ward A	
1	2.18	1.28
2	0.89	−0.56
3	0.88	0.69
4	0.75	0.24
5	1.50	−0.04
6	1.53	0.35
7	2.38	1.14
8	0.69	—*
9	1.81	—*
10	0.07	—*
	Patients originally on ward B	
1	0.94	0.66
2	1.05	0.23
3	0.72	0.25
4	0.61	0.72
5	0.62	−0.23
6	1.18	−0.04
7	1.19	0.66
8	1.37	—*
9	−0.46	—*
	'Newcomers' to merged ward	
1	—	−0.36
2	—	0.50
3	—	0.82
4	—	1.03
5	—	0.56

* Transferred elsewhere.

Table 2 Mean individual care scores

Phase 1	
Ward A	1.27
Ward B	0.80
All patients	1.04
Phase 2	
Patients remaining on ward A	0.44
Patients transferred from ward B	0.32
'Newcomers'	0.51
All patients on merged ward	0.41

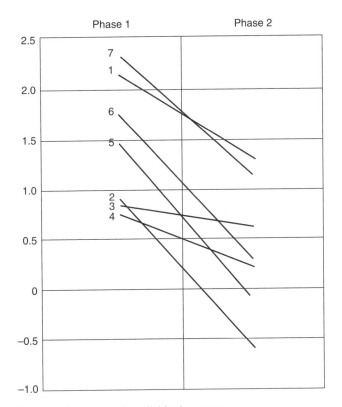

Figure 1 Patients originally on Ward A. Individual care scores.

Originally, the DCQ was designed for heuristic purposes. It must be regarded only as a very crude indicator, and genuine statistical weight cannot be attached to it. However, the figures shown in Table 3 do strongly corroborate the statistically significant results.

Four items of qualitative data, recorded in some detail at the same time as the actual mapping, support these findings.

1. Before the merger the mealtimes on both wards were relaxed, calm and sociable, whereas after the merger they tended to be rushed, with very little social exchange between nurses and patients. The average time spent on dinner was 15 minutes less in phase 2, despite the fact that there were more patients to serve.

2. The quality of physical care before the merger varied, but at least some conversation was made with the more able patients while they were receiving care. After the merger physical care was more hurried, less supportive and sometimes accompanied by critical comments.

3. Staff were more inclined to absent themselves when basic physical care had been carried out. There was even one period of about half an hour when the 'mappers' were left in sole charge of the patients in the day room.

4. Episodes of personal detraction increased in frequency and severity after the

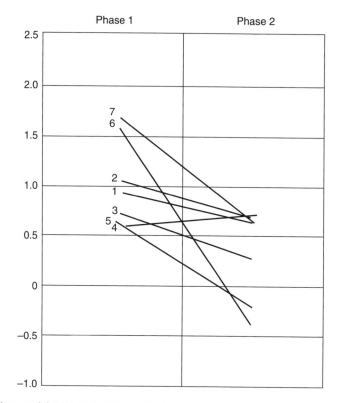

Figure 2 Patients originally on Ward B. Individual care scores.

Table 3

| | Phase 1 | | Phase 2 | |
	GCS	DCQ	GCS	DCQ
Ward A	1.27	54	0.32	17
Ward B	0.81	40	—	—

merger. This can only be asserted in a general way, because at the time of this study the technique that is now in use for converting PD codings into numerical data had not been developed.

Independent corroboration of the decline in quality of care is provided by one small but noteworthy indicator: the prevalence of pressure sores. At the time of phase 1 only one patient out of the total of 19 on both wards had a pressure sore, whereas five had pressure sores at the time of phase 2.

Discussion

Throughout the study the nurses carried out their duties efficiently, and generally with patience, kindness and goodwill. There is strong evidence, however, for a severe decline in patient well-being following the merger. Surprisingly, perhaps, this was somewhat more marked for the patients on the receiving ward, whose initial quality of life had been slightly higher. The evidence for a lower quality of life after the merger is supported by the DCM data for the 'newcomers'; for, as Table 2 shows, their mean ICS was 0.51, whereas the comparable figures for the two wards before the merger were 1.27 (ward A) and 0.80 (ward B). Three hypotheses to explain the decline will now be considered and rejected, and a possible explanation will then be given.

First, the decline might be largely due to the disruptive effects of the relocation itself. Against this being a major factor it should be noted that phase 1 occurred when the relocation was imminent and a sense of disarray was already present; phase 2, however, took place over 3 months later, when most of the disturbance due to the process of change would have died down. Also, if this was an important factor, we might expect the measures to show greater decline for the patients whose lives had been the most disrupted. In fact this was not the case; a serious decline in well-being was noted in both patient groups.

Second, the decline might have been due to changes in policy, management, staffing or care practice. In fact there were no policy revisions at this time, nor did senior management change; consultant responsibility remained the same throughout the whole period. The most significant issue here is probably that around half of the patients were now under a new ward manager, and all patients were faced with some new staff. It is also the case that the patient-to-staff level rose slightly. While these factors may have contributed to the decline, we are disinclined to attach major weight to them in themselves, for reasons that will become apparent.

A third hypothesis is that the neuropathology associated with the patients' dementia might have advanced significantly between the two phases of the study; and that this, together with a decline in physical health, led to lower levels of well-being. There are two arguments against this. First, the advance of neuropathology in the brains of elderly persons is relatively slow (short of vascular accidents or those episodes of sudden deterioration which are known to occur in some cases of multi-infarct dementia). Second, as Table 2 shows, the scores for the 'newcomers' were very similar to those for the patients involved in the merger; it is much more likely, then, that the low level of well-being is a reflection of poor-quality care.

An explanation that is consistent with all of our observations, both quantitative and qualitative, is as follows. Around the time that the merger was proposed, there was a general background insecurity and unsettlement among staff, who had worked hard under difficult conditions and felt that new changes were being forced through for managerial reasons. Their morale was already low and they were highly vulnerable to pressures of any kind. Although morale was not formally assessed in this study, many informal comments made by the nurses support this view. As a result of the merger there was a genuine deterioration in the working conditions, although this in itself was relatively small. In addition, there was a considerable increase in the size of the patient group; regardless of the staffing ratio, this may have been perceived as overwhelming.

Here the DCQ is a useful index, because it compensates for the patient-to-staff ratio. The figures shown in Table 3 testify clearly to a serious decline in the quality of care. The qualitative observations (reported earlier) support this view.

So, while there was a small objective increase in workload, the subjective sense of strain increased greatly. The response of staff was to perform their duties in a less personal way, and to abstain from the kind of 'psychological care work' that goes beyond practical nursing. This is the kind of defensive retreat that has often been noted in the literature on burnout (eg Chernis, 1980). The reactions of staff to their new situation in turn led to an increased depersonalization of the patients, whose quality of life had not been particularly high in any case. Some patients went into a state of almost complete vegetative withdrawal; others manifested their distress through an increase in 'problem behaviours'. Staff responded to the latter with a higher frequency of personal detractions and by neglecting patients who were not 'causing trouble'. And so a cycle of demoralization and depersonalization was set into effect, the needs of both patients and staff being drastically unmet. There were no signs of a reversal of this cycle during phase 2 of the research.

Conclusion

This study adds to the now considerable literature on the damage that can be inflicted on patients as a result of relocation. We do not, however, draw negative or deterministic conclusions from what we have observed. The relocation of patients is sometimes inevitable, for practical and economic reasons. Although in some instances it is forced through at short notice, without proper preparation or briefing, and without a framework of support for either staff or patients, this does not have to be the case. If the necessary preparation, support and guidance are given, the consequences can be very different. We ourselves know of relocations that have been accompanied by relatively benign effects; in one case this is supported by DCM data, not yet published. The issue is a particularly serious one in the case of patients with dementia because of their psychological vulnerability. Also, it has to be recognized that very few nurses have been adequately prepared for carrying out the 'psychological care work' that is necessary for maintaining patients' well-being. There is, then, a background of insecurity in many staff, besides any that arises as a result of organizational changes. The long-stay dementia care situation is often very fragile, and liable to the kind of cycle of demoralization and depersonalization that we have documented here.

At present medical science has very little to offer to patients with dementia. Their well-being, however, is not uniquely determined by the neuropathological process; it is also crucially affected by the quality of psychosocial care. This much neglected area deserves far more attention than it has had hitherto, and there are major training needs that urgently need to be addressed.

Acknowledgements

Thanks are due to the patients included in this study, the staff who allowed their care practice to be observed and to Leeds Healthcare who sponsored this research.

References

Borup, J. H. (1983) Relocation mortality research: Assessment, need to focus on the issue. *Gerontology* 23, 235–242.

Bowie, P. and Mountain, G. (1993) Using direct observation to record the behaviour of long-stay patients with dementia. *Int. J. Geriatr. Psychiat.* 8, 857–864.

Brooker, D. (1995) Looking at them, looking at me. A review of observational studies into the quality of institutional care for elderly people with dementia. *J. Mental Health* 4, 145–156.

Chernis, C. (1980) *Staff Burn-out: Job Stress in the Human Services.* Sage, Beverly Hills.

Dingleton Hospital, Melrose (1993) Senior QASP: Quality assurance for psychiatric wards.

Harré, R. (1993) Rules, roles and rhetoric. *Psychologist* 16, 24–28.

Hutt, S. J. and Hutt, C. (1970) *Direct Observation and Measurement of Behaviour.* Charles Thomas, Illinois.

Kitwood, T. (1990) The dialectics of dementia: With particular reference to Alzheimer's disease. *Ageing Soc.* 10, 177–196.

Kitwood, T. (1992) Quality assurance in dementia care. *Geriatr. Med.*, September, 34–38.

Kitwood, T. (1993) Towards a theory of dementia care: The interpersonal process. *Ageing Soc.* 13, 51–57.

Kitwood, T. and Bredin, K. (1992a) A new approach to the evaluation of dementia care. *J. Adv. Health Nurs. Care* 1, 41–60.

Kitwood, T. and Bredin, K. (1992b) Toward a theory of dementia care: personhood and well-being. *Ageing Soc.* 12, 269–287.

Kitwood, T. and Bredin, K. (1994) *Evaluating Dementia Care: The DCM Method,* 6th edn. Bradford Dementia Research Group, Bradford.

McFayden, M. (1984) The measurement of engagement in institutionalised elderly. In *Psychological Approaches to Care of the Elderly* (I. Hanley and J. Hodge, Eds). Croom Helm, London.

Miesen, B. M. L. (1992) Attachment theory and dementia. In *Caregiving in Dementia* (G. M. M. Jones and B. M. L. Miesen, Eds). Routledge, London.

Robertson, C., Warrington, J. and Eagles, J. M. (1993) Relocation mortality in dementia: The effects of a new hospital. *Int. J. Geriatr. Psychiat.* 8, 521–525.

Sabat, S. and Harré, R. (1992) The construction and deconstruction of self in Alzheimer's disease. *Ageing Soc.* 12, 443–461.

Wilkinson, A. M. (1993) Dementia care mapping: A pilot study of its implementation in a psychogeriatric service (Letter). *Int. J. Geriatr. Psychiat.* 8, 1027–1029.

4.3

Cultures of care: tradition and change (1995)

The historical background to the old culture of care is traced in outline. Ten key points of contrast between the old and the new cultures of dementia care are given and explained.

One of the most striking facts about dementia care at the present time is the tremendous variety of its quality. When we spend some time in a really good care environment, several things are likely to impress us. Those who have dementia are very much alive, responsive, relating to each other, making their presence felt; there is the sense that a lot is going on. The staff seem to be enjoying what they are doing; they are satisfied, relaxed and free. Not all is happiness and peace, of course – but there is vitality, energy, inspiration.

However, we also know environments that are very different from this. There is a sense of deadness, apathy, boredom, gloom and fear; most of those being cared for appear to have given up hope, their last resort being an occasional moan, or shout, or angry outburst. The staff are patronising, cynical, uninvolved, and even relating to each other largely in superficial ways. One way of describing this remarkable difference is to say that it represents two contrasting cultures of care.

The asylum tradition

The uncertainty that so clearly marks the present time has come about, in part, because of the breaking up of ways of dealing with the mentally infirm that were established over 300 years ago.

It was during the 17th century that the foundations of the modern European societies were firmly laid. This was the period when many nation states emerged, with more or less the boundaries we know today, and when a general way of life structured around production, trade and profit began to take form. In the cause of "efficiency" and "rationality" large numbers of obvious misfits – the mad, the deformed, beggars, witches and the flagrantly immoral – were taken out of society and put into a new kind of institution. Later these were called asylums (meaning, paradoxically, a place of safety, to describe a place where all forms of safety were imperilled).

The history of this "great confinement", as the French historian Michel Foucault has called it, unfolds in three main phases (Foucault 1967). The first was one of *bestialisation*, where the inmates were treated very much as animals in an old-fashioned zoo: crowded in wretched cages, left untended, and on view to a sensation-seeking public on high days and holidays.

There followed a phase of *moralisation*, through the main part of the 19th century, with high-minded attempts to re-create the asylum as a place of kindly re-education. Then, around the turn of our own century, came a new phase of *medicalisation*, through which many types of non-conformity were re-classified as disease. The patterns of "uncare" that we know so well in the case of dementia, are largely inherited from these different phases.

Now the asylums have closed or are closing, for reasons that are as much financial as humanistic (Murphy 1991). This does not in itself mean that those with dementia have better life prospects. For the worst possibility is that we might simply see the bad patterns of the past reconstituted: either in new and smaller institutions, many of which are in private hands, or in people's own homes as they await their so-called packages of care. Nothing, then, follows automatically from the sweeping changes that are now taking place. All that can be said is that this is a time of opportunity to do something better. Any success will be achieved through a movement contrary to the shallow, technical and money-obsessed mentality of our times.

The idea of a culture

We could define a culture as "a settled, patterned way of giving meaning to human existence in the world, and of giving structure to action within it" (Williams 1976). Three components of a culture are important for us here. First there are institutions, through which social power is clearly allocated. Second there are norms, meaning standards for behaviour, including that within the main institutions. Third, there are beliefs, both about the nature of what is, and about what ought to be. The power of a culture stems from the fact that when people are immersed in it, the framework that it provides seems self-evident. What nature is to creatures whose lives are governed by instinct, culture is to human beings, who live their lives in a world of meanings.

One point about cultures deserves special attention here. It is often thought that the actions of human beings follow their beliefs, as if by logical deduction. History, however, often gives us another picture: that the institutions arise first, with their ways of establishing power and control; then follow the beliefs, in order to create "facts" that fit in (Henriques & Hollway 1984). The Europeans colonised black peoples in their search for trade and valuable materials; later they defined these peoples as inferior, in justification of the status quo (Fanon 1967). We find such specious rationalisations in every part of human life.

So our understanding of culture needs to be enriched by an idea from psycho-analysis (Becker 1973). This is that each culture has its special way of occluding, or hiding away, parts of the truth about human existence that are too difficult or inconvenient to bear. Some cultures, perhaps, are relatively open, without strong vested interests in obscuring the truth. Others, especially those which have great disparties of power and elaborate forms of control, are deeply repressive.

The "rational", masculine cultures of the Europeans, in which our patterns of so-called care are embedded, are of the latter kind.

A contrast of cultures

I wish now to draw out ten differences between the old and new cultures of dementia care. The emphasis here is on beliefs and attitudes. Behind these lie the organisations, with their power structures and their patterns of status and control.

1. Attitude to dementia care

Old culture: *Dementia care is a backwater, and deservedly so. The demands are high, but the real challenges are few. It is an area of work well suited to those who have low ability, little inspiration and few qualifications.*

Here the shadow of the asylum is clearly visible. People with dementia sometimes resemble wild beasts which cannot be controlled – they simply need "keepers"; they are incapable of receiving moral education; they are afflicted with an incurable disease. There is little that can be done for them, except to wait until they die.

New culture: *Dementia care is one of the richest areas of human work. It requires very high levels of ability, creativity and insight. In our involvement with those who have dementia we are pushing our humanity to its outer limits.*

The change to this view has been taking place for some years now. An increasing number of people are involved in work with those who have dementia because they want to be there, because of a sense of commitment. New forms of training are needed, and a freeing of the personality from defensiveness and restraint.

2. General view of dementia

Old culture: *The primary degenerative dementias are devastating diseases of the central nervous system, in which personality and identity are progressively destroyed.*

In such a definition there is no recognition of the human environment that surrounds a person with dementia. It is as if he or she is left alone and powerless, while the degenerative process takes its course. This deeply pessimistic view is not supported by scientific evidence; it is, rather, a reflection of the kind of institutional setting in which dementia care has traditionally taken place.

New culture: *Dementing illnesses should be seen, primarily, as forms of disability. How a person is affected depends crucially on the quality of care.*

Here there is no denying of the damage that occurs to nervous tissue, or of the consequences for a person's abilities. However, matters are taken out of the negative, deterministic framework that the old culture had created, by placing the emphasis on human action. The focus is on enabling and empowering, through the provision of what is necessary to compensate for disability, and on recognising the unique way in which each person deals with his or her damaged world.

3. Ultimate source of knowledge

Old culture: *In relation to dementia, the people who possess the most reliable, valid and relevant knowledge are the doctors and the brain scientists. We should defer to them.*

Here again we see an almost superstitious belief. It is not based on any systematic review of the findings of medical science, nor an appraisal of its benefits for those who have dementia. It is rather, an inference from the structure of power. If medical science has so much power, if it attracts such vast funding, then it must be important and true; whatever knowledge we have gained through action must be trivial compared to theirs.

New culture: *In relation to dementia, the people who possess the most reliable, valid and relevant knowledge are skilled and insightful practitioners of care.*

The key point here is that those who actually do the caring have a great advantage as researchers, when compared to medical scientists. For one thing, they have far more data, because they know a person over a sustained period, with all the accompanying fluctuations of mood and action. For another, they have data concerning the whole person in everyday life: knowledge, so to speak, of the working of an exceedingly intricate system, taken as a system.

This is more valuable, in many respects, than knowledge about the functioning of minute parts; for with a system, the functioning of the whole is never ascertained by merely analysing the parts. Good caregivers are not necessarily good researchers; they may not have a framework for making sense of their knowledge. The point is that the best database is there for them, and there is no reason for them to be talked out of the knowledge that they have tested in experience.

4. Emphasis for research

Old culture: *There is not much that we can do positively for a person with dementia, until the medical breakthroughs come. Hence much more biomedical research is urgently needed.*

Beliefs of this kind underpin the enormous outlay of money and the great dedication of scientific talent to biomedical research related to dementia. Often we are presented, at a popular level, with the impression that great discoveries are just round the corner.

A closer inquiry, however, suggests that this is far from being the case. Research itself has often been allied to commercial interests, or driven by the pursuit of what is "technically sweet". Inferences drawn from research at a popular level are full of fallacy and half-truths.

New culture: *There is a great deal that we can do now, through the amplification of human insight and skill. This is the most urgent matter for research.*

The new culture certainly welcomes the genuine discoveries of brain science, when the surrounding garbage has been cleared away. It does, however, suggest that the priorities of the last 40 years have been inept, often governed more by vested interests than a concern with truth or the relief of suffering. The social psychology of dementia – how a person relates, communicates, compensates, makes sense, responds to change – is only in its infancy. Yet even now we have sufficient ground for believing that this is where many great new breakthroughs will come.

5. Us and them

Old culture: *Those who have dementia are significantly different from the rest of us, because of their "organic mental disorder". Hence there is a legitimacy in staff having different styles of clothing, meals, crockery, chairs, toilets, etc.*

Again we see beliefs that reflect the form of life of the institution, rather than an inference from sound research. The old-time asylum, with its imposition of power and its imperative of control, could only function by creating a massive difference between staff and inmates. If there was too much "fraternisation", all legitimacy for the system would collapse.

New culture: *Those who have dementia are equal members of the human race with the rest of us. We are all persons, and all, fundamentally, in the same boat. This should be reflected in our practice.*

The new culture, then, works to minimise difference. Let us be clear that this does not, in any sense, mean a grading down of competent people. It does, however, require all of us to own up to our areas of damage and deficit, not hiding behind a professional facade; and, on the other side, to perceive, honour, and nurture the qualities of each person with dementia, however seemingly damaged or unattractive they may be.

6. What caring involves

Old culture: *Care is concerned primarily with such matters as providing a safe environment, meeting basic needs (food, clothing, toileting, warmth, cleanliness, adequate sleep, etc), and giving physical care in a competent way.*

In other words, the old culture is involved primarily with what is obvious, external, easily managed. This was the emphasis placed in the training of several generations of nurses. Their expertise lies here. If they did in fact engage with persons, it was not on the official agenda.

New culture: *Care is concerned primarily with the maintenance and enhancement of personhood. Providing a safe environment, meeting basic needs and giving physical care are all essential, but only part of the care of the whole person.*

So the new culture sets a much larger, more interesting, more personally demanding agenda. The maintenance and enhancement of another's personhood is something that requires very delicate sensitivities, very highly developed skills, and hence new forms of preparation and training. The care of the whole person, moreover, requires carers to be whole persons too, cured of their mania for control.

7. Priorities for understanding

Old culture: *It is important to have a clear and accurate understanding of a person's impairments, especially those of cognition. The course of a dementing illness can be charted in terms of stages of decline.*

The old culture feeds on deficits, both neurological and psychological, and a tremendous amount of money, time and energy has been expended in discovering what people with dementia cannot do. All this might be helpful if it led to forms of action that would bring about improvement. Generally, however, this is not the case, and the main consequence is often further labelling. Much the same applies to those stage theories that chart a person's decline: assuming (without clear evidence) that this decline is due solely to the degeneration of nervous tissue. Stage theories are linked to scenarios of gloom and doom; it is hard to find any instance where they have led to better forms of care.

New culture: *It is important to have a clear and accurate understanding of a person's abilities, tastes, interests, values, forms of spirituality. There are as many manifestations of dementia as there are persons with dementia.*

The key point here is that while we all have deficits and impairments of some kind, we also have a marvellous capacity for overcoming them. So the new culture is concerned primarily with what a person can do and wants to do, and finding the conditions under which he or she can thrive even in the face of disability. From this perspective the classification of deficits, or placing a person in a stage sequence, has a very minor place. One has, rather, a sharpened sense of the uniqueness of the individual, each with his or her personality and life-history. Disability is fitted into that pattern, and not the other way round.

8. "Problem behaviours"

Old culture: *When a person shows problem behaviours, these must be managed skillfully and efficiently.*

Notice the language here; it is the language of control, spoken by those who have power about those who do not. It would be refreshing to hear people talk about managing the behaviour of the royalty, or our political leaders, or the super-rich tycoons and landlords. Managing the behaviour of another means a disregard of that person's own frame of reference, their struggle for life and meaning.

New culture: *All so-called problem behaviours should be viewed, primarily, as attempts at communication, related to need. It is necessary to seek to understand the message, and so to engage with the need that is not being met.*

The first thing, then, is to drop the concept of behaviour, and replace it by the concept of action. This is to recognise that each person (even when carrying severe cognitive impairments), looks for the meaning of the situation, formulates an intention, and then tries to make something happen in line with that intention.

When we re-frame the so-called problem-behaviours in this way, again and again we find that they have meaning; perhaps at first we were too narrow-minded to see it.

There is no denying that we may be disturbed and annoyed by what a person with dementia is doing – and with good reason. But the new culture points to a way of finding solutions that meet the needs of all concerned.

9. Carers' feelings

Old culture: *In the process of care the key thing is to set aside our own concerns, feelings, vulnerabilities, etc, and get on with the job in a sensible, effective way.*

One great difficulty with this is that it seems to require carers to be less than the fully human beings they really are. The old culture actually encouraged people to hide behind a professional mask, to avoid facing the truth about themselves. For many carers, then, their anxiety, depression, impotence and rage remained hidden away in the shadow – exerting a negative influence but in unacknowledged ways. It is not surprising that the old culture produced so much abuse, both physical and psychological, and was accompanied by such a high degree of burn-out.

New culture: *In the process of care the key thing is to be in touch with our concerns, feelings, vulnerabilities, etc, and transform these into positive resources for our work.*

The new culture encourages us to use every part of our being. If I know my own feelings, I can engage my feeling self when I am caring for another; if I know my vulnerabilities, I can lovingly take care of these, and draw on my self-knowledge as a basis for empathy. There is no question here of a carer being overwhelmed by his or her own emotions, and so being rendered ineffectual. It is simply the invitation to be real, whole people, knowing who we are and what we bring.

10. Personhood of staff

Old culture: *Direct care staff are "servants of the organisation". It is not on the agenda of the organisation to take them really seriously, or to engage with their psychological needs.*

This view goes along naturally with the old institutions and their distribution of power. The care worker was to be some kind of combination of zoo-keeper, guard, moral tutor and medical orderly – reflecting the different phases of the asylum tradition. And since those with dementia had the lowest status of all inmates, little was either required of or given to those who looked after them.

New culture: *Direct care staff are persons. Respect for their personhood is as much on the agenda of the organisation as respect for the personhood of those who have dementia.*

This point is absolutely crucial, and recognition of it still lags far behind. Some organisations that are committed to the new culture are only part-way there: they acknowledge the need to recognise the personhood of the clients, but do not perceive accurately the necessary conditions for bringing this about. Staff can only give person-centred care to others, in the long term, if their own personhood is acknowledged and nurtured. Where this is not the case, they will revert to lower aspirations and less committed forms of practice – except for a few lonely heroes who place themselves in grave danger of exhaustion and burn-out.

The new culture, however, fosters a realistic long-term commitment, providing the means of personal renewal in the face of difficult and demanding work.

Great contrasts

The contrasts, then, between the old culture and the new appear to be very great. Sometimes when I make comparisons in this kind of way I wonder if I am exaggerating. It is all too easy to set up a "straw man" and then demolish it in order to score points.

However, just after I finished the basic preparation of what I have written here, and while I was having some doubts, an article appeared on my desk. It was from a popular magazine. The headline was *Alzheimer's – No Cure, No Help, No Hope*. There followed the dreadful story of a man who had developed a dementing illness around the age of 40, and of the burden and anguish of his wife and family. This account offered not a single ray of hope at the human level, but ended with an invitation to donate to a particular fund for neuroscientific research. Virtually every feature of the old culture, as I have set it out here, was displayed at some point in this article.

I do not wish in any way to make light of the suffering that surrounds dementia, both for those who have it and for their families and friends. But I have to say that what the article contained was not the truth as I know it, even in instances of early dementia that are just as severe. It was not the truth; it was a representation that used the concepts of the old culture. The new culture, also, does not provide "the truth"; but it does provide a very different representation, grounded in a richer range of evidence and experience.

Coming home

What, then, lies at the core of the difference between the two cultures? I think it is this. The old culture is one of alienation and estrangement. Through it we are distanced from our fellow human beings, deprived of our insight, cut off from our own vitality. The old culture is one of domination, technique, evasion and buck-passing. To enter the new culture is like coming home. We can now draw close to other human beings, accepting all that we genuinely share. We can recover confidence in our power to know, to discover, to give, to create, to love. And this homecoming is a cause for joy and celebration.

References

Foucault M (1967) *Madness and Civilization*. English Translation by Richard Howard. Tavistock, London.
Murphy E (1991) *After the Asylums*. Faber, London.
Williams R (1976) *Keywords: A Vocabulary of Culture and Society*. Fontana, London.
Henriques J, Hollway W, Urwin C, Venn C, Walkerdine V (1984) *Changing the Subject*. Methuen, London.
Fanon F (1967) *Black Skin, White Masks*. Grove Press, New York. English Translation by Charles Markmann.
Becker E (1973) *The Denial of Death*. The Free Press, New York.

4.4

Some notes on personhood and deformation (1997)

When I first met Ralph Ruddock I was working on my Ph.D., and I was struggling with a complex conceptual problem: "what does it mean, in terms of social science, if we say that a person has or holds certain values?". I was extremely sceptical about the conventional answers given by mainstream academic psychology, which generally said that a person's values, in operational terms, are the responses he or she gives to a values questionnaire. I was vaguely aware that people 'have values' in different ways: for example, with varying degrees of conscious awareness and commitment. It was also conceivable that some people might not 'have values' at all – but this was a possibility that psychological methods of 'measurement' did not allow. What I needed in order to resolve my problem and to make sense of the data I was collecting, was a theory or model of the person that was truly developmental, and that covered many aspects of our personal and social being.

A colleague of mine had been to some of Ralph's seminars, and suggested that I might get help from a book which he had edited: *Six Approaches to the Person*. When I read his article "Conditions of Personal Identity" I immediately felt that there was a framework here that I could use in my research. I wrote to Ralph, explaining my problem to him, and outlining how I thought I might draw on his ideas, so long as I had understood him rightly. He invited me over to Manchester to see him, and we had a most enjoyable time together. There was an immediate accord, both on the personal and intellectual levels. Ralph said that I had understood his position well, and encouraged me to develop my thinking along the lines I had outlined in my letter. Not long afterwards I wrote an article entitled 'What Does "Having Values" Mean?', which drew explicitly on his model.

Ralph gave me much more than academic guidance on that day of our first meeting, which was during the winter of 1975/1976. He gave me friendship too – a friendship which has gone on for over twenty years. I was a newcomer to postgraduate study, and inclined to be overawed by academia. It was not easy to challenge established positions in psychology, and even to disagree with some of my tutors. Ralph had a breadth and humanism which I found very inspiring, a refreshing contrast to the superficial and over-ambitious culture that I had been surprised to find in university life.

After that first encounter Ralph and I continued to meet, usually at intervals of about three months. Each time we have been together our conversations have been wide-ranging, covering numerous topics of shared interest, and also bringing in many aspects of our personal lives. We have talked about Freud and Jung, about the nature of social science, the problems of medicine, Third World development and under-development, democracy, collaboration, lifelong education, Laing's anti-psychiatry, technology, Beethoven, dialectics. We have even touched on Chinese philosophy, where Ralph has a high regard for Confucius and I am a disciple of Lao Tzu.

The times that I have spent with Ralph have been an important part of my 'formation' – to use a term that he has espoused. I am especially grateful to him for two things, beyond the ordinary bounds of friendship. First, Ralph has sometimes seen areas of imbalance or uneven development in my work, and has gently jogged me to look again. For example, in my research on dementia he suggested a few years ago that I would do well to move beyond the personal and interpersonal aspects, and give more attention to the organisational frameworks within which care is delivered. Now that I have begun to do so, I am convinced that he is right. Second – and this is what I value most – Ralph has given me constant encouragement, and helped me when my self-esteem in academic work was fragile. As in the case of 'having values', there have been other times when I was developing an unorthodox point of view. I have always felt that Ralph supported me in my efforts, however tentative and amateurish they may have been at first.

As my academic contribution to this book I would like to return to the model of the person which Ralph set out in 1972. Recently I asked him whether he would now wish to modify it in any way. His reply was that he would try to show more clearly how society 'bears down upon the person'. In other words, even if the model as he first presented it was appropriate for 25 years ago, it now appears too liberal, too opti-mistic. We are painfully aware of the new inequalities of society, and the way in which individuals have been damaged as a result. So I wish here to take up Ralph's agenda, and use his model to present some ideas about the deformation of persons. Finally I shall make some brief comments about the relevance of all this to our thinking about the future, as we look beyond the philistinism that has dominated our culture in recent years.

Social science and the person

The strength of Ralph's model of personhood was its eclecticism: its use of several bodies of theory at the same time. In social science the custom has generally been to play safe, and stay within familiar boundaries of expertise; retaining conceptual and empirical precision, perhaps, but sacrificing broader humanistic concerns. As a result, there have been too many sectarian divisions, too many failures of communica-tion and vision. In particular, there has often been a sharp divide between psycholo-gists and sociologists, even though there is, in fact, such a high degree of overlap in their subject-matter. Anyone who dares to draw heavily on both psychological and sociological theory runs the danger of being unrecognisable as a valid member of either academic community, and thenceforward of having no clear reference group. Ralph took that risk, and it proved thoroughly worthwhile, as witness the great success of his *Roles and Relationships*, which provided the basis for his later model (Ruddock 1969).

From sociology he elaborated the concept of *role*, viewing this as the primary link between the person, taken as an individual, and the society of which he or she is a member of some kind. From mainstream psychology he took the concept of *personality*, using a geological metaphor: personality might be viewed as a set of layered deposits from past experience, especially the performance of roles. This view is strikingly similar to that which was developed, a few years later, by the ethogenic social psychologists (Harré 1993). The concept of personality has often been trivialised in psychology, and become a system of bland descriptions based on simple ideas of traits. Ralph, however developed his ideas with much more insight, and drew on the depth psychologies of both Freud and Jung. Thus the person was viewed as having both a conscious and an unconscious mental life, and a concern about the future as well as the past. The future aspect is even more strongly expressed in the concept of the *project*, taken principally from existentialism. Here there is a recognition that each person is in a process of becoming, and that some will attempt to shape their lives according to a larger purpose.

In order to deal with interpersonal processes Ralph brought in ideas from the phenomenological and symbolic interactionist traditions, and focused on the concept of *perspective*: essentially what a person learns through the reflected appraisals of others. The operative agent in the model is the *self*: approximating to the I in Mead's account of social action and the ego of Freudian theory. The self is pure subjectivity: that which undergoes experience and is the source of action. Finally, the person has the problem of how to create a sense of coherence, how to be consistent, from time to time and from place to place. This is conceptualised as the issue of *identity*. It is recognised, then, people differ in the extent to which they achieve an identity, and the manner in which they do so.

When I consulted Ralph about his model, I suggested that it might be helpful to draw also on the German microsociological tradition, particularly the work of Schutz, and include the concept of *lebenswelt*; usually translated as '*social life-world*' – a zone where meanings are shared. For part of the existential problem, in the industrialised world at least, is that of the 'pluralization of life worlds' (Berger *et al.* 1974). Most people have to 'make out' in several different zones of meaning, and the meanings do not necessarily agree. Part of the problem of identity, then, is finding a way to hold the meanings together. I incorporated this idea in my paper on 'having values' (Kitwood 1977).

How persons are deformed

Not long after his theory of personhood was published, Ralph began to examine the idea of *formation*, seeing it as a central concept for developing a theory of adult education (Ruddock 1980). He also noted some of the parallel terms: *deformation, reformation, transformation, information*. Ralph's first ponderings were later developed in his article written with Colin Fletcher (Ruddock and Fletcher 1986). Two chapters in this book bear witness to the fruitfulness of those early deliberations. The concept of deformation, however, was never thoroughly explicated.

As soon as we use a 'deficit' concept such as this, there is an implied standard in the background: in this case, an ideal of well-developed personhood. If we take Ralph's model as portraying possible paths of personal development, we might come to the conclusion that the latent ideal is of someone who is very well integrated into society, highly competent in several major social roles; someone whose life has an overarching purpose that is intrinsically worthwhile; whose personality is well-balanced, based on a rich life-history; who is inwardly at ease, and very open to experience; whose self-esteem is high; and who is congruent, rather in the sense used by Rogers (1961) – there is a consistency between what he or she undergoes object-ively, feels subjectively and presents to other people. This is a fine ideal indeed. We must recognise, of course, that it is grounded in western humanism, and that each culture fashions its concept of a fully human life in its own particular way.

So what can we learn by exploring the processes of deformation, and what kind of prospect is suggested for the psychological future of societies like our own? Method-ologically, two main tactics are available. The first is to tackle the subject historically, as was done by Fromm in the *Fear of Freedom* (1941). Here capitalism is portrayed as bringing profound and class-based deformations. The somewhat earlier psycho-historical work of Reich, first published in 1933, is less well known. It is even more radical in its analysis, and suggests that both property and patriarchy set powerful deformations in train; capitalism was but a latter-day instantiation (Reich 1946). The second tactic is rather less ambitious, and involves looking at aspects of individual development in a particular period. That will be my method here, using Ralph's model as a basis.

If we follow Ralph's thinking, and take a view of personality that includes the key developmental ideas of depth psychology, we might infer that the process of deform-ation can occur very early in life. Two conditions seem to be necessary for a child to acquire a robust and healthy sense of self. The first is an environment of acceptance and nurturance, one which is safe enough for the child to experience and 'work through' such emotions as rage, grief, fear, hatred, envy, disappointment, and to deal with feelings of ambivalence. The child must come to realise that these are part of the human condition, and that love is stronger and more enduring than them all. The second condition is that the child must develop a sense of agency, of inner vitality: knowing that he or she has the ability to influence others, and to make a mark upon the world. A child who has the first condition, but not the second, is likely to be somewhat dependent, and may develop a pattern of life that tends to over-adaptation. A child who has the second condition, but not the first, is likely to have psychopathic tendencies: to be skilled in action, but devoid of feeling or concern for others. A child for whom both conditions are lacking is in danger of becoming psychotic: that is, the sense of self cannot hold up. We might imagine little flashes of self-realisation in infancy gradually joining up to make the continuing line of selfhood that constitutes normal experience, very much as Ralph described. In childhood psychosis that line is never properly formed; and in adult psychosis the line, such as it is, breaks in its weakest place.

As psychoanalytic theory has been assimilated into our culture, the injuries inflicted on children have become far more widely recognised. The contemporary psychotherapist John Bradshaw (1990) has even gone so far as to suggest that the 'wounded child' is the new archetype of our time; emerging into consciousness as the many abuses of children – physical, sexual, emotional, commercial, spiritual – have gradually been exposed. So it is at least possible that fewer children are being deformed in their earliest months and years, as compared with previous generations.

With regard to the schooling of children and adolescents, there is little ground for optimism at the present time. The education systems of the western world have always had a considerable part in the deformation of persons – with the possible exception of playschool. Principally this is because there has been such a strong emphasis on the intellect and such a gross neglect of the sensibilities. In the training of the scientist, of course, a rigorous abstinence from feeling has become the norm. Another deforming tendency is competition, which has persisted despite many efforts to make education a more truly co-operative process. Over the last twenty years or so both the intellectualising and the competitive tendencies have been increased, as our political masters have elevated achievement (defined in an extremely narrow way), and turned the system of inspection into a kind of inquisition. The formation of a person who is kind, fair, sensitive, tolerant, aware and socially concerned, does not really feature on the formal educational agenda. The sociology of education has persistently brought forward evidence that schooling mirrors society, and serves to impede the development of the majority of people, at different stages that correspond to socially available positions. In other words, it implements deformation in a systematic and structural way.

Moving on now to further and higher education, more students are involved in these sectors than ever before. If we look at the range of courses on offer, many involve a rather narrow view of 'competence', and this might be seen in part as a way of minimising reflection; it may also be a ruse to keep down the statistics on unemployment. Furthermore, there can be no doubt, in Britain at least, that we have a system of 'education on the cheap' with its own deforming tendencies: a disastrous lack of personal contact, for example, and many people living under severe stress as they struggle both to complete their studies and find the means of economic survival. Despite these and other difficulties, there are several very encouraging signs. One is that, compared with 20 or 30 years ago, far more women are continuing their education beyond the end of schooling; and evidently succeeding, even in such traditionally masculine fields as engineering and computer science. Another is the presence of more mature students than ever before, particularly from a cohort of women who did not continue their studies after school. Despite so many structural and economic difficulties, we are now witnessing the beginnings of a system of lifelong education.

In the world of work the overall picture is far from hopeful, if our concern is with the formation and deformation of persons. In Britain now only about 30% of the potential workforce have jobs that might be described, even euphemistically, as 'permanent', thus offering the prolonged development of personhood in a socially valued role. Many of these jobs, however, have now become extremely stressful, as economic conditions have become more stringent and the demands for so-called productivity have increased. In the major professions there can be no doubt that far fewer people actually enjoy their work as compared to a generation ago; often early retirement is considered as a relief, and even redundancy is sometimes seen as a blessing in disguise.

A large proportion of people are now employed in temporary or part-time work, or in some marginal form of self-employment. The climate here is one of extreme insecurity, which for many people erodes the reserves of personality. Many of the jobs in this occupational sector are low paid, and some involve naked exploitation, where employees have neither holiday pay nor sick pay, and no formal way for grievances to be given a fair hearing. Here we see the so-called 'business culture' at work, operating an even more devastating 'principle of systematic deformation' than the one which Ralph described in his article of 1980. Now it is not only "Do not give any employee a training beyond the operational requirements of the work role", but also "Do not give any employee a rate of pay or a form of job security that places more than minimal demands upon the organisation". Tragically, this even applies in many areas of care work. Employees have little option but to become cynical and self-protective in their attempt to minimise the process of personal deformation, perhaps reserving trust and commitment only for the arena of private life.

Then there is the problem of unemployment, where the true picture is far more serious than the official statistics imply. Immense harm to personhood is inflicted by depriving people of an occupational role. They are in many respects alienated from the mainstream of society; self-esteem is damaged; the sense of personal efficacy is crippled; human potential cannot develop, because of lack of opportunity. New roles do, of course, emerge through unemployment, but many of these are marginal and undervalued.

In the present situation it is hard to develop long-term projects, either in work or leisure. Many people who are in full-time jobs (read 'over-employed') face huge work-loads, and do not have sufficient scope for self-direction. Those who are in temporary or part-time work simply do not have the security to make long-term commitments. Unemployment provides ample time, but the poverty trap sets its own severe limitations. Economic survival from one week to another can hardly be considered as a project.

With regard to the 'pluralization of life-worlds', and the general problem of finding meaning, we are now in a new era. It has been described as post-modern, and its key characteristics are transitoriness and fragmentation. It is now extremely difficult for many people to find or create a coherent framework of meaning, or a genuine value base for personal existence. The most common solution is not even to make the attempt, and to live in a generally good-natured way; following the prevailing patterns of hedonism and consumerism. A small minority find a very different solution, and take refuge in a sect or cult. Here a meaningful basis for living is indeed guaranteed, but at enormous cost: critical awareness has to be permanently suspended, and any broader social involvement cut to the barest minimum.

One of the greatest causes for encouragement at the present time is a growth in awareness of the processes of deformation, and the discovery of forms of remedial action; mostly, as Ralph might have put it, at the level of interpersonal perspectives. A new humanism is gradually making its presence felt in many areas of contemporary life; more committed, grounded and pragmatic than anything that has ever gone before. It is manifested in the involvement of many people in counselling and psycho-therapy; in the huge interest in psychology courses and psychology training; in the collective efforts of women (and, more recently, also of men), to free themselves from the limitations of traditional gender ascriptions. In these and many other ways we see signs of a new attempt to rectify the effects of long-standing and deep-seated deformations. Even in such a cinderella field as the one I have made my own speciality – dementia care – there can be no doubt that a sea-change is slowly occurring. Perhaps we are just beginning to take on Erich Fromm's agenda, and learning how to love.

The last concept in Ralph's model was identity. If my brief sketch contains at least some truth, the conclusion seems to be this. As compared with twenty years ago, the raw materials obviously available for constructing an identity are fewer and flimsier today. There are not so many stable occupational roles; there is less opportunity for forming long-term projects; there is a greater confusion of meaning. Perhaps more people than before are living without having solved 'the problem of personal identity' – at least at a conscious level. However, it is possible that some, at least, are developing a greater psychological resilience, an experiential frame that is more at ease with the life of the emotions, and an integrity that has deep unconscious roots.

Looking ahead

In this impressionistic and extremely incomplete account of deformation, I have made a few suggestions about the trends of our time, both positive and negative. What grounds for hope are there – if any – as we look towards the twenty first century? In his last seminar at Manchester Ralph was extremely pessimistic, but perhaps part of his intention was to provoke us to think more deeply.

If we look at the 'state of the world', as Ralph did, the picture is a gloomy one indeed. One part of the globe after another is being overtaken by the advance of a rapacious capitalism which wrecks culture and creates poverty on a massive scale. Political tyranny is probably still on the increase. There has been no cessation of war, and the weapons of destruction are becoming ever more efficacious. The first signs of the breakdown of our ecosystem are now becoming clear. In the 1970s several well-researched reports were published, predicting catastrophe in the mid-twenty-first century if existing trends continued. The fact that we have not yet departed from those trends is one mark of the extent of our collective deformation.

If there is any real hope for humankind, almost certainly it will not come from the western world. In political terms, we are too enmeshed in the disastrous system that we have created. The best that we can offer at this point is a change at the psychological level, as we begin to undo that profound deformation that set the global system into disarray. There was never a golden age in Europe. The deformations go back one, two, four, six thousand years – perhaps (as Reich suggested) to the time when property was first invented, and our forbears felt such strong imperatives to protect what they had grabbed. 'Civilisation' was simply a veneer, covering over these deformations. For one generation after another people have acceded to exploitation, slavery, class oppression, colonial conquest, plunder, torture: culminating in the collective madness of the first world war, several genocides and the coming of the nuclear age. The missing word in our psychological vocabulary is *conformation*: a process of making people into conformists, beginning in the very earliest months of life.

Perhaps we are now seeing the very first signs of a reversal of the psychological processes which led to such conformation, as the personhood of children is recognised more strongly, and as the injusticies of gender, class, ethnicity and ageism begin to be corrected. Although the social and economic prospects for the rising generation are so bleak, it is possible that, compared to their parents and grandparents, a far greater number have essentially sound psychological foundations.

So the sum of my argument is this. If we go back one or two generations, to what may now appear to have been a sunnier age, there is much evidence of superficial well-being; but it is possible that this was often superimposed on deformations of the most disastrous kind. On the surface the problems of personal identity looked capable of resolution; but the deeper psychological problems, related to conformation and psychopathy – were largely left untouched. When the psychopaths flexed their muscles, there was not the collective strength to give them opposition. Now the problems are more obvious, and on the surface it seems almost impossible for many people to create a sound identity. Perhaps the superficial chaos is the emergence of what has been deeply repressed for generations. Whether the new humanism can overtake the political and economic forces of destruction, no one can know. But at least here there is a basis for action and a ground for hope.

References

Berger, P.L., Berger, B. and Kellner, H. (1974) *The Homeless Mind*. Harmondsworth: Penguin.

Bradshaw, J. (1990) *Homecoming*. London: Piatkus.

Fromm, E. (1941) *The Fear of Freedom*. New York: Avon Books.

Harré, R. (1993) Rules, Roles and Rhetoric. *Psychologist*, 16(1), pp.24–28.

Kitwood, T. (1977) What Does 'Having Values' Mean? *Journal of Moral Education*, 6, pp.81–89.

Reich, W. (1946) *The Mass Psychology of Fascism*. London: Souvenir Press (first German edition 1933).

Rogers, C.R. (1961) *On Becoming a Person*. Boston: Houghton Mifflin.

Ruddock, R. (1969) *Roles and Relationships*. London: Routledge and Kegan Paul.

Ruddock, R. (1972) Conditions of Personal Identity. In: RUDDOCK, R. (ed) (1972) *Six Approaches to the Person*. London: Routledge and Kegan Paul, pp.93–125.

Ruddock, R. (1980) *Beyond Vocational Training*. International Conference Proceedings Nottingham University.

Ruddock, R. and Fletcher, C.L. (1986) Key Concepts for an Alternative Approach to Adult Education. *Convergence: an International Journal of Adult Education*, 19(2), pp.41–48.

4.5

Professional and moral development for care work: some observations on the process (1998)

Abstract

Several aspects of the professional education of those who work in caring roles are discussed, with particular reference to dementia. Three experiential learning exercises are described, together with the opportunities they provide for moral development. Suggestions are made about the moral demands of care work, and general inferences are drawn for the practice of moral education.

The topic of care has had a significant place on the agenda of moral education for some time now. After a period when a Platonist methodology was dominant, with its preference for form over content, for thought over feeling, for stasis over flux, there has been a renewal of interest in more Aristotelian approaches, grounded in the realities of everyday life. This has involved making close inquiry into the nature of people's lived morality; as, for example in the research of Kohn (1990) on altruism and empathy, that of Taylor (1992) on the experience of schoolchildren, or that of Haste (1996) and others on the nature of community. It has also involved a revival of interest in the idea of moral character (Knowles & McLean, 1986; Lickona, 1996). The moral agent is one who can engage consistently in right action, even in the face of countervailing pressures; moral character is learned primarily through practice, by facing up to real opportunities, difficulties and dilemmas. It is clear from many studies that the closer we come to everyday life, the more salient become the issues related to care.

For our purposes here, three ideas about care are particularly significant. First, it implies beneficent involvement with particular others, who are known in their uniqueness, and with whom (in most instances) there is a long-term involvement. Second, it implies a concern that is deeply felt; probably it is grounded in the human instinct-like propensity for attachment. Third, care is expressed in a cultural context—a *lebenswelt*; it is bound up with a cluster of other meanings, created over time, and it is expressed in forms of action that are typical of that context.

Among those who have brought the topic of care into the forefront, the work of Gilligan (1982) is of special significance. As part of her project to enable the concerns of women to be defined and heard she showed that, typically, her female respondents defined themselves not so much as individuals, but as people living in a web of "given" attachments and obligations. Whereas many men had a moral outlook that focused on justice, many women had one that focused on care. These findings must, of course, be interpreted sociologically, in the light of the fact that traditional gender roles have often drawn women into patterns of life where specific ties and relationships form the central focus of their day-to-day existence (Wilkinson, 1997). One of the enduring contributions of this whole body of work, however, is the recognition that the morality of care is different from that of justice. It has a different basic validation, it has its own form of progression and its own developmental goal. Both justice and care make their moral claims upon us, and maturity entails the recognition of them both.

It is remarkable how little attention has been given as yet to the topic of providing a moral education for those who will work, or who are already working, in the so-called caring professions: for example, nurses, social workers, occupational therapists and staff at all grades in residential settings (significantly, the majority of these people are women). Here the word "care" designates primarily a type of task, which might be better described by a term such as "tending". Whether or not it is done with care, in the stronger sense of a felt concern for the other, is a different matter; it is simply a variable that depends both on the person and the context. Many people enter these professions very poorly prepared, in moral terms, for the tasks that they will face; often nursing assistants and care assistants have had no preparation at all. In this paper I shall refer to all who work in so-called caring roles—whatever place they have in the status system—simply as "careworkers", and assume that many of the issues related to their moral development are held in common.

Here we will focus particularly on those who work with men and women who have some kind of dementia, where professionals at all levels are often disastrously ill-prepared. The dementing conditions, of which Alzheimer's disease is the best known, have an astonishingly high prevalence in all the industrialised societies: currently estimated, for example, at between half and three-quarters of a million people in the United Kingdom, and around two-and-a-half million in the United States—the majority of whom are in the older age range. All the dementias are characterised by a progressive loss of cognitive functions such as memory, orientation and problem-solving capability, making a person increasingly dependent on the help provided by others.

For a long time the task of care in institutional settings was defined primarily as that of attending to basic physical needs, while the disease processes in the brain took their inexorable course. In recent years, however, many discoveries have been made about how to enable people with dementia to maintain some degree of well-being in the face of advancing cognitive impairment (Kitwood, 1997a). The achievements of new drug treatments thus far are negligible in comparison. As the awareness of what is possible has grown, roles that were formerly despised and trivialised have begun to be reframed, with an appreciation of the awareness and skill that they entail. The work involves an orientation both to justice and to care; it is thus a moral project, and of the most exacting kind. The issues that arise here are present, to some degree, in all contexts where people are highly dependent on others; dementia simply presents one of the most poignant examples. For here the matter of personhood is pressed, both conceptually and practically, to its outer limits, and the demands on a caregiver's personal resources are extreme.

Considering that dementia care work has been so undervalued, it is not surprising that the related issues of education and professional development have been disastrously trivialised and neglected. In recent years, however, many attempts have been made to rectify this deficit. Bradford Dementia Group, for example, has designed several courses for people at different levels, including a Higher Education programme that amounts to one-third of a degree. With a pervasive emphasis on the personal rather than the technical, and its detailed social psychology of interaction, this is undoubtedly a form of moral education, if that term is taken in its broadest sense.

In this paper I shall describe three of the 70 or so experiential learning exercises that my colleagues and I have designed for use in short courses intended for care-workers who are involved with dementia. I have chosen these three partly because they illustrate different kinds of learning task, and partly because they require different levels of personal engagement and impose progressively greater degrees of psychological threat. I shall then make some suggestions about the moral requirements of care work, and offer some more general reflections about the nature and process of moral education.

First example: exploring a family problem

This exercise requires the participants to look at the predicament of a married couple, one of whom has dementia, as described below:

Mr Mildon (Harry) is 82 years old, and Mrs Mildon (Betty) is 84. They have been married for 48 years. Harry had been married previously; his wife died tragically from tuberculosis in 1938. The only child from this marriage (Janet) is now 59 and lives in Australia. She lost her husband 9 months ago through a sudden heart attack. Her children are grown up and she is due to retire in a few months' time. She last saw Harry and Betty when they visited her in Australia eight years ago, but has expressed her willingness to come and help after she has retired.

The Mildons live in a small terraced house in a friendly neighbourhood. The house is warm and comfortable, but most of the appliances have seen better days. Harry still drives a car—a 10-year-old Fiesta. Harry had been a textile worker before World War II, and after the war worked mainly as a truck driver. Betty had a traditional role as a home-maker, and had also worked for about 20 years as an office cleaner.

Five years ago Betty was diagnosed as having Alzheimer's Disease. Now she is very confused, and often incontinent. Harry looks after her at home, and she goes to a day centre 3 days a week. Harry is determined to carry on caring for Betty at home, if possible right to the end. He himself, however, is not in the best of health. He has chronic back pain, and a hernia which is being "contained" by an uncomfortable truss. Also he often gets very tired. The only help he has had at home thus far has been from one of his neighbours (Ivy), a widow aged 74. She often gets his shopping, and drops in two or three times each week.

Harry has been on the hospital waiting list for some time, and he has now been called for his hernia operation in just over 6 weeks. The prognosis is good, if he can get the necessary rest. Decisions have to be made now about what to do.

The participants first work in groups of 3–5 people. They are invited to read the description carefully, and then undertake two tasks. The first is to discuss, and note down, what appear to be the main strengths and needs of each of the individuals in the scenario. The second is to envisage at least three ways in which the problem might be resolved. Finally, in a plenary discussion, the participants are asked to reflect on the process in which they have been engaged.

The exercise usually evokes a high level of interest. The story is based on a real case, and it often has resonances with the experience of those who have worked in some way in community care. The first task seems, at the outset, to be fairly simple, but grows in complexity as it develops. In doing the second task most groups easily emerge with three solutions, and some are able to envisage as many as seven. It is in the final discussion, however, that the learning most aligned to moral development is likely to occur, around three main issues.

(i)   Participants become aware that in this exercise, as in real life, many assumptions are made about other people, often without a strong evidential base. We do not know, for example, how resilient Betty might be in Harry's absence, or the extent to which Harry's intentions as a carer are realistic. Ageist attitudes may have corrupted the discussion, and Betty's own understanding may have been radically discounted. Some participants become aware that they have assimilated this case to others with which they have been involved, and see how dangerous this can be. The conclusion that emerges is that it is essential to explore each situation with a very open mind. The social context with which a moral dilemma arises is generally uncharted, and often insecure.

(ii) There is a sober recognition that in "community care" there are no perfect solutions. This fact is well known to those who have been involved in social work, but is often not fully appreciated by those who work in residential or hospital settings. Resources are scarce, and subject to budgetary ebbs and flows; many of the needed services (for example, for good respite relief) do not exist, there is a kind of social Darwinism, in which only those who fight and shout get what they need, and those who have no one to shout for them are tragically neglected. Thus any concept of an idealised, disembodied "ought" is irrelevant. Often, in situations such as this, it is impossible to find the right course of action, because all realistic possibilities are morally flawed; the least wrong will have to suffice. The demands of justice cry out, as well as those of care.

(iii) Some participants realise that their approach to the exercise has been very prescriptive, and that this may reflect the way they handle their occupational role. Some may have actually decided what Harry should do. As the discussion continues, it becomes clear that the careworker's task is not to make decisions for other people, but to enrich and catalyse their decision-making, for example by providing accurate information, by enlarging their understanding of alternatives and exploring the probable consequences of particular choices. Respect for individuals, in community care work as elsewhere, entails giving them the freedom to decide, but with the greatest possible clarity. This is a position that those with a highly moralistic disposition may find very hard to adopt in practice.

Second example: preparing a life history

One of the anomalies in the care of older people, especially in residential settings, is that there is often virtually no knowledge of how they have lived their lives. This exercise requires a careworker to discover something of the life history of one person, and relate it to care practice. In one version the instructions are as follows.

> Take one resident with whom you are involved in providing care.
> 1. Over 3–5 shifts, keep notes about what is going well and not so well for this person.
> 2. Find out as much as you can about this person's past, through conversation with any relatives whom you can contact. Explain that you are doing this so that the care can be made better.
> 3. In the light of what you have discovered suggest up to five ways in which the quality of life of this person might be improved.
> Present your findings in a clearly written account, giving about 300–500 words to each section.

Although the task takes a good deal of time, and often presents practical difficulties, those who undertake it usually show a remarkable commitment. The collection of the data typically involves spending several hours with the residents' relatives, who are in most cases very willing to provide any information that would lead to better care. Those who complete the exercise are often able to see very positive changes in the quality of life of the person whose life history they have prepared, particularly through richer communication and through providing more meaningful occupations.

In relation to the broader issues of moral development, learning seems to occur in three main areas.

(i) The resident is seen as a real person, perhaps for the first time ever. Up to the point of preparing a life history the careworker may have responded with kindness and sincerity, but in many respects this was done blindly; stereotypes and superficial banter had often been used to fill the empty spaces in their knowledge. A relationship that had been largely instrumental now becomes more personal. "Caring for" is enriched with "caring about". Furthermore, some of the statements which the resident had made, and which had been framed as delusion or confabulation, are reappraised. One woman, for example, claimed repeatedly that she had rowed for England, and this had been dismissed as ridiculous. Her relatives confirmed, however, that this was true, and that she had been a pioneer of competitive rowing among women. A depth is thus given to the careworker's recognition of the residents. There is greater regard for their achievements, a fuller acceptance of their needs, a richer compassion for what they have endured. That respect for people which lies at the heart of the Kantian ethic becomes more of a lived reality; and once this has happened with one man or woman, there is a sense of unease about the way many others are being treated: a desire is engendered that the same respect should be shown in all cases.

(ii) There is a greater awareness of the way members of a family frame the problem of dementia in someone they have known in better times. In almost every case there is a profound sense of loss—a kind of bereavement, often this is compounded with feelings of guilt at having had to resort to residential care. One husband, for example, had vowed to his wife that he would never "have her put away", but then had to face the fact that the task of looking after her at home was beyond him. One of the hardest things that a person doing this exercise may have to face is the anger of relatives, particularly if this is displaced onto the inadequacies of the care setting. On the positive side there are often strong expressions of gratitude, and an acknowledgement of the difficult task that staff are undertaking. Compared to the complexity of the family members' emotions surrounding the resident, those of the careworker are relatively simple. He or she is confronted with the co-existence of two very different "moral worlds", and has to learn how to negotiate between them.

(iii) This exercise, like many others we have devised, provokes a critical awareness of prevailing patterns of care practice. If the failure of existing provision, and the possibilities for something far better, are so clearly exposed in one case, the inference is inescapable that similar considerations apply to others. Thus arises a different overall vision of how to engage with this area of human need, and a deep dissatisfaction with the ineptitude and neglect to which so many people with dementia are subjected. The loss of personhood that so often accompanies dementia is no longer to be simplistically attributed to an advancing pathology in the brain. So long as the residents remain as stereotypes, without a history and without a context, this awareness and the moral responsibility that it entails can be avoided, or covered over with specious rationalisations. When, however, the awareness has come, for most people there can be no possibility of returning. Thus those who complete exercises of this kind come to understand that moral categories do not simply apply to interpersonal actions; they apply also to the entire social context—its power structure, its reward system, its role demarcations and its existential beliefs. A whole culture is in need of change (Kitwood, 1995).

Third example: role-play of a person with dementia

Being close to dementia can be deeply disturbing: it is liable to arouse fears concerning frailty, dependence, madness, dying and death. This exercise is designed to help workers to come to terms with their fears, and to draw closer to those whom they are looking after. It involves taking on the persona of an imagined older man or woman, and "being" that person in two role plays. I have myself been through this process many times.

The nature of the exercise is explained several days beforehand, so that participants can make a clear choice whether or not to take part. In preparation they are asked to create a fictitious life history, based on their real knowledge, and to bring one or two props—items of clothing or specific objects—to identify the person they will play. The first enactment consists of each person, in role, giving a brief life history, at a point when memory for the distant past is still intact. The second enactment is a simulation of about half an hour of life in a residential setting; where some of the group are "being" people with dementia and some of the others are careworkers, operating at their present level of skill. The exercise is only done when plenty of psychological support is available, and when there has been time for trust to have developed: typically during a residential course. Great care is taken over the final shedding of the role; there is also a thorough de-briefing.

The first role-play has an unexpected poignancy. One study after another depicts life-changes, illness, suffering and bereavement, an almost palpable atmosphere of melancholy pervades the room. The losses that accompany later life are understood more deeply, and there is a new appreciation of the courage with which many older people live through their last years.

For most participants, however, the second role play is the more powerful of the two. Those who are able to engage in it with sincerity may be coming closer to dementia than they have ever done before, perhaps recruiting to their role some of their buried memories of dementia-like experiences. They assimilate a minute sample of the daily life of a residential setting: its loneliness, its boredom, its frustration; its sheer impersonality; and, on the other side, the reality of simple pleasures and the joy of human contact when it does occur. A surprising range of feelings are aroused, such as an urgent, overpowering need for comfort, a childlike sense of freedom, the desire to escape, the urge to destroy. The sense of chaos and disorganisation is some-times near-to-overwhelming, even if the simulated care practice is good by present standards.

Some participants find that they are able to give themselves wholeheartedly to this exercise, daring to expose themselves to the experience. Others, however, are not able to engage so fully. Various tactics are used in order to create a distance; such as offering a wooden imitation of one of their own clients, minimal participation or actual escape. One or two decide, at the last minute, not to take part, and prefer to be spectators. Whatever a person's response he or she has something to learn from it, as both the briefing and the de-briefing make clear.

An exercise of this kind has much to contribute to a careworker's moral develop-ment, principally along two lines.

(i)   It is a powerful way of transcending that existential divide which so often separ-ates people with dementia from the rest of humankind: for developing a deeper level of empathy. There are limits to how close we come to the experience of another, if our part is simply that of a receptive listener. The role-play can enable a richer understanding, grounded in emotion and bodily movement. In his theory of stagecraft Stanislavsky suggested that a good actor is able to relax the con-straints of ordinary behaviour, and draw freely on his or her emotional memories so as to create an authentic part (Margashack, 1961). Something remarkably similar seems to occur in good caregiving.

(ii) The exercise is an encounter with the defence processes that so often get in the way of authentic moral engagement, creating distance and impersonality. Those defences have a function, of course, in protecting the psyche from forms of awareness that it cannot bear. Some participants are ready to allow their defences to be lowered a little, going forward on a path that will lead to much greater efficacy in their work. As they progress they tend to experience themselves as more vulnerable than before, but they also find a greater poise and resilience.

Those who distanced themselves from the role in some way may have the chance to learn more about their defence processes, developing new awareness of what it is that they fear. The same is true for any who chose simply to be observers; paradoxically, it may be these who are in the greatest need of support, because their competence has been implicitly challenged.

The moral requirements of care work

The three examples I have given here are sufficient to provide a glimpse of what caregiving in dementia involves in moral terms. Many of the exercises that we have designed are a practical induction into an ethic of respect for persons; the great moral principle of universalisability is grasped gradually, by inference from real engagement. A good careworker should be able to act fluently, spontaneously, using his or her feelings and intuitions, combining a heightened sensitivity with mundane practical skill. Moral judgements are, for the greater part, made subliminally and intuitively, and in the flux of everyday life.

The moral situation, however, in care work as in many other contexts, is not simply a Kantian one. For each person working in a care environment has also to be some kind of utilitarian, endeavouring to maximise—or rather, optimise—the well-being of a number of people simultaneously. It can be a source of great discomfort to feel an intense moral commitment to one individual, while at the same time having to attend to several others. This point is demonstrated in the first of the exercises, where the needs of several people have to be considered simultaneously. It emerges even more clearly in the second, after life history work has intensified the concern for particular individuals. It is experienced inversely, and in a powerful and immediate way in the third, through enacting the role of a person with dementia in a simulated care setting; perhaps through discovering the scarcity of close attention in a time of need.

Thus a careworker has to live with an uneasy tension between two rival and irreconcilable moral imperatives, and endure the consequences of being able to meet neither in an adequate way. The problem is compounded by the fact that staffing ratios in many care settings are still disgracefully low: often one worker to eight or ten highly dependent recipients of care. A manager may experience extremes of dissonance at those times when it seems necessary to compromise the well-being of one person for the sake of the others. The hardest decision of all is to arrange for a person to be transferred elsewhere, almost certainly against his or her best interests, because neither the other residents nor the staff can cope with his or her behaviour. It must be said that these crises of conscience become less frequent as the quality of care improves, although they are unlikely to disappear altogether.

The developmental process

In this final section, I wish to draw back a little, and suggest some broader inferences from the work that I have been describing.

One thing is certain. These attempts to promote professional and moral development in care work are not "training", in the ordinary sense of the word—although that is the term that is commonly used. The concept of training is far too mechanistic and behaviouristic; it allows no place for theory or critique, it does not recognise that *prise de conscience* that is of the essence of all highly skilled practice. In a double sense the idea of training de-moralises both the careworker and the work. That is to say, it can easily detract from personal confidence and courage, and it devalues a sensitive and reflexive concern for others.

The concept that best describes the process exists in the Latin-based languages, but not in those with an Anglo-Saxon base, in French the term is *formation*, and in Spanish *formación*. It is in the work of Ralph Ruddock, one of Britain's leading figures in adult education during the last 30 years, that we find the clearest exposition. Formation, so Ruddock (1980) suggests, is both a psychological and a sociological concept. It implies the preparation of a person for a particular occupational role, one which involves responsibility and integrity. Psychologically, it points to a differential growth in capability: out of all the possible ways in which a person might develop, one broad line is taken, while others are necessarily laid aside. There is a concomitant reintegration of the personality, because the psyche functions holographically, not as a mere assemblage. For example, that sensitivity to others' experience that is essential in care work is taken into relationships elsewhere, and becomes an enduring trait. Then, as the person takes on the role and learns how to perform well in it, a new sense of identity emerges. Sociologically, the idea of formation suggests that a good society will provide a rich variety of such roles, all of which are well structured and properly rewarded. The social tragedy of unemployment and low-grade labour is that of widespread deformation (Kitwood, 1997b).

Formation, then, can never be simply a matter of promoting change in individuals. It is necessarily connected to the way roles are socially defined, and to the culture that exists in each work setting. In any field an enduring transformation is more likely to occur when whole staff groups are taken through a process of professional education and where personal development is accompanied by a supporting culture. Each person is unique, of course, in the way he or she participates in the developmental process, or blocks it off through psychological defences, but at least there is a social framework for promoting positive change. If this matter is not addressed it is likely that those who have caught a glimpse of something different, perhaps through going on a course as individuals, will later be re-assimilated into the existing culture; or, if they have great ability and clear vision, they will find that the workplace is now intolerable and they will leave.

For moral education in general one main inference is that we would do well to continue in the Aristotelian mode. We should become more sociological in our emphases, and engage with the power structures and subcultures that already shape people's lives. We need to come much closer to the life-worlds of real occupations: nursing, medicine, social work, the police force, the prison service, trade unions, the media, management and so on. Each one of these arenas has its social practices and shared assumptions; each *lebenswelt* is in need of a specific form of moral education. If the subject of "professional ethics" is taught at all, it tends to focus on particular issues that come to the surface and crystallise, while the details of how people relate to each other in everyday life remain unexamined. Thus, as I have argued elsewhere, we need an "ethic of process", so that the entire pattern of everyday life is subjected to a profound moralisation (Kitwood, 1998). It is this that our own attempt to promote personal development in care work is intended to achieve.

References

Gilligan, C. (1982) *In a Different Voice* (Cambridge, Harvard University Press).

Haste, H. (1996) Communitarianism and the social construction of morality, *Journal of Moral Education*, 25, pp. 47–56.

Kitwood, T. (1995) Cultures of care: tradition and change, in: T. Kitwood & S. Benson (Eds) *The New Culture of Dementia Care* (London, Hawker Publications).

Kitwood, T. (1997a) *Dementia Reconsidered* (Buckingham, Open University Press).

Kitwood, T. (1997b) Some notes on personhood and deformation, in: C.L. Fletcher (Ed.) *The Spirit of Adult Learning: essays in honour of Ralph Ruddock* (Wolverhampton, University of Wolverhampton).

Kitwood, T. (1998) Towards a theory of dementia care: ethics and interaction, *Journal of Clinical Ethics*, 9, 1, pp. 23–34.

Knowles, R.T. & McLean, G.F. (Eds) (1986) *Psychological Foundations of Moral Education and Character Development* (Lanham, MD, University Press of America).

Kohn, A. (1990) *The Brighter Side of Human Nature: Altruism and Empathy in Everyday Life* (New York, Basic Books).

Lickona, T. (1996) Eleven principles of effective character education, *Journal of Moral Education*, 25, pp. 93–100.

Margashack, D. (Ed.) (1961) *Stanislavsky on the Art of the Stage* (London, Faber).

Ruddock, R. (1980) Beyond Vocational Training, International Conference on Adult Education, Nottingham University.

Taylor, M.J. (1992) Learning fairness through empathy: pupils' perspectives on putting policy into practice, in: M. Leicester & M.J. Taylor (Eds) *Ethics, Ethnicity and Education* (London, Kogan Page).

Wilkinson, S. (1997) Feminist psychology, in: D. Fox & I. Prilleltensky (Eds) *Critical Psychology* (London, Sage).

Annotated Bibliography

This bibliography is intended to help readers follow up the themes and issues raised in the critical reviews of Kitwood's work. As such it is not a comprehensive bibliography – we have chosen to include only those works that are in English and are either related specifically to dementia or are cited in our commentaries. We have provided very brief comments on each entry to help the reader locate it in the context of Kitwood's work as a whole.

Kitwood, T. (1970) *What is Human?* London: Inter-Varsity Press.

Written from a specifically Christian perspective, when he was still an ordained minister. Kitwood explores three versions of what it means to be human: existentialist, humanist and Christian. Traces of the ideas in this book can be found throughout Kitwood's later writings.

Kitwood, T. (1980) *Disclosures to a Stranger: Adolescent values in an advanced industrial society.* London: Routledge & Kegan Paul.

Based on Kitwood's doctoral thesis, this book reports on empirical research carried out to explore the development of 'self-values' among adolescents.

Kitwood, T. (1987). Dementia and its pathology: in brain, mind or society?, *Free Associations*, 8(April): 81–93.

While essentially a review of *Another Name for Madness* by Marion Roach, here, Kitwood begins to explicate his thoughts on the social and psychological aspects of dementia, clearly taking a social constructionist stance on the aetiology of dementia.

Kitwood, T. (1987) Explaining senile dementia: the limits of neuropathological research, *Free Associations*, 10: 117–140.

A detailed critique of four papers, three of which are held to be definitive in the field of neuropathological research. Kitwood details the limits of such research and its mythological character. This critique formed the basis of Kitwood's development of an alternative theory of dementia.

Kitwood, T. (1988) The contribution of psychology to the understanding of senile dementia, in Gearing, B., Johnson, M. and Heller, T. (eds) *Mental Health Problems in Old Age: A reader.* Chichester: John Wiley & Sons.

This is essentially a reiteration of many of the points made in the previous two articles, with some slightly enhanced emphasis on the contribution of psychology to understanding dementia.

Kitwood, T. (1988) Sentient being, moral agent, *Journal of Moral Education*, 17(May): 83–91.

A presentation of a theory of what it means to be a sentient being and its implications for moral theory. Drawing on depth psychology, Kitwood argues that feelings and emotions play an important part in our moral lives.

Kitwood, T. (1988) The technical, the personal and the framing of dementia, *Social Behaviour*, 3(2): 161–179.

Kitwood critiques the view that dementia can be understood in terms of neuropathology alone. He argues that the evidence does not support this view and offers reasons for why this view, despite its shortcomings, has become the prevalent view of dementia. He then contrasts the technical with the personal view of dementia based on theories from psychoanalysis and psychotherapy.

Kitwood, T. (1989) Brain, mind and dementia: with particular reference to Alzheimer's disease, *Ageing and Society*, 9(1): 1–15.

Kitwood starts to develop his theory of dementia as a function between brain and mind, within the parameters set by the brain's developmental and pathological aspects. He also introduces the notion of 'rementia'.

Kitwood, T. (1990) *Concern for Others: A new psychology of conscience and morality*. London: Routledge.

In this non-dementia-related book, Kitwood propounds the theory of psychology as a 'moral science of action'. He argues that the practices of counselling and therapy epitomise a form of moral action lacking in contemporary western society. Chapter 6 is particularly relevant to the development of Kitwood's later thinking on organizational culture in dementia care.

Kitwood, T. (1990) The dialectics of dementia: with particular reference to Alzheimer's disease, *Ageing and Society*, 10(2): 177–196.

Here Kitwood presents his new theory of the dementing process in old age, focusing on the dialectical interplay between neurological and social–psychological factors.

Kitwood, T. (1990) Psychotherapy and dementia, British Psychological Society, *Psychotherapy Section Newsletter*, 8: 40–56.

Kitwood explains how the principles of psychotherapy can be applied in dementia care practice.

Kitwood, T. (1990) Psychotherapy, postmodernism and morality, *Journal of Moral Education*, 19(1): 3–13.

This paper is not specifically related to dementia care. In it, Kitwood suggests that a form of psychotherapy, based on co-counselling, which involves the exchange of free attention, offers a model of interpersonal morality that transcends the 'grand narratives' of much western moralism.

Kitwood, T. (1990) Understanding senile dementia: a psychobiographical approach, *Free Associations*, 19: 60–76.

An application of the psychobiographical approach to a single case study – exploring how a person's past can contribute to the development of senile dementia. One of the clearer statements by Kitwood regarding dementia as a function of social relations in late capitalism.

Kitwood, T. (1992) How valid is validation therapy?, *Geriatric Medicine*, 22(4): 23.

While critical of validation therapy in terms of its methodology, Kitwood is generally supportive of its psychotherapeutic stance.

Kitwood, T. (1992) Quality assurance in dementia care, *Geriatric Medicine*, 22(9): 34–38.

A very brief description of Dementia Care Mapping and its usefulness in quality assurance.

Kitwood, T. (1993) Discover the person, not the disease, *Journal of Dementia Care*, 1(1): 16–17.

A brief outline of Kitwood's social–psychological approach to dementia, using the 'equation' D = P + B+ H + NI + SP, aimed at practitioners rather than academics.

Kitwood, T. (1993) Frames of reference for an understanding of dementia, in Johnson, J. and Slater, R. (eds) *Ageing and Later Life*. London: Sage.

A further reiteration of how dementia has been framed by medical science and a brief outline of the contribution that social psychology might make to our understanding of dementia.

Kitwood, T. (1993) Person and process in dementia, *International Journal of Geriatric Psychiatry*, 8(7): 541–545.

Here Kitwood introduces further social and psychological factors (personality, biography, and health) into his formulation of the dementing process and outlines some of the features that would be required by a sustained inquiry into the social psychology of dementia.

Kitwood, T. (1993) Towards the reconstruction of an organic mental disorder, in Radley, A. (ed.) *Worlds of Illness*. London: Routledge.

A bringing together of the critique of neuropathological research, a focus on social–psychological factors in the dementing process and the need to maintain personhood through dementia care.

Kitwood, T. (1993) Towards a theory of dementia care: the interpersonal process, *Ageing and Society*, 13(1): 51–67.

This is a detailed description of interpersonal processes in dementia, introducing the concepts of facilitation and the 'culture of dementia' based on observation of interactions between people with dementia and caregivers and between people with dementia themselves.

Kitwood, T. (1994). The concept of personhood and its implications for the care of those who have dementia, in Jones, G. and Miesen, B. (eds) *Caregiving in Dementia*, Vol. II. London: Routledge.

A development of Kitwood's theory of personhood, based on Buber's I–Thou relationship and stressing the importance of the uniqueness of each person, subjectivity and relatedness, each of which challenges modern ways of being in the world.

Kitwood, T. (1994) Lowering our defences by playing the part, *Journal of Dementia Care*, 2(5): 12–14.

Kitwood discusses the use of role play in deepening our understanding of the experience of dementia and overcoming the defences that separate us from people with dementia.

Kitwood, T. (1995) Cultures of care: tradition and change, in Kitwood, T. and Benson, S. (eds) *The New Culture of Dementia Care*. London: Hawker.

Kitwood briefly discusses the concept of a 'culture' and then goes on to identify 10 points of difference between the 'old' and 'new' cultures of dementia care.

Kitwood, T. (1995) Dementia: social section – part II, in Berrios, G. and Porter, R. (eds) *A History of Clinical Psychiatry: The origin and history of psychiatric disorders*. London: Athlone.

In this chapter from an academic textbook, Kitwood challenges the way in which orthodox psychiatry has narrowed down the definition of dementia. The disease category 'dementia' is problematized with reference to prevalence, psychological and social factors and developments in care practice.

Kitwood, T. (1995) Exploring the ethics of dementia research: a response to Berghmans and ter Meulen: a psychosocial perspective, *International Journal of Geriatric Psychiatry*, 10(8): 655–657.

In responding to Berghmans and ter Meulen, Kitwood criticizes their justification of non-therapeutic research involving people with dementia and argues that ethical considerations apply not only to the 'what' of 'research' (the subject under scrutiny) but also the 'how' (the research process itself).

Kitwood, T. (1995) Positive long-term changes in dementia: some preliminary observations, *Journal of Mental Health*, 4(2): 133–144.

Kitwood presents evidence of the restoration of personality and personal growth from observations of 49 persons with dementia and speculates on the conditions necessary to promote such positive changes.

Kitwood, T. (1995) Studies in person-centred care: building up the mosaic of good practice, *Journal of Dementia Care*, 3(5): 12–13.

An introduction to a series of articles – in subsequent issues – on person-centred care. These case studies are, Kitwood argues, essential as a preliminary to formal research and illustrative of the uniqueness and variety of experiences of living with dementia.

Kitwood, T. (1996) A dialectical framework for dementia, in Woods, R.T. (ed.) *Handbook of the Clinical Psychology of Ageing*. London: John Wiley & Sons.

A further iteration of Kitwood's critique of the standard paradigm and the role of psychology in understanding dementia, but developing the concept of dementia as a dialectical process.

Kitwood, T. (1996) The psychology of caring, *Journal of Dementia Care*, 4(4): 11.

An edited transcript of an interview by Anthony Clare for the BBC programme *All in the Mind*. The interview is focused on the nature of relationships in dementia care.

Kitwood, T. (1996) Some problematic aspects of dementia, in Heller, T., Reynolds, Gomm, R., Muston, R. and Pattison, S. (eds) *Mental Health Matters*. Basingstoke: Macmillan.

An outline of four problematic issues in the narrow biomedical model of dementia, focusing on the prevalence of dementia, research on psychological and social factors associated with the dementing process, the rise of the 'Alzheimer culture' and approaches to dementia care.

Kitwood, T. (1997) *Dementia Reconsidered: The person comes first*. Buckingham: Open University Press.

Kitwood's best-known book, drawing together many of the ideas found in earlier articles. Here, he argues that we need to rethink our approach to people with dementia and put the person before the disease. Neuropathology is only one aspect of the dementia experience and there is much that can be done to alleviate the negative aspects of dementia and promote positive, creative care for those living with dementia.

Kitwood, T. (1997) *Evaluating Dementia Care: The DCM method* (7th edn). University of Bradford: Bradford Dementia Group.

A manual providing explanation of the key principles and philosophy of the DCM method, giving detailed instruction on its coding frames and operational rules. This edition of the DCM manual has now been superseded by the 8th edition.

Kitwood, T. (1997) The experience of dementia, *Aging and Mental Health*, 1(1): 13–22.

Stressing the uniqueness of persons, six routes to understanding the experience of dementia are discussed and comments made on the psychological needs of people with dementia.

Kitwood, T. (1997) Personhood, dementia and dementia care, in Hunter, S. (ed.) *Research Highlights in Social Work*, Vol. 31. London: Jessica Kingsley.

A positive review of advances in dementia care and the focus on person-centred care. This chapter brings together arguments made previously about personhood and the need for a social–psychological approach to dementia care.

Kitwood, T. (1997) The profound lessons dementia can teach us, *Journal of Dementia Care*, 5(2): 26–27.

A brief reflection by Kitwood on his work and the publication of *Dementia Reconsidered*.

Kitwood, T. (1997) Some notes on personhood and deformation, in Fletcher, C.L. (ed.) *The Spirit of Adult Learning: Essays in honour of Ralph Ruddock*. Wolverhampton: University of Wolverhampton Press.

Kitwood pays tribute to the influence of Ruddock's work on personal identity on his own thinking. The chapter is not dementia specific but makes reference to the part played by social factors in bringing about a 'deformation' of personhood.

Kitwood, T. (1997) The uniqueness of persons in dementia, in Marshall, M. (ed.) *The State of the Art in Dementia Care*. London: Centre for Policy on Ageing.

A brief reiteration of what is necessary to fully appreciate the uniqueness of persons, namely, personal knowledge and empathy. Uniqueness is seen as an important part of maintaining personhood.

Kitwood, T. (1998) Professional and moral development for care work: some observations on the process, *Journal of Moral Education*, 27(3): 401–411.

This paper discusses the professional education of those who work in caring roles, with specific reference to dementia care. Three experiential learning exercises are discussed in terms of their potential for bringing about the moral development of care workers.

Kitwood, T. (1998) Towards a theory of dementia care: ethics and interaction, *The Journal of Clinical Ethics*, 9(1): 23–34.

A discussion of how the ethical concerns that arise in day-to-day dementia care practice lie outside the parameters of conventional ethical discourses. Kitwood advances a theory of the 'ethics of the context' in which 'positive person work' has much to offer.

Bredin, K., Kitwood, T. and Wattis, J. (1995) Decline in quality of life for patients with severe dementia following a ward merger, *International Journal of Geriatric Psychiatry*, 10(11): 967–973.

Empirical data from Dementia Care Mapping is put forward to demonstrate that quality of life for patients on long-stay wards deteriorated following a ward merger. This deterioration is attributed to the effects of the merger on staff morale.

Capstick, A. and Kitwood, T. (1999) Dementia and nursing – part 2: person-centred care, *Journal of Nursing Care*, 2(2): 4–6.

A basic core curriculum for pre- and post-registration nurse education is outlined, focusing on the interpretation of behaviour, communication and maintenance of physical health. A model of learning that matches person-centred care with student-centred learning is proposed.

Kitwood, T. and Benson, S. (eds) (1995) *The New Culture of Dementia Care*. London: Hawker.

This edited collection of short articles addresses a range of issues involved in establishing and maintaining the 'new culture' of dementia care: communication, sexuality, spirituality, supporting carers, volunteering, occupation and activities and training and organizational change. The articles draw on both professional practice and empirical research and are aimed at those who work in residential settings and day centres.

Kitwood, T. and Bredin, K. (1992) A new approach to the evaluation of dementia care, *Journal of Advances in Health and Nursing Care*, 1(5): 41–60.

A general description of the method of Dementia Care Mapping and a discussion of some of the possible criticisms of the method. Implications for our understanding of dementia and dementia care are also discussed.

Kitwood, T. and Bredin, K. (1992) *Person to Person: A guide to the care of those with failing mental powers*. Loughton: Gale.

Still regarded as a seminal text, this short book outlines the basic principles of the person-centred approach in an accessible way intended for care staff and family members.

Kitwood, T. and Bredin, K. (1992). Towards a theory of dementia care: personhood and well-being, *Ageing and Society*, 12(3): 269–287.

In this article, the authors lay some of the foundations for a social–psychological theory of dementia, focusing on the centrality of personhood. Personhood is seen in social rather than individual terms and the key task of dementia care is seen as maintaining that personhood.

Kitwood, T. and Bredin, K. (1994) Charting the course of quality care, *Journal of Dementia Care*, 2(3): 22–23.

A brief account of the history and development of the Dementia Care Mapping method. The authors explain how their experience of carrying out detailed observations of care settings led them to abandon the view that there are stages of dementia resulting directly from the advance of degenerative processes in the brain.

Kitwood, T. Buckland, S. and Petre, T. (1995) *Brighter Futures: A report on research into provision for persons with dementia in residential homes, nursing homes and sheltered housing*. Kidlington: Anchor Housing Association.

A report on empirical research bringing together two different studies: one on the well-being and ill-being of people with dementia in residential care and one on factors affecting continued residency for people with dementia in sheltered housing.

Kitwood, T. and Capstick, A. (1999) Dementia and nursing – part 1: educational strategy, *Journal of Nursing Care*, 2(1): 10–12.

An outline of the educational deficit in preparing nurses for working with people with dementia is presented in relation to current and projected prevalence rates.

Kitwood, T. and Fox, L. (1997) *Evaluation of a Day Centre by Use of Dementia Care Mapping*. Bradford: Bradford Dementia Group.

An unpublished report on the evaluation of a specific care setting using an early version of Dementia Care Mapping.

Kitwood, T. and Woods, R.T. (1997) *Training and Development Strategy for Dementia Care in Residential Settings*. Bradford: Bradford Dementia Group.

Initially produced as an advisory document for a charitable organization opening its first dementia specialist nursing home, this report outlines some of the fundamental considerations for a staff development strategy.

Loveday, B., Kitwood, T. and Bowe, B. (1998) *Improving Dementia Care: A resource for training and professional development*. London: Hawker.

A resource pack for staff development in dementia care, which includes a trainer manual and wide range of exercises that can be used to introduce the basic principles of the person-centred approach.

References

Adams, T. (1996) Kitwood's approach to dementia and dementia care: a critical but appreciative review, *Journal of Advanced Nursing*, 23(5): 948–953.

Adams, T. and Bartlett, R. (2003) Constructing dementia, in Adams, T. and Manthorpe, J. (eds) *Dementia Care*. London: Arnold.

Adelman, R.C. (1995) The Alzheimerization of aging, *The Gerontologist*, 38(4): 526–532.

Age Concern. (1998) News release, 10 October.

Althusser, L. (1970) Ideology and ideological state apparatuses (notes towards an investigation), in *Lenin and Philosophy and Other Essays*. London: New Left Books.

Alzheimer's Australia. (2004) Tests used in diagnosing dementia, update sheet. Available from http://www.alzheimers.org.au (accessed 10 January 2007).

Balfour, A. (2006) Thinking about the experience of dementia: the importance of the unconscious, *Journal of Social Work Practice*, 20(3): 329–346.

Bartlett, R. and O'Connor, D. (2007) From personhood to citizenship: broadening the conceptual base for dementia practice and research, *Journal of Aging Studies*, 21(2): 107–118.

Barton, L. (1993) The struggle for citizenship: the case of disabled people, *Disability, Handicap and Society*, 8(3): 235–248.

Beauchamp, T.L. (1999) The failures of theories of personhood, in Thomasma, D.C., Weisstub, D.N. and Herve, C. (eds) *Personhood and Health Care*. Dordrecht: Kluwer Academic Publishers.

Beauchamp, T.L. and Childress, J.F. (2001) *Principles of Biomedical Ethics* (5th edn). New York: Oxford University Press.

Bender, M. (2003) *Explorations in Dementia: Theoretical and research studies into the experience of remediable and enduring cognitive losses*. London: Jessica Kingsley.

Bentham, J. (1789) *An Introduction to the Principles of Morals and Legislation* (J.H. Burns and H.L.A. Hart (eds) (1970)). Oxford: Clarendon Press.

Bloom, H. (1973) *The Anxiety of Influence: A theory of poetry*. New York: Oxford University Press.

Bond, J. (1992) The medicalization of dementia, *Journal of Aging Studies*, 6(4): 397–403.

Bradford Dementia Group. (1997) *The Dementia Care Mapping Manual* (7th edn). Bradford: University of Bradford Press.

Brane, G., Karlsson, I., Kohlgren, M. and Norberg, A. (1989) Integrity-promoting care of demented nursing home patients: psychological and biochemical changes, *International Journal of Geriatric Psychiatry*, 4(3): 165–172.

Bredin, K., Kitwood, T. and Wattis, J. (1995) Decline in quality of life for patients with severe dementia following a ward merger, *International Journal of Geriatric Psychiatry*, 10(11): 967–973.

Brock, D. (1993) *Life and Death: Philosophical essays in biomedical ethics*. Cambridge: Cambridge University Press.

Brooker, D. (2003) Maintaining quality in dementia care practice, in Adams, T. and Manthorpe J. (eds) *Dementia Care*. London: Arnold.

Brooker, D. and Surr, C. (2005) *Dementia Care Mapping: Principles and practice*. Bradford: University of Bradford Press.

Bruce, E. (2004) Social exclusion and inclusion in care homes, in Innes, A., Archibald, C. and Murphy, C. (eds) *Dementia and Social Inclusion: Marginalized groups and marginalized areas of dementia research, care and practice*. London: Jessica Kingsley.

Bruce, E., Tibbs, M. and Downs, M. (2002) Moving towards a special kind of care for people with dementia living in care homes, *Nursing Times Research*, 7(5): 335–347.

Burkitt, I. (1993) *Social Selves*. London: Sage.

Burns, A., Howard, R. and Pettit, W. (1995) *Alzheimer's Disease: A medical companion* (1st edn). Oxford: Blackwell Science Ltd.

Cantley, C. and Bowes, A. (2004) Dementia and social inclusion: the way forward, in Innes, A., Archibald, C. and Murphy, C. (eds) *Dementia and Social Inclusion: Marginalized groups and marginalized areas of dementia research, care and practice*. London: Jessica Kingsley.

Capstick, A. (2003) The theoretical origins of dementia care mapping, in Innes, A. (ed.) *Dementia Care Mapping: Applications across cultures*. Baltimore, MD: Health Professions Press.

Capstick, A. and Kitwood, T. (1999) Dementia and nursing – part 2: person-centred care, *Journal of Nursing Care*, 2(2): 4–6.

Chaudhury, H. (1999) Self and reminiscence of place: a conceptual study, *Journal of Aging and Identity*, 4(4): 231–253.

Chaudhury, H. (2002) Journey back home: recollecting past places by people with dementia, *Journal of Housing for the Elderly*, 16(1/2): 85–106.

Chaudhury, H. (2003) Remembering home through art, *Alzheimer's Care Quarterly*, 4(2): 119–124.

Cheston, R. (1996) Review of *The New Culture of Dementia Care*, *PSIGE Newsletter*, 58(October): 37.

Davies, B. and Harré, R. (1990) Positioning: the discursive production of selves, *Journal of the Theory of Social Behavior*, 20(1): 43–63.

Davis, D.H. (2004) Dementia: sociological and philosophical constructions, *Social Science and Medicine*, 58(2): 369–378.

Davis, H.T.O. and Nutley, S.M. (2000) Organisational culture and quality of health care, *Quality in Health Care*, 9(2): 111–119.

Deleuze, G. and Guattari, F. (2004) *A Thousand Plateaux: Capitalism and schizophrenia*. London: Continuum.

Downs, M. (1997) The emergence of the person in dementia research, *Ageing and Society*, 17(5): 597–607.

Downs, M. (2000) Dementia in a socio-cultural context: an idea whose time has come, *Ageing and Society*, 20(3): 369–375.

Featherstone, M., Hepworth, M. and Turner, B.S. (1991) *The Body, Social Process and Cultural Theory*. London: Sage.

Fleischer, T.E. (1999) The personhood wars, *Theoretical Medicine and Bioethics*, 20(3): 309–318.

Flicker, L. (1999) Review of *Dementia Reconsidered*, *British Medical Journal*, 318(7187): 880.

Foucault, M. (1967) *Madness and Civilization*. London: Tavistock.

Fox, P. (1989) From senility to Alzheimer's disease: the rise of the Alzheimer's disease movement, *Milbank Quarterly*, 67(1): 58–102.

Frank, J. (2005) Semiotic use of the word 'home' among people with Alzheimer's disease: a plea for selfhood?, in Rowles, G.D. and Chaudhury, H. (eds) *Home and Identity in Late Life: International perspectives*. New York: Springer.

Fromm, E. (1941) *The Fear of Freedom*. New York: Avon Books.

Gaston, L. (1995) Common factors exist is reality but not in our theories, *Clinical Psychology: Science and Practice*, 2(1): 83–86.

Gibson, F. (1997) Review of *Dementia Reconsidered, Journal of Dementia Care*, 5(4): 29.

Goldsmith, M. (1996) *Hearing the Voice of People with Dementia: Opportunities and obstacles*. London: Jessica Kingsley.

Griffin, J. (1986) *Well Being*. Oxford: Clarendon Press.

Gubrium, J.F. (1986) *Old Timers and Alzheimer's*. Greenwich, CT: JAI Press.

Hamilton, G. (2005) Epilogue: the prism, the soliloquy, the couch and the dance – the evolving study of language and Alzheimer's disease, in Davis, B.H. (ed.) *Alzheimer Talk, Text and Context: Enhancing communication*. Basingstoke: Palgrave Macmillan.

Harding, N. and Palfrey, C. (1997) *The Social Construction of Dementia: Confused professionals?* London: Jessica Kingsley.

Harré, R. and van Langenhove, L. (1991) Varieties of positioning, *Journal of the Theory of Social Behaviour*, 21 (4): 393–407.

Hohl, U., Tiraboschi, P., Hansen, L.A., Thal, L.J. and Corey-Bloom, J. (2000) Diagnostic accuracy of dementia with Lewy bodies, *Archives of Neurology*, 57(3): 347–351.

Hughes, J.C. (2001) Views of the person with dementia, *Journal of Medical Ethics*, 27(2): 86–91.

Hulko, W. (2002) Making the links: social theories, experiences of people with dementia, and intersectionality, in Leibing, A. and Scheinkman, L. (eds) *The Diversity of Alzheimer's Disease: Different approaches and contexts*. Rio de Janeiro: CUCA-IPUB.

Hurka, T. (1993) *Perfectionism*. New York: Oxford University Press.

Ibbotson, T. and Goa, K.L. (2002) Management of Alzheimer's disease: defining the role of donepezil, *Disease Management and Health Outcomes*, 10(1): 41–54.

Innes, A., Archibald, C. and Murphy, C. (eds) (2004) *Dementia and Social Inclusion: Marginalized groups and marginalized areas of dementia research, care and practice*. London: Jessica Kingsley.

Jacques, A. (1988) *Understanding Dementia*. Edinburgh: Churchill Livingstone.

Karlawish, J.H., Bonnie, R.J., Appelbaum, P.S., Lyketsos, C., James, B., Knopman, D., Patusky, C., Kane, R. and Karlan, P. (2004) Addressing the ethical, legal and social issues raised by voting by persons with dementia, *Journal of the American Medical Association*, 292(11): 1345–1350.

Karlsson, I., Brane, G., Melin, E., Nyth, A.-L. and Rybo, E. (1988) Effects of environmental stimulation on biochemical and psychological variables in dementia, *Acta Psychiatrica Scandinavica*, 77(2): 207–213.

Killick, J. and Allan, K. (2001) *Communication and the Care of People with Dementia*. Buckingham: Open University Press.

Kittay, E.F. (2005) At the margins of moral personhood, *Ethics*, 116(1): 100–131.

Kitwood, T. (1970) *What is Human?* London: Inter-Varsity Press.

Kitwood, T. (1980) *Disclosures to a Stranger: Adolescent values in an advanced industrial society*. London: Routledge & Kegan Paul.

Kitwood, T. (1987a) Dementia and its pathology: in brain, mind or society?, *Free Associations*, 8: 81–93.

Kitwood, T. (1987b) Explaining senile dementia: the limits of neuropathological research, *Free Associations*, 10: 117–140.

Kitwood, T. (1988a) The contribution of psychology to the understanding of senile dementia, in Gearing, B., Johnson, M. and Heller, T. (eds) *Mental Health Problems in Old Age: A reader*. Chichester: John Wiley & Sons.

Kitwood, T. (1988b) The technical, the personal and the framing of dementia, *Social Behaviour*, 3(2): 161–179.

Kitwood, T. (1988c) Sentient being, moral agent, *Journal of Moral Education*, 17(May): 83–91.

Kitwood, T. (1989) Brain, mind and dementia: with particular reference to Alzheimer's disease, *Ageing and Society*, 9(1): 1–15.

Kitwood, T. (1990a) The dialectics of dementia: with particular reference to Alzheimer's disease, *Ageing and Society*, 10(2): 177–196.

Kitwood, T. (1990b) Understanding senile dementia: a psychobiographical approach, *Free Associations*, 19: 60–76.

Kitwood, T. (1990c) *Concern for Others: A new psychology of conscience and morality*. London: Routledge.

Kitwood, T. (1990d) Psychotherapy, postmodernism and morality, *Journal of Moral Education*, 19(1): 3–13.

Kitwood, T. (1993a) Towards the reconstruction of an organic mental disorder, in Radley, A. (ed.) *Worlds of Illness*. London: Routledge.

Kitwood, T. (1993b) Frames of reference for an understanding of dementia, in Johnson, J. and Slater, R. (eds) *Ageing and Later Life*. London: Sage.

Kitwood, T. (1993c) Person and process in dementia, *International Journal of Geriatric Psychiatry*, 8(7): 541–545.

Kitwood, T. (1993d) Towards a theory of dementia care: the interpersonal process, *Ageing and Society*, 13(1): 51–67.

Kitwood, T. (1994) The concept of personhood and its implications for the care of those who have dementia, in Jones, G. and Miesen, B. (eds) *Caregiving in Dementia*. London: Routledge.

Kitwood, T. (1995a) Cultures of care: tradition and change, in Kitwood, T. and Benson, S. (eds) *The New Culture of Dementia Care*. London: Hawker.

Kitwood, T. (1995b) Positive long-term changes in dementia: some preliminary observations, *Journal of Mental Health*, 4(2): 133–144.

Kitwood, T. (1996a) A dialectical framework for dementia, in Woods, R.T. (ed.) *Handbook of the Clinical Psychology of Ageing*. London: John Wiley & Sons.

Kitwood, T. (1996b) Some problematic aspects of dementia, in Heller, T., Reynolds, J. Gomm, R., Muston, R. and Pattison, S. (eds) *Mental Health Matters*. Basingstoke: Macmillan.

Kitwood, T. (1997a) *Dementia Reconsidered*. Buckingham: Open University Press.

Kitwood, T. (1997b) Personhood, dementia and dementia care, in Hunter, S. (ed.) *Research Highlights in Social Work*. London: Jessica Kingsley.

Kitwood, T. (1997c) The uniqueness of persons in dementia, in Marshall, M. (ed.) *The State of the Art in Dementia Care*. London, Centre for Policy on Ageing.

Kitwood, T. (1997d) The experience of dementia, *Aging and Mental Health*, 1(1): 13–22.

Kitwood, T. (1997e) Some notes on personhood and deformation, in Fletcher, C.L. (ed.) *Values in Adult Education*. Wolverhampton: University of Wolverhampton Press.

Kitwood, T. (1998a) Professional and moral development for care work, *Journal of Moral Education*, 27(3): 401–411.

Kitwood, T. (1998b) Towards a theory of dementia care: ethics and interaction, *The Journal of Clinical Ethics*, 9(1): 23–34.

Kitwood, T. and Benson, S. (eds) (1995) *The New Culture of Dementia Care*. London, Hawker.

Kitwood, T and Bredin K. (1992a) Towards a theory of dementia care: personhood and well-being, *Ageing and Society*, 12(3): 269–287.

Kitwood, T. and Bredin, K. (1992b) *Person to Person: A guide to the care of those with failing mental powers*. Loughton: Gale.

Kitwood, T., Buckland, S. and Petre, T. (1995) *Brighter Futures: A report on research into provision for persons with dementia in residential homes, nursing homes and sheltered housing*. Kidlington: Anchor Housing Association.

Kitwood, T. and Capstick, A. (1999) Dementia and nursing – part 1: educational strategy, *Journal of Nursing Care*, 2(1): 10–12.

Knopman, D.S., DeKosky, S.T., Cummings, J.L., Chui, H., Corey-Bloom, J., Relkin, N., Small, G.W., Miller, B. and Stevens, J.C. (2001) Practice parameter: diagnosis of dementia (an evidence-based review), *Neurology*, 56(9): 1143–1153.

Kontos, P.C. (2004) Ethnographic reflections on selfhood: embodiment and Alzheimer's disease, *Ageing and Society*, 24(6): 829–849.

Kontos, P.C. (2005) Embodied selfhood in Alzheimer's disease: rethinking person centred care, *Dementia: International Journal of Research and Practice*, 4(4): 553–570.

Lakatos, I. (1970) Falsification and the methodology of scientific research programmes, in Lakatos, I. and Musgrave, A. (eds) *Criticism and the Growth of Knowledge*. London: Cambridge University Press.

Leder, D. (1990) *The Absent Body*. Chicago, IL: Chicago University Press.

Leonard, P. (1984) *Personality and Ideology: Towards a materialist understanding of the individual*. London: Macmillan.

Lyman, K.A. (1989) Bringing the social back in: a critique of the biomedicalization of dementia, *The Gerontologist*, 29(5): 597–605. [Reprinted in Gubrium, J.F. and Holstein, J.A. (eds) (2000) *Ageing and Everyday Life*. Oxford: Blackwell.]

Malloy, D.C. and Hadjistavropoulos, T. (2004) The problem of pain management among persons with dementia, personhood, and the ontology of relationships, *Nursing Philosophy*, 5(2): 147–159.

Mental Capacity Act. (2005) Norwich: The Stationery Office.

Menzies, I. (1972) The functioning of social systems as a defence against anxiety, in Menzies-Lyth, I. (ed.) (1988) *Containing Anxiety in Institutions: Selected essays*, Vol. 1. London: Free Association Books.

Mischel, W. (1977) The interaction of person and situation, in Magnusson, D. and Endler, N.S. (eds) *Personality at the Crossroads: Current issues in interactional psychology*. Hillsdale, NJ: Lawrence Erlbaum.

Moniz-Cook, E., Stokes, G. and Agar, S. (2003) Difficult behaviour and dementia in nursing homes: five cases of psychosocial intervention, *Clinical Psychology and Psychotherapy*, 10(3): 197–208.

Müller, N. and Guendouzi, J.A. (2005) Order and disorder in conversation: encounters with dementia of the Alzheimer's type, *Clinical Linguistics and Phonetics*, 19(5): 393–404.

Murphy, C.J. (1997) Review of *Brighter Futures, Ageing and Society*, 17(1): 102–104.

Netten, A. (1992) The effect of the social environment on demented elderly people in residential care, in Morgan, K. (ed.) *Gerontology: Responding to an ageing society*. London: Jessica Kingsley.

Nichol, B. and Raye, L. (2001) Anxiety and work. Available from http://www.healthyplace.com/Communities/Anxiety/work.asp (accessed 12 January 2007).

Nolan, M., Ryan, T., Enderby, P. and Reid, D. (2002) Towards a more inclusive vision of dementia care practice and research, *Dementia: International Journal of Research and Practice*, 1(2): 193–211.

O'Connor, D. (2007) Self-identifying as a caregiver: exploring the positioning process, *Journal of Aging Studies*, 21(2): 165–174.

O'Connor, D.L. and Phinney, A. (2006) Contextualizing the dementia experience: a unique case study exploring social location. Paper presented at the British Society of Gerontology 35th Annual Scientific Meeting, Bangor, Wales.

O'Connor, D.L., Phinney, A., Smith, A., Small, J., Purves, B., Perry, J., Drance, E., Donnelly, M., Chaudhury, H. and Beattie, L. (forthcoming) Personhood in dementia: developing a research agenda for broadening the vision, *Dementia: International Journal of Research and Practice*.

Oxford Paperback Dictionary. (2001) New York: Oxford University Press Inc.

Phillipson, C. (1982) *Capitalism and the Construction of Old Age*. London: Macmillan.

Phinney, A. and Brown, P. (2004) Developing visual methods for studying everyday life of people with dementia. Research plenary paper presented at the Annual Conference of the Alzheimer Society of Canada, Montreal, Canada, April.

Phinney, A. and Chesla, C.A. (2003) The lived body in dementia, *Journal of Aging Studies*, 17(3): 283–299.

Post, S.G. (1995) *The Moral Challenge of Alzheimer's: Ethical issues from diagnosis to dying*. Baltimore, MD: Johns Hopkins University Press.

Purves, B. (2006) Family voices: analyses of talk in families with Alzheimer's disease or a related disorder. Unpublished doctoral dissertation, University of British Columbia, Vancouver, Canada.

Reich, W. (1946) *The Mass Psychology of Fascism*. London: Souvenir Press.

Richards, G. (1996) *Putting Psychology in its Place: An introduction from a critical historical perspective*. London: Routledge.

Roach, M. (1985) *Another Name for Madness*. Boston, MA: Houghton-Mifflin.

Rockwood, K., Wallack, M. and Tallis, R. (2003) The treatment of Alzheimer's disease: success short of cure, *Lancet Neurology*, 2(10): 630–633.

Rogers, C.R. (1951) *Client-centered Counseling*. Boston, MA: Houghton-Mifflin.

Rogers, C.R., Stevens, B., Gendlin, E.T., Shlien, J.M. and Van Dusen, W. (1967) *Person to Person: The problem of being human*. Lafayette, CA: Real People Press.

Rose, S. (1997) *Lifelines – Biology, Freedom, Determinism*. London: Penguin.

Ryan, E., Byrne, K. Spykerman, H. and Orange, J.B. (2005) Evidencing Kitwood's personhood strategies: conversation as care in dementia, in Davis, B.H. (ed.) *Alzheimer Talk, Text and Context: Enhancing communication*. Basingstoke: Palgrave Macmillan.

Sabat, S. (2003) Malignant positioning and the predicament of people with Alzheimer's disease, in Harré, R. and Moghaddam, F. (eds) *The Self and Others: Positioning individuals and groups in personal, political and cultural contexts*. Westport, CT: Praeger.

Sabat, S.R. (2001) *The Experience of Alzheimer's Disease: Life through a tangled veil*. Oxford: Blackwell.

Sève, L. (1978) *Man in Marxist Theory and the Psychology of Personality*. Hassocks: Harvester.

Shabahangi, N.R. (2005) Redefining dementia: between the world of forgetting and remembering. Available from http://www.pacificinstitute.org/events/nader_dementia.pdf (accessed June 2007).

Sheard, D. (2004) Person-centred care: the emperor's new clothes, *Journal of Dementia Care*, 12(2): 22–24.

Shotter, J. (1993) Psychology and citizenship: identity and belonging, in Turner, B. (ed.) *Citizenship and Social Theory*. London: Sage.

Sixsmith, A., Stilwell, J. and Copeland, J. (1993) 'Rementia': challenging the limits of dementia care, *International Journal of Geriatric Psychiatry*, 8(12): 993–1000.

Sloan, T. (1997) Theories of personality, in Fox, D. and Prilleltensky, I. (eds) *Critical Psychology: An introduction*. London: Sage.

Smail, D. (1984) *Illusion and Reality*. London: Dent.

Smail, D. (1993) *The Origins of Unhappiness: A new understanding of personal distress*. London: HarperCollins.

Small, J.A., Geldart, K., Gutman, G., and Clarke Scott, M. (1998) The discourse of self in dementia, *Ageing and Society*, 18(3): 291–316.

Spence, D.P. (1986) Narrative smoothing and clinical wisdom, in Sarbin, T. (ed.) *Narrative Psychology: The storied nature of human conduct*. New York: Praeger.

Thomas, D. (1951) Do not go gentle into that good night, in *Dylan Thomas: Collected poems 1934–1953*. London: Everyman.

Tune, P. and Bowie, P. (2000) The quality of residential and nursing home care for people with dementia, *Age and Ageing*, 29(4): 325–328.

Turner, S., Iliffe, S., Downs, M., Wilcock, J., Bryans, M., Levin, E., Keady, J. and O'Carroll, R. (2004) General practitioners' knowledge, confidence and attitudes in the diagnosis and management of dementia, *Age and Ageing*, 33(5): 461–467.

Walker, A. (1993) *Possessing the Secret of Joy*. London: Vintage.

Wilkinson, H. (2002) *The Perspectives of People with Dementia: Research methods and motivations*. London, Jessica Kingsley.

Williams, R. (1976) *Keywords: A vocabulary of culture and society*. London: Fontana.

Woods, B. (1999) Editorial: the legacy of Kitwood: Professor Tom Kitwood 1937–1998, *Aging and Mental Health*, 3(1): 5–7.

Index

A HANDBOOK OF DEMENTIA CARE

Caroline Cantley (ed.)

Recently, professional understanding of dementia has broadened and has opened up new thinking about how we can provide more imaginative, responsive and 'person-centred' services for people with dementia. Against this background *A Handbook of Dementia Care* provides a wide-ranging, up-to-date overview of the current state of knowledge in the field. It is comprehensive, authoritative, accessible and thought-provoking. It asks:

- How do different theoretical perspectives help us to understand dementia?
- What do we know about what constitutes good practice in dementia care?
- How can we improve practice and service delivery in dementia care?
- How do policy, organizational issues and research impact on dementia care?

This handbook provides a unique, multidisciplinary and critical guide to what we know about dementia and dementia care. It is written by leading academics, practitioners and managers involved in the development of dementia care. It demonstrates the value of a wide range of perspectives in understanding dementia care, reviews the latest thinking about good practice, and examines key ethical issues. It explores the way organizations, policy and research shape dementia care, and introduces a range of approaches to practice and service development.

A Handbook of Dementia Care is an essential resource for students and professionals in such fields as gerontology, social work, nursing, occupational therapy, geriatric medicine, psychiatry, mental health, psychology, social services and health services management, social policy and health policy.

Contents
Introduction – Part one: Understanding dementia – Bio-medical and clinical perspectives – Psychological perspectives – Sociological perspectives – Philosophical and spiritual perspectives – The perspectives of people with dementia, their families and their carers – Part two: Practice knowledge and development – Understanding practice development – Assessment, care planning and care management – Living at home – Communication and personhood – Therapeutic activity – Working with carers – Care settings and the care environment – Ethical ideals and practice – Part three: Policy, organizations and research – Understanding the policy context – Understanding people in organizations – Developing service organizations – Developing quality in services – Involving people with dementia and their carers in developing services – Research, policy and practice in dementia care – Conclusion: The future development of dementia care – Glossary – References – Index.

400pp   0 335 20383 3 (Paperback)   0 335 20384 1 (Hardback)

DEMENTIA RECONSIDERED
THE PERSON COMES FIRST

Tom Kitwood

For some years now, Tom Kitwood's work on dementia care has stood out as the most important, innovative and creative development in a field that has for too long been neglected. This book is a landmark in dementia care; it brings together, and elaborates on, Kitwood's theory of dementia and of person-centred care in an accessible fashion, that will make this an essential source for all working and researching in the field of dementia care.

Robert Woods, Professor of Clinical Psychology, University of Wales

Over the last ten years or so Tom Kitwood has made a truly remarkable contribution to our understanding of dementia, and to raising expectations of what can be achieved with empathy and skill. This lucid account of his thinking and work will communicate his approach to a yet wider audience. It is to be warmly welcomed.

Mary Marshall, Director of the Dementia Services Development Centre, University of Stirling

- What is the *real* nature of the dementing process?
- What might we reasonably expect when dementia care is of very high quality?
- What is required of organizations and individuals involved in dementia care?

Tom Kitwood breaks new ground in this book. Many of the older ideas about dementia are subjected to critical scrutiny and reappraisal, drawing on research evidence, logical analysis and the author's own experience. The unifying theme is the personhood of men and women who have dementia – an issue that was grossly neglected for many years both in psychiatry and care practice.

Each chapter provides a definitive statement on a major topic related to dementia, for example: the nature of 'organic mental impairment', the experience of dementia, the agenda for care practice, and the transformation of the culture of care.

While recognizing the enormous difficulties of the present day, the book clearly demonstrates the possibility of a better life for people who have dementia, and comes to a cautiously optimistic conclusion. It will be of interest to all professionals involved in dementia care or provision, students on courses involving psychogeriatrics or social work with older people, and family carers of people with dementia.

Key features:

- One of the few attempts to present the whole picture.
- Very readable – many real-life illustrations.
- Offers a major alternative to the 'medical model' of dementia.
- Tom Kitwood's work on dementia is very well known.

Contents

Series editor's preface – Brian Gearing – Acknowledgements – Introduction – On being a person – Dementia as a psychiatric category – How personhood is undermined – Personhood maintained – The experiences of dementia – Improving care: the next step forward – The caring organization – Requirements of a caregiver – The task of cultural transformation – References – Index.

176pp   0 335 19855 4 (Paperback)   0 335 19856 2 (Hardback)